T0332280

Analyzing Longitudinal Clinical Trial Data

A Practical Guide

Chapman & Hall/CRC Biostatistics Series

Editor-in-Chief

Shein-Chung Chow, Ph.D., Professor, Department of Biostatistics and Bioinformatics,
Duke University School of Medicine, Durham, North Carolina

Series Editors

Byron Jones, Biometrical Fellow, Statistical Methodology, Integrated Information Sciences,
Novartis Pharma AG, Basel, Switzerland

Jen-pei Liu, Professor, Division of Biometry, Department of Agronomy,
National Taiwan University, Taipei, Taiwan

Karl E. Peace, Georgia Cancer Coalition, Distinguished Cancer Scholar, Senior Research Scientist
and Professor of Biostatistics, Jiann-Ping Hsu College of Public Health,
Georgia Southern University, Statesboro, Georgia

Bruce W. Turnbull, Professor, School of Operations Research and Industrial Engineering,
Cornell University, Ithaca, New York

Published Titles

Published Titles

Published Titles

Published Titles

Chapman & Hall/CRC Biostatistics Series

Analyzing Longitudinal Clinical Trial Data
A Practical Guide

Craig Mallinckrodt

Eli Lilly Research Laboratories

Indianapolis, Indiana, USA

Ilya Lipkovich

Quintiles

Durham, North Carolina, USA

CRC Press is an imprint of the
Taylor & Francis Group, an **informa** business

A CHAPMAN & HALL BOOK

CRC Press
Taylor & Francis Group
6000 Broken Sound Parkway NW, Suite 300
Boca Raton, FL 33487-2742

Printed on acid-free paper
Version Date: 20161025

International Standard Book Number-13: 978-1-4987-6531-2 (Hardback)

Library of Congress Cataloging-in-Publication Data

Names: Mallinckrodt, Craig H., 1958- | Lipkovich, Ilya.
Title: Analyzing longitudinal clinical trial data / Craig Mallinckrodt and Ilya Lipkovich.
Description: Boca Raton : CRC Press, 2017. | Includes bibliographical references.
Identifiers: LCCN 2016032392 | ISBN 9781498765312 (hardback)
Subjects: LCSH: Clinical trials--Longitudinal studies.
Classification: LCC R853.C55 M33738 2017 | DDC 615.5072/4--dc23
LC record available at https://lccn.loc.gov/2016032392

Visit the Taylor & Francis Web site at
http://www.taylorandfrancis.com

and the CRC Press Web site at
http://www.crcpress.com

Printed and bound in the United States of America by Sheridan

Contents

Section I Background and Setting

Section II   Modeling the Observed Data

Section III   Methods for Dealing with Missing Data

Section IV   A Comprehensive Approach to Study Development and Analyses

Preface

The statistical theory relevant to analyses of longitudinal clinical trial data is extensive, and applying that theory in practice can be challenging. Therefore, this book focuses on the most relevant and current theory, using practical and easy-to-implement approaches for bringing that theory into routine practice. Emphasis is placed on examples with realistic data, and the programming code to implement the analyses is provided, usually in both SAS and R.

While this book focuses on analytic methods, analyses cannot be considered in isolation. Analyses must be considered as part of a holistic approach to study development and implementation. An industry working group recently proposed a study development process chart that begins with determining objectives, followed by choosing estimands, design, and analyses and assessing sensitivity (Phillips et al. 2016). This book is oriented in accordance with that process. Early chapters focus on objectives, estimands, and design. Subsequent chapters go into detail regarding analyses and sensitivity analyses. The intent of this book is to help facilitate an integrated understanding of key concepts from across the study development process through an example-oriented approach. It is this holistic approach to analysis planning and a focus on practical implementation that sets this text apart from existing texts.

Section I includes an introductory chapter along with chapters discussing estimands and key considerations in choosing them, study design considerations, introduction of the example data sets, and a chapter on key aspects of mixed-effects model theory. Section II covers key concepts and considerations applicable to modeling the observed data, including choice of the dependent variable, accounting for covariance between repeated measurements, modeling mean trends over time, modeling covariates, model checking and validation, and a chapter on modeling categorical data. Section III focuses on accounting for missing data, which is an inevitable problem in clinical trials. Section IV integrates key ideas from Sections I to III to illustrate a comprehensive approach to study development and analyses of realistic data sets.

Throughout this book, example data sets are used to illustrate and explain key analyses and concepts. These data sets were constructed by selecting patients from actual clinical trial data sets and manipulating the observations in ways useful for illustration. By using small data sets, readers can more easily understand exactly what an analysis does and how it does it. For the comprehensive study development and analysis example in Section IV, two data sets contrived from actual clinical trial data are used to further illustrate key points for implementing an overall analytic strategy that includes sensitivity analyses and model checking.

Craig Mallinckrodt
Eli Lilly Research Laboratories, Indianapolis, Indiana

Ilya Lipkovich
Quintiles, Durham, North Carolina

Acknowledgments

We would like to thank the Drug Information Association Scientific Working Group on missing data. We have benefited significantly from many discussions within the group and from our individual discussions with other group members. In this book, we have frequently cited work from the group and from its individual members. We especially thank Lei Xu, James Roger, Bohdana Ratitch, Michael O'Kelly, and Geert Molenberghs for their specific contributions to this book.

List of Tables

List of Figures

List of Code Fragments

Section I

Background and Setting

Section I begins with an introductory chapter covering the settings to be addressed in this book. Chapter 2 discusses trial objectives and defines and discusses estimands. Study design considerations are discussed in Chapter 3, focusing on methods to minimize missing data. Chapter 4 introduces the data sets used in example analyses. Chapter 5 covers key aspects of mixed-effects model theory.

Some readers may at least initially skip Chapter 5 and refer back to it as needed when covering later chapters. Other readers may benefit from this review of mixed-effect models prior to moving to later chapters.

1

Introduction

The evidence to support new medicines, devices, or other medical interventions is based primarily on randomized clinical trials. Many of these trials involve assessments taken at the start of treatment (baseline), followed by assessments taken repeatedly during the treatment period. In some cases, such as cancer trials, the primary outcome is whether or not some important event occurred during the assessment intervals. These outcomes can be summarized by the time to the event, or as a percentage of patients experiencing the event at or before some landmark time point. Alternatively, the multiple post-baseline assessments can all be used in a longitudinal, repeated measures framework, which can either focus on a landmark time point or consider outcomes across time points. This book focuses on the longitudinal, repeated measures framework.

With multiple post-baseline assessments per subject, linear mixed-effects models and generalized linear mixed-effect models provide useful analytic frameworks for continuous and categorical outcomes, respectively. Important modeling considerations within these frameworks include how to model the correlations between the measurements; how to model means over time; if, and if so, how to account for covariates; what endpoint to choose (actual value, change from baseline, or percent change from baseline); and how to specify and verify the assumptions in the chosen model. In addition, missing data is an incessant problem in longitudinal clinical trials. The fundamental problem caused by missing data is that the balance provided by randomization is lost if, as is usually the case, the subjects who discontinue differ in regards to the outcome of interest from those who complete the study. This imbalance can lead to bias in the comparisons between treatment groups (NRC 2010).

Data modeling decisions should not be considered in isolation. These decisions should be made as part of the overall study development process, because how to best analyze data depends on what the analysis is trying to accomplish and the circumstances in which the analysis is conducted. Therefore, study development decisions and data modeling decisions begin with considering the decisions to be made from the trial, which informs what objectives need to be addressed. Study objectives inform what needs to be estimated, which in turn informs the design, which in turn informs the analyses (Garrett et al. 2015; Mallinckrodt et al. 2016; Phillips et al. 2016).

The decisions made from a clinical trial vary by, among other things, stage of development. Phase II trials are typically used by drug development decision makers to determine proof of concept or to choose doses for subsequent studies. Phase III, confirmatory, studies typically serve a diverse audience and therefore must address diverse objectives (Leuchs et al. 2015). For example, regulators render decisions regarding whether or not the drug under study should be granted a marketing authorization. Drug developers and regulators must collaborate to develop labeling language that accurately and clearly describe the risks and benefits of approved drugs. Payers must decide if/where a new drug belongs on its formulary list. Prescribers must decide for whom the new drug should be prescribed and must inform patients and care givers what to expect. Patients and care givers must decide if they want to take the drug that has been prescribed.

These diverse decisions necessitate diverse objectives and therefore diverse targets of estimation, and a variety of analyses. For example, fully understanding a drug's benefits requires understanding its effects when taken as directed (efficacy) and as actually taken (effectiveness) (Mallinckrodt et al. 2016). As will be discussed in detail in later chapters, different analyses are required for these different targets of estimation.

It is important that the study development process be iterative so that considerations from downstream aspects can help inform upstream decisions. For example, clearly defined objectives and estimands lead to clarity in what parameters are to be estimated, which leads to clarity about the merits of the various analytic alternatives. However, an understanding of the strengths and limitations of various analytic methods is needed to understand what trial design and trial conduct features are necessary to provide optimum data for the situation at hand. Moreover, for any one trial, with its diverse objectives and estimands, only one design can be chosen. This design may be well-suited to some of the estimands and analyses but less well-suited to others.

Therefore, an integrated understanding of objectives, estimands, design, and analyses are required to develop, implement, and interpret results from a comprehensive analysis plan. The intent of this book is to help facilitate this integrated understanding among practicing statisticians via an example-oriented approach.

2

Objectives and Estimands—Determining What to Estimate

2.1 Introduction

Detailed discussion of estimands is relatively new to clinical trial literature, but very important. Estimands bridge the gap between study objectives and statistical methods (Phillips et al. 2016). The importance of estimands was highlighted in the National Research Council's (NRC) expert panel report that was commissioned by the Food and Drug Administration (FDA) (NRC 2010). Although the report focused on the problem of missing data, their recommendations set forth an overarching framework for the analysis of longitudinal clinical trial data.

Until recently, many protocols had general objectives such as "To compare the efficacy and safety of...." Such statements give little guidance to the designers of the studies and can lead to statistical analyses that do not address the intended question (Phillips et al. 2016). Estimands link study objectives and the analysis methods by more precisely defining what is to be estimated and how that quantity will be interpreted (Phillips et al. 2016). This provides clarity on what data needs to be collected and how that data should be analyzed and interpreted.

Conceptually, an estimand is simply the true population quantity of interest (NRC 2010); this is specific to a particular parameter, time point, and population (also sometimes referred to as the intervention effect).

Phillips et al. (2016) used an example similar to the one below to illustrate the key considerations in defining the intervention effect component of estimands. Consider a randomized, two-arm (Drug A and Drug B) trial in patients with type 2 diabetes mellitus. The primary endpoint is mean change from baseline to Week 24 in HbA1c levels. Assessments are taken at baseline and at Weeks 4, 8, 12, 16, and 24. For ethical reasons, patients are switched to rescue medication if their HbA1c values are above a certain threshold. Regardless of rescue medication use, all patients are intended to be assessed for the 24-week study duration.

TABLE 2.1

Three Estimands of Interest in an Example Trial

Estimand	Intervention Effect
1	Population-average effect regardless of what treatment was actually received; i.e., effect of treatment policy. Includes data after initiation of rescue treatment
2	Population-average effect attributable to the initially randomized medications; i.e., free from the confounding effects of rescue medication, and which accounts for reduction or loss of effect after discontinuation of the randomized treatment
3	Population-average effect if all patients remain on the initially randomized treatment throughout the study; i.e., effect if patients who switched to rescue would have remained on their randomized treatment

Table 2.1 outlines three of the estimands that can be defined for this trial. Each estimand is based on all randomized patients at the planned endpoint of the trial. However, as detailed in subsequent sections, each estimand implies different data to be included and potentially different analysis methods. Simply specifying the objective as assessing mean change from baseline to Week 24 does not distinguish between these three estimands.

Although estimands are often discussed in the literature as part of dealing with missing data, the above considerations exist even if all the data intended to be collected were indeed observed. However, further complexity does arise from the missing data caused by patients failing to adhere to the protocol specified procedures. Patients may fail to adhere on an intermittent basis, being compliant with protocol procedures and having outcome assessments during some treatment intervals, but not all. Early discontinuation (dropout) from the trial and the missing data that can result from it is a more frequent and more troublesome problem. Missing data issues are covered in detail in Section III.

With the diversity in medical research and the many clinical trial scenarios that exist, consensus on a universally best estimand is neither realistic nor desirable. Therefore, attention has turned to how to choose estimands (Mallinckrodt et al. 2016). Phillips et al. (2016) proposed a study development process chart similar to the one depicted in Figure 2.1. As the chart illustrates, choice of the primary estimand is informed by the decisions to be made from the trial and the objectives needed to inform these decisions. Although the general approach is to move from the top of the chart to the bottom, the arrows point in both directions. The study development process proceeds in an iterative manner so that interactions between the various components can be considered (Phillips et al. 2016). Importantly, the chart makes clear that in order to determine how best to analyze clinical trial data, it is important to first consider the trial objectives and the estimands needed to be estimated in order to address those objectives.

Trial objectives are typically driven by the decisions to be made from the trial results (Mallinckrodt et al. 2016). In Chapter 1, it was noted that the decisions to be made from a trial depend in part on stage of development. Phase II trials

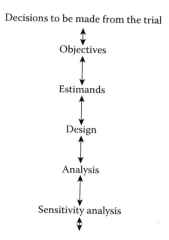

FIGURE 2.1
Study development process chart.

typically inform drug development decisions. Phase III, confirmatory studies typically inform a diverse audience, including the sponsor, multiple regulatory agencies, dozens of disparate health technology assessment groups (payers), prescribers, patients, journal editors and reviewers, along with other researchers (Leuchs et al. 2015; Mallinckrodt et al. 2016).

Specific estimands are as numerous and varied as the clinical trials scenarios in which they are applied. However, estimands can be grouped in several meaningful ways. For example, at the most conceptual level, estimands can be divided into two general categories based on adherence to protocol-defined interventions: (1) Efficacy is the effects of the drug if taken as directed; that is, the effects if patients adhere to the protocol-defined interventions. (2) Effectiveness is the effects of the drug as actually taken; that is, the effects without regard to adherence to the protocol-defined interventions (Mallinckrodt et al. 2012, 2014; Leuchs et al. 2015). However, the efficacy and effectiveness nomenclature does not make sense for safety outcomes. Therefore, a more general terminology is de jure (if taken as directed) and de facto (as actually taken) (Carpenter et al. 2013). The estimands introduced in Table 2.1 can be categorized according to this nomenclature. Again, each of these estimands involves the difference versus control in change to the planned endpoint of the trial, in all randomized patients.

- *Estimand 1* is the change due to the treatments as actually taken, a de facto (effectiveness) estimand. The inference target is the treatment regimens; that is, Drug A plus rescue versus Drug B plus rescue.
- *Estimand 2* is the change due to the initially randomized treatments as actually taken, a de facto (effectiveness) estimand. The inference

target is the initially randomized treatments; that is, Drug A versus Drug B.

- *Estimand 3* is the change due to the initially randomized treatments if taken as directed, a de jure (efficacy) estimand. The inference target is the initially randomized treatments.

It is important to differentiate estimand 3, which is based on all randomized patients, from a similar de jure estimand that is based on completers—that is, conditional on having been adherent. The completers estimand is limited for inference because it does not preserve the initial randomization. In contrast, estimand 3 includes all randomized patients. Therefore, inferences and parameter estimates apply to all patients in the population, not merely to those who were doing well enough to remain adherent, as is the case for compeleters analyses.

2.2 Fundamental Considerations in Choosing Estimands

Given the diversity in clinical settings and decisions to be made from clinical trial data, no universally best primary estimand exists, and therefore multiple estimands are likely to be of interest for any one trial (Mallinckrodt et al. 2012, 2014, 2016; Garrett et al. 2015; Leuchs et al. 2015; Phillips et al. 2016).

Each of the three estimands defined in Section 2.1 have strengths and limitations. Estimand 3, the de jure estimand, can be considered hypothetical (i.e., counterfactual) for groups of patients because treatment effects are assessed as if taken as directed when in any meaningfully sized group some patients will not adhere (NRC 2010). Therefore, de jure estimands assess what is possible to achieve in a group of patients, not what actually was achieved. However, de jure estimands assess what to expect if patients are adherent—and in most clinical settings the majority of patients are adherent (Mallinckrodt et al. 2014). In addition, patients are advised to take their medication as directed; therefore, it is important to assess what would happen if a medication were taken as directed so that optimal directions can be developed (Mallinckrodt et al. 2016).

De facto estimands can be considered counterfactual for individual patients because treatment effects are assessed from a mix of adherent and nonadherent patients, but each patient is either adherent or not adherent, no patient is both. On the other hand, de facto estimands can provide useful estimates of what to expect from the group as a whole (CHMP 2010; NRC 2010).

Most of the discussion on de jure and de facto estimands has been in the context of assessing drug benefit. However, estimands for assessing drug risk are also important. Consider a drug that has the adverse effect of increasing blood pressure. Some patients may become hypertensive and discontinue study medication and/or take medication to treat the high blood pressure, with subsequent return to normal blood pressure. De facto estimands would reflect the patients' return to normal, thereby suggesting no change at the planned endpoint of the trial. De jure estimands would not reflect a return to normal and would reflect increases at endpoint because had the patients been adherent they would likely have continued to be hypertensive (Mallinckrodt et al. 2016).

2.3 Design Considerations in Choosing Estimands

2.3.1 Missing Data Considerations

Universal agreement exists that clinical trials should aim to minimize missing data, thereby maximizing the portion of the intended data that was actually collected. The intent is to maximize adherence to the initially assigned treatments in order to minimize reliance of inferences on untestable assumptions about the missing data (Verbeke and Molenberghs 2000; Molenberghs and Kenward 2007; CHMP 2010; NRC 2010; Mallinckrodt 2013; Ratitch and O'Kelly 2014). These considerations have often been in the context of de jure estimands. However, the impact of maximizing retention on de facto estimands is also important (Leuchs et al. 2015; Mallinckrodt et al. 2016).

Increasing adherence is likely to increase benefit from the drug as actually taken, thereby resulting in more favorable outcomes for de facto estimands. If the measures used to engender adherence in the clinical trial are not feasible in clinical practice the trial could yield biased estimates of effectiveness relative to the conditions under which the drug would be used.

Specifically, assessment of de facto estimands often entail using adherence as part of the primary outcome. For example, patients that discontinue study drug can be considered a treatment failure regardless of the observed outcomes. Therefore, it is important to consider the degree to which treatment adherence decisions in the clinical trial match adherence decisions in clinical practice. These generalizability considerations may be especially important in trials with placebo and/or blinding because these factors are never present in clinical practice (Mallinckrodt 2013; Mallinckrodt et al. 2016).

2.3.2 Rescue Medication Considerations

Whether or not data should be collected after discontinuation of initially randomized study medication or initiation or rescue medication, and whether that data should be included in an analysis are critically important considerations.

Use of rescue medications for patients not adequately responding to the initially randomized medications has been suggested because this provides an assessment of pragmatic effectiveness and can reduce dropout (NRC 2010; Fleming 2011; Permutt 2015a). The need for rescue therapy is also partly motivated by arguments for ethical patient care, especially in placebo-controlled trials. However, rescue medications can mask or exaggerate the efficacy and safety effects of the initially assigned treatments, thereby biasing estimates of the effects of the originally assigned medication (Buncher and Tsay 2005; Holubkov et al. 2009; Henning 2011; Mallinckrodt et al. 2012, 2014; Leuchs et al. 2015). In placebo-controlled trials, if rescue therapy is beneficial and post-rescue data are included in the analysis, the treatment effect is likely to be substantially diminished compared to the effect if post-rescue data are not included (Mallinckrodt et al. 2016).

Another consideration is that readily available rescue medications may reduce study discontinuation, but could increase discontinuation from the initially randomized medication, which would of course be counter to the primary goal of maximizing retention on the initial medications (Mallinckrodt 2013). This issue may be particularly important in placebo-controlled trials where patients are aware that they may be randomized to an ineffective treatment but switching to rescue guarantees use of an effective treatment (Mallinckrodt et al. 2016).

With estimand 1 (de facto, treatment regimens), data after discontinuation of the initially randomized medication and/or addition of rescue medication are included in the analyses. The study protocol should specify the rescue treatment(s) and how they are administered, or specify that rescue treatment is at the discretion of the investigator. The protocol should also specify if rescue treatment is provided by the sponsor or if marketed product is to be used.

As noted above, estimand 1 is with regard to treatment policies or regimens (NRC 2010; Mallinckrodt et al. 2012; Leuchs et al. 2015). Estimand 1 is often seen as an assessment of pragmatic effectiveness (Permutt 2015a). As with estimand 2, generalizability must be considered. For estimand 1, a design comparing an experimental drug plus rescue versus a standard of care plus rescue may be appropriate. However, designs with placebo control (e.g., experimental drug plus rescue versus placebo plus rescue) may be less appropriate in some settings. Decisions regarding adherence and need for rescue in double-blind, placebo-controlled settings may not be as applicable to general clinical practice as the decisions made when all patients receive active medication. Simply put, placebo is never used in general clinical settings; therefore, when assessing pragmatic effectiveness, placebo control may not be ideal (Mallinckrodt et al. 2016). Moreover, the most relevant questions in early research and initial regulatory reviews, especially for placebo-controlled trials, are often about the effects of the investigational drugs, not treatment policies (Mallinckrodt et al. 2012; Mallinckrodt 2013).

The ICH E9 guidance is often cited when justifying choice of a primary analytic approach (http://www.ich.org/fileadmin/Public_Web_Site/ICH_Products/Guidelines/Efficacy/E9/Step4/E9_Guideline.pdf). This guidance emphasizes the ITT principle, which is defined as "the principle that asserts that the effect of a treatment policy can be best assessed by evaluating on the basis of the intention to treat a subject (i.e., the planned treatment regimen) rather than the actual treatment given. It has the consequence that subjects allocated to a treatment group should be followed up, assessed and analyzed as members of that group irrespective of their compliance to the planned course of treatment."

Thus, ITT has two parts, the patients to include and the data for each patient to include (Permutt 2015a; Mallinckrodt et al. 2016). Some deviations from one or both aspects of the intent-to-treat principles are routinely accepted (Permutt 2015a). The guidance is clear on the need to include all randomized patients and that all data should be included, but it does not specifically address data after initiation of rescue treatment.

Rescue therapy is specifically addressed in ICH E10, Section 2.1.5.2.2 (http://www.ich.org/fileadmin/Public_Web_Site/ICH_Products/Guidelines/Efficacy/E10/Step4/E10_Guideline.pdf). In referring to trials with rescue, E10 states: "In such cases, the need to change treatment becomes a study endpoint." Thus, according to E10, post-rescue data need not be included in the primary analysis.

It is important to recognize that the ICH guidance was developed before the NRC report (NRC 2010) that focused on the need for clarity on estimands. The E9 guidance refers to ITT as the best way to assess treatment policies/regimens. It does not address inference for the initially randomized medications. Considerations of estimands today are often more nuanced than anticipated by the 1998 ICH guidance. An addendum to the E9 guidance specific to choices of estimands is anticipated in 2016 or soon thereafter.

A reasonable approach is to maintain the principles of ITT, but employ a slight modification to address the need for greater specificity (Mallinckrodt et al. 2016). In this modified approach to ITT, all randomized patients are again included, thereby maintaining consistency with the first tenant of ITT. The second tenant of ITT is modified to mean that all data—*relevant to the estimand*—are included. For example, when evaluating estimand 2 (de facto, initially randomized treatments) and estimand 3 (de jure, initially randomized treatments), post-rescue data are not relevant and are therefore not included in the analysis, thereby avoiding the confounding effects of rescue medication.

O'Neill and Temple (2012) noted that estimand 1 may be a more common choice for the primary estimand in outcomes trials where the presence/absence of a major health event is the endpoint and/or the intervention is intended to modify the disease process. Symptomatic trials (symptom severity is the endpoint) often use a primary estimand where the inferential target is the initially randomized treatments. In these scenarios the confounding from rescue medications is avoided by excluding data after discontinuation of study medication/initiation of rescue from the primary analysis.

2.4 Analysis Considerations

To understand the analytic implications in choice of estimand, first consider estimand 3, the de jure effects of the initially randomized medication. The intent of estimand 3 is to assess drug effects if all randomized patients were adherent, even though in any realistically sized trial there will be some patients who do not adhere. Although failure to adhere can be manifest in many ways, the most common scenario is that of missing data. Patients may discontinue the study and all study-related procedures prior to the planned time of the primary assessment. Patients may also discontinue the randomized study medication but remain in the study for follow-up assessments.

For estimand 3, data after discontinuation of the initially randomized study medication are not needed. That is, post-rescue/post-discontinuation data are not included, thereby avoiding the potentially confounding effects of rescue medication. However, some data intended to be collected are not available. Moreover, the reason(s) data are not available are usually related to outcome. That is, patients with poor outcomes are more likely to be missing than patients with good outcomes. This selection process means that the observed data are not a random sample of the data intended to be collected. Therefore, analysis of estimand 3 requires estimates of what would have happened if all patients were adherent, but this cannot be based on only those patients who *were* adherent.

Common analytic approaches for estimand 3 involve the assumption that data are missing at random (MAR). This assumption and other missing data considerations are covered in detail in Section III. Missing at random essentially means that conditional on the observed data, the statistical behavior (means, variances, etc.) of the unobserved data is the same as the observed data. Put another way, the unobserved data can be predicted in an unbiased manner from the observed data. Analytic approaches valid under MAR include likelihood-based analyses, multiple imputation of missing values followed by an analysis that would have been appropriate had the data been complete, and weighted generalized estimating equations. These analyses are covered in detail in Section III.

Given the reliance of these methods on assumptions about the missing data, which of course cannot be verified since the data are missing, sensitivity analyses are required to assess the degree to which inferences are dependent on the assumptions (Verbeke and Molenberghs 2000; NRC 2010; Mallinckrodt 2013).

Estimand 1 can be evaluated using analyses similar to estimand 3, with the exception that estimand 1 requires including post-rescue data (Permutt 2015a).

This has several important implications. First, the confounding effects of the rescue medication necessitate that inference is on the treatment regimens, not the individual treatments to which patients were randomized. In addition, including the post-rescue data means less data will be missing compared with that same scenario when not including post-rescue data.

Approaches to assessing estimand 2 often entail ascribing unfavorable outcomes to patients who discontinue the initially randomized medication or who need rescue medication, regardless of what outcomes were actually observed while the patients were adherent (Carpenter et al. 2013; Mallinckrodt 2013; Permutt 2015a). This approach has the compelling benefit of resulting in no missing data. And for symptomatic treatments that do not change the underlying disease process, it is intuitively sensible to assume that if patients can not adhere to a drug they will not benefit from it in the long run (O'Neill and Temple 2012).

However, the generalizability considerations noted in the section on design considerations are particularly important. Fully satisfactory assessments of effectiveness from clinical trials may be problematic (NRC 2010). Adherence decisions in the clinical trial setting must sufficiently match the decisions in clinical practice for the estimand to be useful. Placebo control and blinding in a clinical trial may result in adherence decisions different from what would be seen in clinical practice (Mallinckrodt et al. 2016).

Another consideration is exactly what value(s) to impute as unfavorable outcomes for nonadherent patients. Such imputations for continuous endpoints have historically been done using baseline observation carried forward (BOCF). However, single imputation approaches such as BOCF have a number of disadvantages that are discussed in Chapters 12 and 13, and more principled approaches are gaining favor (Kenward and Molenberghs 2009; Carpenter et al. 2013; Mallinckrodt 2013; Mallinckrodt et al. 2014).

Multiple imputation-based approaches to estimate parameters for and test hypotheses about de facto estimands have come into the literature recently. These methods have been referred to as controlled imputation or more specifically reference-based controlled imputation. See Chapter 18 for detailed descriptions of these approaches. However, the general approach is to use multiple imputation in a manner that accounts for the change in/discontinuation of treatment. In so doing, patients that discontinue from an experimental arm have values imputed as if they were in the reference (e.g., placebo arm). Depending on the exact implementation, imputed values can either reflect no pharmacologic benefit from the drug immediately upon discontinuation/rescue, a decaying benefit after discontinuation/rescue, or a constant benefit after discontinuation/rescue (Carpenter et al. 2013; Mallinckrodt et al. 2014).

For categorical endpoints, nonresponder imputation (NRI) has often been used, wherein all patients that discontinue initially randomized medication and/or initiate rescue medication are considered nonresponders, regardless of the observed outcome. The term NRI is somewhat of a misnomer.

The name implies explicit imputation of repeated (binary) measurements. In this context, NRI would have the same disadvantages as BOCF. However, NRI as commonly used does not involve imputation of repeated measures. Rather, there is a single endpoint per patient, reflecting treatment success or failure. Patients that remain adherent to the protocol-specified intervention and achieve the predefined level of response are considered a treatment success (responder) and patients that either fail to achieve the needed level of response or who deviate from the protocol-specified intervention are considered treatment failures.

As with continuous endpoints, the advantage of the treatment success/failure approach is that it yields complete data; and, the important caveat is that adherence decisions in the trial must be similar to the decisions that would be made in clinical practice if results are to be generalizable.

2.5 Multiple Estimands in the Same Study

The multifaceted nature of clinical trials is important to appreciate when considering estimands (Leuchs et al. 2015; Mallinckrodt et al. 2016). Within a trial, diverse objectives are often needed to inform the decisions of the diverse stakeholders (multiple regulatory agencies, dozens of health technology assessors/payers, prescribers, patients, caregivers, sponsors, other researchers, etc.). Even for a single stakeholder in a single trial it is often important to know what happens when a drug is taken as directed (de jure estimand) and to know what happens when the drug is taken as in actual practice (de facto estimand). Therefore, no single estimand is likely to best serve the interests of all stakeholders and de jure and de facto estimands will both be of interest (Mallinckrodt et al. 2012; Leuchs et al. 2015; Mallinckrodt et al. 2016).

The following example first described in Mallinckrodt et al. (2012) illustrates the benefits of assessing both de jure and de facto estimands in the same trial. Drug A and Drug B (or Dose A and Dose B of a drug) have equal effectiveness, but drug A has superior efficacy and Drug B has greater adherence. Even if effectiveness is the primary estimand, de jure estimands are needed to understand the differences in clinical profiles.

Dose/Drug A might be the best choice for patients with more severe illness because it has greater efficacy. Dose/Drug B might be best for patients with less severe illness and/or safety and tolerability concerns because it has greater adherence resulting from fewer side effects. A more nuanced understanding of efficacy and adherence could lead to additional investigation that could lead to more optimized patient outcomes. For example, subgroups of patients who especially benefit from or tolerate the high dose might be identified from the existing data or from a new trial (nonresponders to low dose).

Or, alternate dosing regimens that might improve the safety/tolerability of the high dose, such as titration, flexible, or split dosing (40 mg every 2 weeks rather than 80 mg every 4 weeks), could be investigated in subsequent trials (Mallinckrodt et al. 2016).

One approach to evaluating multiple estimands in the same study is to have some outcomes geared toward assessing a certain estimand(s) while other outcomes address other estimand(s). However, study designs and the data generated from them are often such that multiple estimands can be evaluated from the same outcome measure.

For example, estimand 1 could be assessed by including post-rescue data in the analysis in order to provide an evaluation of pragmatic effectiveness. Estimand 2 could be evaluated in the same trial by not including post-rescue data and defining discontinuation of the initial study medication or the need for rescue medication as treatment failure. Estimand 3 could also be evaluated from the same trial by not including post-rescue data and applying an appropriate analysis.

The ability to assess multiple estimands from the same outcome variable reinforces the need for clarity as to which estimand is addressed by each analysis. This in turn highlights the need for clarity on the assumptions, strengths, and limitations of analyses, which can vary from one estimand to another.

Even though multiple estimands can be assessed from the same outcome, the internal validity and external generalizability of those results will vary. Some designs are better suited to certain estimands than others. Therefore, choice of the primary estimand has a particularly important influence on choice of design.

2.6 Choosing the Primary Estimand

Historical precedent, especially for trials submitted to regulatory authorities in support of marketing authorizations, can influence choice of the primary estimand. However, fundamental understanding of key considerations should be the primary driver in choice of primary estimands.

In the iterative study development process outlined in Section 2.1, design and analysis considerations can influence objectives and estimands. For example, consider a short-term, acute phase clinical trial where extensive efforts to maximize adherence are expected to yield 95% of patients remaining on the initially assigned study medication. Given this highly controlled setting and strong adherence, a de jure primary estimand may be most relevant. However, in a long-term trial in an otherwise similar setting, the design may need to be more similar to clinical practice, with open-label treatment, rescue therapy, etc., in order to enroll patients willing to participate in a long-term study. The more pragmatic intent and design of the long-term study, along with the inevitable loss of adherence over time, are more consistent with a de facto primary estimand than a de jure primary estimand (Mallinckrodt et al. 2016).

Mallinckrodt et al. (2016) detailed another example of how other factors can influence choice of primary estimand. Consider a trial where focus is on effectiveness, but interest is in both estimand 1 and estimand 2; that is, results with and without post-rescue data are relevant. Also consider that in this scenario it is important to keep the sample size as small as possible either because patients are hard to recruit, or for ethical reasons it is important to limit exposure to placebo. Use of estimand 2 as the primary estimand is likely to result in greater power, which translates into smaller sample sizes and reduced exposure to placebo. If estimand 2 was chosen as the primary estimand, estimand 1 with post-rescue data may still be collected and used secondarily.

2.7 Summary

An iterative process should be used to choose estimands, beginning with the objectives required to address the needs of diverse stakeholders. No single estimand is likely to meet the needs of all stakeholders. De jure (efficacy) and de facto (effectiveness) estimands each have strengths and limitations, and fully understanding a drug's effects requires understanding results from both families of estimands.

Whether or not data after initiation of rescue medication should be included in the primary analysis depends on the estimand to be tested and the clinical setting. Including versus not including post-rescue data can have an important impact on results, and therefore sample size implications and total exposure to placebo must be carefully considered.

There are many important nuances to understand about various analyses as they are applied to different estimands. These nuances are the focus of Sections II, III, and IV. However, one factor is common to all analyses for all estimands: the analysis must either entail modeling assumptions about missing data or use the fact that data are missing to ascribe an outcome. Therefore, minimizing missing data reduces sensitivity to missing data assumptions for de jure estimands, but it is also important to consider generalizability of results for de facto estimands if efforts to maximize adherence in the trial are not feasible in clinical practice. The next chapter discusses trial design and conduct for limiting missing data.

3

Study Design—Collecting the Intended Data

3.1 Introduction

The trial design element of the study development process depicted in Figure 2.1 can be parsed into two distinct components: (1) determining what data is to be collected and (2) ensuring the intended data is collected. The intent of this chapter is not to provide a broad discussion of both components. This chapter addresses the second component of ensuring that the intended data is collected. The focus is on practical aspects of preventing missing data, which is important regardless of the specific design—regardless of what data was intended to be collected. For general texts on clinical trial design, see Piantadosi (2005).

The consequences of even moderate amounts of missing data can be noteworthy and the impact of higher rates of missing data can be profound (Mallinckrodt 2013). Therefore, maximizing the number of participants who are maintained on the protocol-specified interventions until the outcome data are collected is the single most important thing that can be done to mitigate the impact of missing data (NRC 2010). That is, the best way to handle missing data is to prevent it.

Studies with more missing data than expected are suspect for poor conduct in general (LaVange and Permutt 2015). These authors noted that from a regulatory perspective, aberrantly high rates of missing data raise questions about what else may have gone awry. If a surprising number of patients miss their scheduled visits, then other aspects of patient compliance or study conduct in general may be questioned. Similarly, if a surprising number of patients are lost to follow-up with little attempt at finding out why or encouraging those still willing to participate to reconsider a decision to drop out, the study objectives may not have been adequately explained to the patients at the time of their consent, or the enrollment criteria may have been applied inconsistently, with some patients enrolled that should not have been and vice versa. A key component of study planning is to anticipate the eventualities of missed visits and attrition during the treatment and follow-up periods (LaVange and Permutt 2015).

However, minimizing missing data is not easy. Strategies for maximizing retention are difficult to study directly and what evidence there is comes from between study comparisons that are subject to confounding factors that can mask or exaggerate differences in retention due to a design feature or trial conduct strategy (Mallinckrodt 2013).

Mindful of these limitations, recent guidance on preventing and treating missing data (NRC 2010; Hughes et al. 2012; LaVange and Permutt 2015) provided a number of suggestions on ways to minimize missing data. An overview of these suggestions is provided in the following sections. Additional details on these approaches can be found elsewhere (Mallinckrodt 2013).

3.2 Trial Design

Some of the trial design options to limit missing data considered by the NRC expert panel (NRC 2010) include:

- Run-in periods and enrichment designs
- Randomized withdrawal studies
- Choice of target population
- Titration and flexible dosing
- Add-on studies
- Shorter follow-up
- Rescue medications
- Definition of ascertainable outcomes

One of the complicating aspects of lowering rates of missing data is that design options to maximize retention often entail trade-offs. A design feature that reduces the probability of dropout is likely to have consequences in other aspects of the trial. Understanding and managing the trade-offs is key to picking appropriate options for a particular scenario. The following discussion focuses on general aspects of these trade-offs. Given the idiosyncratic nature of missing data and its impacts, it is important to assess the pros and cons of the various options in the specific situation at hand.

Treatments typically do not work equally well in all patients. If there is a systematic trend for some groups of patients to have better outcomes, this knowledge can be used to reduce dropout by testing the treatment in the subpopulation with the most favorable outcome or greatest likelihood of adherence/compliance.

Selecting participants prior to randomization that are thought to have more favorable responses or other attributes is termed "enrichment" (NRC 2010). Run-in designs have an initial (run-in) period in which a subset of patients is selected based on initial response. The key difference between run-in and enrichment designs is that the active treatment is used to identify the subset of participants in a run-in design whereas prior knowledge is used in enrichment designs (NRC 2010). The trade-off with enrichment and run-in designs is that inference is restricted to the subset of patients meeting randomization criteria. Inferences do not apply to the general population because the patients available for randomization are expected to have more favorable responses than the population as a whole. For additional information on and descriptions of run-in periods and enrichment designs, see Fedorov and Liu (2007) and Temple (2005).

A randomized withdrawal design is a specific form of run-in design, typically having a longer run-in phase because the goal is to identify patients that sustain an adequate efficacy response and to then test whether or not continued treatment is needed. However, many of the same design considerations and trade-offs apply to both randomized withdrawal and run-in designs (Mallinckrodt 2013).

Protocols that allow flexible dosing to accommodate individual differences in response may reduce the frequency of dropout due of adverse events or inadequate efficacy (NRC 2010). Dose titration is when patients initially take a drug at a dose lower than the target or posited optimal dose in order to reduce adverse events and improve initial tolerability, which can reduce dropout. Flexible dosing may include dose titration, but also allows subsequent dosing adjustments. The basic idea is to set a target dose that patients may titrate to or begin initially. Dose increases above the target dose are allowed for patients with inadequate initial response, and decreases below the target dose are allowed if safety or tolerability concerns emerge (Mallinckrodt 2013).

In titration and flexible dose trials, inference is on the dosing regimen(s), not on specific doses. Hence, flexible dosing is most applicable to those situations in which inferences on dose response or specific doses are not required. However, flexible dosing may more accurately reflect actual clinical practice in many scenarios (Mallinckrodt 2013).

Add-on studies include designs for which in addition to receiving a standard of care, patients are randomized to an experimental drug versus control (usually placebo). Add-on designs may reduce dropout due to lack of efficacy and in many instances may reflect actual clinical practice (NRC 2010). However, inference is on the dosing regimen, not on the experimental drug as mono-therapy. In addition, add-on designs generally target a subset of the population with inadequate response to the standard of care because patients doing well on the background treatment are not good candidates to assess the benefits of the experimental drug (NRC 2010).

Shorter follow-up periods may lead to lower dropout rates compared with longer follow-up periods, because patients have less opportunity to experience those events that lead to dropout. In addition, shorter follow-up reduces the overall burden on patients because the number of clinical visits may be reduced, thereby fostering greater compliance with the planned assessments (Mallinckrodt 2013).

However, shorter follow-up may not be feasible because trials of specific duration are often required. In addition, shorter follow-up periods may be less efficient in those instances where the treatment benefits increase over time and are therefore larger as the duration of assessment increases (Mallinckrodt 2013). Use of shorter follow-up is essentially trading off participants who respond more slowly to study treatment with participants who drop out early. Past experience from similar trials can guide evaluation of this trade-off (NRC 2010). A potential compromise is to have the primary assessment based on shorter follow-up, but patients continue in the trial and assessments at subsequent times are secondary (NRC 2010).

Use of rescue medication was cited by the NRC expert panel (NRC 2010) as a potential means to reduce missing data. However, this approach has important implications for what estimands can be evaluated. For a complete discussion on the considerations for use of rescue medications, see Chapter 2. Importantly, if rescue medication is provided as part of the protocol, care must be taken so that availability of rescue medication does not increase discontinuation of randomized study medication (Mallinckrodt et al. 2016).

Another highlighted recommendation from the NRC guidance (NRC 2010), closely linked to use of rescue medications, was collecting follow-up data. Specifically, the panel recommended that: "Trial sponsors should continue to collect information on key outcomes on participants who discontinue their protocol-specified intervention in the course of the study, except in those cases for which compelling cost-benefit analysis argues otherwise, and this information should be recorded and used in the analysis."

The NRC guidance goes on to state that benefits of collecting follow-up data include being able to assess the impact of subsequent treatments on outcomes, to assess adverse events after discontinuation of the trial, and to help verify assumptions made about what outcomes would have been had treatment continued. If the primary estimand is to test treatment regimens that include the experimental medication and rescue medication, follow-up data is part of the primary estimand.

Given the idiosyncratic nature of missing data and its consequences, it is important to consider the specific circumstances of a trial. Following patients to monitor resolution of adverse effects is clearly necessary for ethical and scientific reasons, and is already done routinely. Sponsors should consider whether patients who discontinue due to adverse effects should be given a full assessment battery, only safety assessments, or some reduced assessment battery including safety and some efficacy outcomes (Mallinckrodt 2013). For assessing the effects of rescue treatments on outcomes, the follow-up data will often be of an observational nature—not arising from randomized comparisons. Therefore, constructing meaningful statistical comparisons may not be straightforward (Mallinckrodt 2013).

It is important to recognize that collecting follow-up data does not reduce the amount of missing data for some estimands. Therefore, collecting follow-up data should not be seen as a substitute for the most important objective of retaining as many patients as possible on the initially randomized medications (Mallinckrodt 2013).

Primary outcome measures that require invasive procedures (e.g., liver biopsies, endoscopies) are likely to result in significant missing data, and such outcome measures should be avoided whenever possible (NRC 2010). Missing data can also arise from the use of outcomes that are undefined for some patients. Therefore, primary outcomes that are ascertainable for all randomized participants should be used (NRC 2010).

One approach that may be useful in a variety of settings is to define a composite outcome that includes adherence as part of the outcome; for example, outcomes that incorporate death, or study drug discontinuation or the need for rescue medication as part of the outcome (NRC 2010; LaVange and Permutt 2015). The composite outcome may have as one component an ordinal or continuous outcome. The death and adherence components of the composite can be incorporated by ranking a continuous outcome score in a manner that assigns bad outcomes to applicable patients, regardless of the outcomes that were observed (LaVange and Permutt 2015).

Another common approach is to dichotomize the continuous outcome based on criteria for a clinically meaningful response. Patients that meet the response criteria and are adherent to study medication are considered a treatment success. Patients that did not meet response criteria, or who discontinue study medication, are considered treatment failures (LaVange and Permutt 2015).

These approaches are appealing in that they result in no missing data. However, composite outcomes should not be used to avoid the missing data if it compromises the clinical relevance of the outcome (Fleming 2011).

As detailed in Chapter 2, when including adherence as part of an outcome, it is important that the generalizability of the results is justified. For example, in a double-blind and placebo-controlled study, the decisions patients and doctors make about adhering to randomized medication may not reflect the effectiveness of the medication that will be seen in actual clinical practice. Hence, the estimator may be a biased estimate of the intended effectiveness estimand.

3.3 Trial Conduct

Trial conduct approaches to limit missing data include:

- Limiting trial burden on participants
- Providing incentives to patients and investigative sites for trial completion

- Train and educate sites and patients on the importance of complete data
- Monitoring and reporting completion rates during the trial
- Do not discontinue non-compliant patients

Trials should limit participants' burden and inconvenience in data collection. However, collecting less data means getting less information. Therefore study teams need to balance the conflicting goals of getting the most information possible from a trial and reducing patient burden in order to increase retention (NRC 2010).

Some ways to reduce patient burden include: (1) minimize the number of visits and assessments; (2) avoid redundant data collection and collect the minimum amount of information needed to address study objectives; (3) gather data efficiently using user-friendly case report forms and direct data capture (that does not require a clinic visit) whenever feasible; and, (4) allow sufficiently large time windows for assessments (NRC 2010; Mallinckrodt 2013).

Clinic visits can be made less burdensome by making the overall experience more pleasant via a welcoming environment, friendly staff that respects participant's time, provisions for transportation and availability of on-site diversions for children and/or provisions for child care. Sending visit reminders, as is routinely done in clinical practice, can also help avoid missed visits (NRC 2010).

Retention may also be increased by providing incentives for completing treatment. Some possible incentives include providing effective treatments or extension phases to participants that complete the trial (NRC 2010).

Other trial conduct features to consider include basing site/investigator selection on rates of complete data while patients are in the trial and in rates of patients who complete the trial (NRC 2010). Training provided to sites and patients on the study procedures should emphasize the importance of complete data. In those instances when follow-up data are collected, also emphasize the difference between discontinuing the study treatment and discontinuing data collection (NRC 2010).

Data completeness can be improved by monitoring and reporting it during the course of the trial. The NRC guidance (NRC 2010) suggested that the information from these assessments be available at investigator meetings and on study websites in order to create a climate that encourages study completion. Monitoring can also identify poorly performing sites and the need for remediation or site closure (Mallinckrodt 2013).

Patient education should include how their data is important to overall scientific knowledge. This information could be included in a patient video that also covers key study procedures. Participant engagement and retention can be enhanced through newsletters, regularly updated websites, study-branded gifts, regular expressions of thanks, and solicitation of input regarding relevant issues of study conduct (NRC 2010; Mallinckrodt 2013).

Investigator payments can be structured to reward completions. The NRC guidance (NRC 2010) notes that it is acceptable and generally advisable to link a final payment to completion of forms at a study closeout visit. However, the guidance goes on to caution that it is unethical for patients to continue a study if it exposes them to undue risk. But if there are minimal risks to the participant associated with data collection, it may be acceptable to provide financial incentives to continue to collect data, whether or not the participant continues treatment.

The NRC guidance (NRC 2010) also summarized what investigators and site personnel can do to reduce the amount of missing data. Suggestions included emphasizing the importance of completion (and follow-up data, if relevant) during informed consent and informed withdrawal of consent, and providing appropriate incentives for participants. The Code of Federal Regulations requires that study participant compensation is neither coercive nor at the level that would present undue influence (21CFR 50.20). Most institutional review boards allow cash payments that are slightly back-loaded, retaining a small proportion as an incentive for completion (NRC 2010).

Often, trial sponsors discontinue patients who are not compliant, justifying this practice on grounds that non-compliant patients are not useful in evaluating the effects of the drug (LaVange and Permutt 2015). However, this can unnecessarily increase the amount of missing data. Alternatively, a variable can be created in the database to note compliance status. Data can be analyzed for all patients and for compliant patients only. Whatever the reason for the protocol violation, if the patient's safety is not at risk, then encouraging discontinuation should not be necessary (LaVange and Permutt 2015)

Again, the most important aspect is to prevent missing data. Replacing language encouraging discontinuation of protocol violators with strategies for encouraging compliance and minimizing attrition would go a long way to improving study conduct and optimizing data analysis (LaVange and Permutt 2015).

3.4 Summary

Objective evidence on how trial design and trial conduct alternatives influence rates of missing data is scarce. Nevertheless, recent literature provides general recommendations that are practical to implement and consistent with good science, even if their impact on missing data rates is not certain. Although minimizing missing data is important, trials cannot be designed with this lone goal in mind. Design features to maximize retention often involve trade-offs, and these trade-offs must be considered carefully.

After choosing a design that is appropriate for the study objectives and primary estimands, appropriate investigators and patients can be chosen and trained. Trial conduct can proceed mindful of conditions and strategies to maximize retention. Progress is monitored toward study-specific goals. Reasons for dropout other than adverse events and lack of efficacy can include patient decision, physician decision, protocol violation, and loss to follow-up. These reasons leave doubt about treatment-related causality and the impact the missing data may have on treatment comparisons. The ideal trial may be one in which the only reasons for discontinuing the initially randomized study drug are lack of efficacy, adverse events, and withdrawal of consent. Depending on the goals of the study, follow-up data after discontinuation of the initial study drug and/or initiation of rescue medications might be collected.

To achieve such disposition results, proper processes, case report forms, informed consents, data capture procedures, minimal patient burden, patient accommodations, etc., need to be in place. However, trial sponsors, sites, and patients also need to believe in the importance of complete data. Rigorous selection of sites and patients, combined with education, monitoring, and incentives can help in this regard. As LaVange and Permutt (2015) noted, a key in minimizing missing data is creating a culture wherein the importance of complete data is recognized.

Importantly, changing attitudes and behaviors regarding missing data will likely help increase retention in drug groups and control groups, whereas enrichment designs, flexible dosing and other design features may have greater impact on drug groups than on the placebo groups.

4

Example Data

4.1 Introduction

Throughout this book, analyses are illustrated using various example data sets. Data sets are chosen for particular scenarios to match data characteristics with the points and principles to be illustrated. A "hand-sized" data set of four subjects is used primarily in Chapter 5 to illustrate the mixed model equations to be solved for various longitudinal models. "Small" data sets of 50 subjects (25 per arm) with three post-baseline assessments are used to illustrate the actual implementations of those analyses. Two "large" data sets are used to illustrate the analyses in real settings, one where the rate of missing data was low and one where it was high. The following sections provide more details on each data set and how they were created.

4.2 Large Data Sets

The two large data sets were based on actual clinical trial data but were somewhat contrived to avoid implications for marketed drugs tested in those studies. Nevertheless, the key features of the original data were preserved. The original data were from two nearly identically designed antidepressant clinical trials that were originally reported by Goldstein et al. (2004) and Detke et al. (2004). Each trial had four treatment arms with approximately 90 subjects per arm. The treatment arms included two doses of an experimental medication (subsequently granted marketing authorizations in most major jurisdictions), an approved medication, and placebo.

Assessments on the HAMD17 (Hamilton 17-item rating scale for depression; Hamilton 1960) were taken at baseline and Weeks 1, 2, 4, 6, and 8 in each trial. The Patient Global Impression of Improvement (PGI; Guy 1976) was taken at Weeks 1, 2, 4, 6, and 8 in each trial. The HAMD is a continuous variable. The PGI has 7 ordered categories from very much improved = 1, to very much worse = 7, with not improved = 4.

All subjects from the original placebo arm were included along with a contrived drug arm that was created by randomly selecting 100 subjects from the non-placebo arms. In addition to including all the original placebo-treated subjects, additional placebo-treated subjects were randomly re-selected so that there were also 100 subjects in the contrived placebo arms. A new identification number was assigned to the re-selected placebo-treated subjects and outcomes were adjusted to create new observations by adding a randomly generated value to each original observation.

These trials are referred to as the low and high dropout large data sets. In the high dropout data set, completion rates were 70% for drug and 60% for placebo (see Table 4.1). In the low dropout data set, completion rates were 92% in both the drug and placebo arms. The dropout rates in the contrived data sets closely mirrored those in the corresponding original studies. The design difference that may explain the difference in dropout rates between these two otherwise similar trials was that the low dropout data set came from a study conducted in Eastern Europe that included a 6-month extension treatment period after the 8-week acute treatment phase, and used titration dosing. The high dropout data set came from a study conducted in the US that did not have the extension treatment period and used fixed dosing.

Visit-wise mean changes for subjects that completed the trials versus those who discontinued early are summarized in Figures 4.1 and 4.2 for the low and high dropout data sets, respectively. In the high dropout data set, subjects who discontinued early had less favorable outcomes than completers. With only a few dropouts at each visit in the low dropout data set, trends were not readily identifiable.

4.3 Small Data Sets

Two versions of the small data set were created. The first version (complete data) had complete data where all subjects adhered to the originally assigned study medication. The second version (missing data) was identical to the first except some data were missing data such as would arise

TABLE 4.1

Number of Observations by Week in Large Data Sets

	High Dropout					Low Dropout				
Week	1	2	4	6	8	1	2	4	6	8
Placebo	100	92	85	73	60	100	98	98	95	92
Drug	100	91	85	75	70	100	98	95	93	92

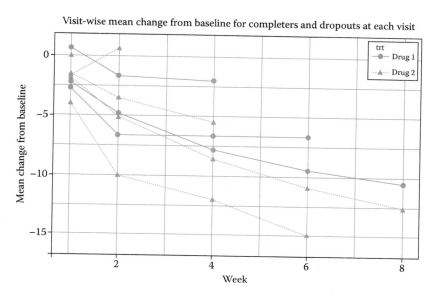

FIGURE 4.1
Visit-wise mean changes from baseline by treatment group and time of last observation in the low dropout large data set.

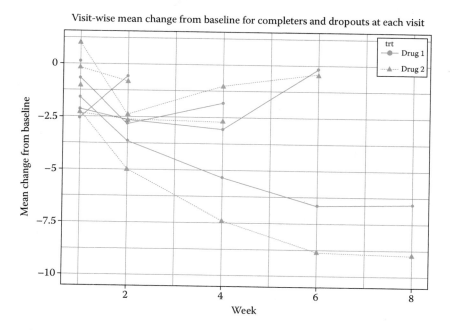

FIGURE 4.2
Visit-wise mean changes from baseline by treatment group and time of last observation in the high dropout large data set.

from subject dropout. Each data set had 50 subjects, 25 per arm, and 3 post-baseline assessments. A complete listing of these data sets is provided at the end of this chapter.

The complete data set was created from the large, low dropout data set. All subjects that completed the trial and were from the investigational site with the largest enrollment were selected. Additional subjects were selected to provide 25 subjects per arm. These additional subjects were chosen based on gender and outcome in order to yield a data set that had a significant treatment effect at endpoint and was not balanced by gender across treatments. Only data from Weeks 2, 4, and 8 were included, and then renamed as Time 1, Time 2, and Time 3. The number of observations by treatment and gender are summarized in Table 4.2. The most notable feature of the data is that the percentage of males was greater in Treatment 1 than in Treatment 2.

Baseline and visit-wise means by treatment are summarized for the complete data set in Table 4.3, and correlations between the baseline and post-baseline assessments are summarized in Table 4.4. Mean baseline values were similar across treatments. Post-baseline changes increased over time in both treatments (negative changes indicate improvement), with greater changes in Treatment 2. Baseline values had moderate to weak negative

TABLE 4.2

Number of Subjects by Treatment and Gender in Small Example Data Set

Treatment	n (%) Female	n (%) Male	Total
1	10(40)	15(60)	25
2	19(76)	6(24)	25
Total	29(58)	21(42)	50

TABLE 4.3

Baseline Means by Treatment and Visit-Wise Means by Treatment in Complete Data

Treatment	Time	N	Mean	Median	Standard Deviation
1	Baseline	25	19.80	20	3.06
1	1	25	−4.20	−4	3.66
1	2	25	−6.80	−6	4.25
1	3	25	−9.88	−10	4.85
2	Baseline	25	19.32	20	4.89
2	1	25	−5.24	−6	5.49
2	2	25	−8.60	−8	5.39
2	3	25	−13.24	−13	5.54

TABLE 4.4

Simple Correlations between Baseline Values and
Post-Baseline Changes in Small Example Data Set

	Baseline	Time 1	Time 2	Time 3
Baseline	1.00	-0.26	-0.32	-0.03
Time 1		1.00	0.76	0.52
Time 2			1.00	0.71
Time 3				1.00

TABLE 4.5

Number of Subjects
by Treatment and Time in
Small Data Set with Dropout

	Time		
Treatment	1	2	3
1	25	20	18
2	25	22	19
Total	50	42	37

correlations with post-baseline changes, such that subjects with greater symptom severity at baseline tended to have greater post-baseline improvement. Post-baseline values had strong positive correlations across time.

The small data set with (monotone) dropout had 18 completers for Treatment 1, the "placebo" group, and 19 completers for Treatment 2, the "experimental" group. Observations were deleted from the complete data set as follows: For Treatment 1, if change from baseline on the HAMD17 total score at Time 1 was less than an 8-point improvement, the probability of dropout was 30%; and, if the improvement at Time 2 was less than 10 points, the probability of dropout was 40%. For Treatment 2, if change at Time 1 was less than a 12-point improvement, the probability of dropout was 20%; and, if the improvement at Time 2 was less than 12 points, the probability of dropout was 25%. In all instances, the value that triggered the dropout was included in the data. The number of subjects by treatment and time is summarized in Table 4.5.

Visit-wise means by treatment are summarized for the data set with dropout in Table 4.6.

In contrast to the complete data set, the difference between treatments in mean change at Time 3 based on the observed data was somewhat smaller in the data with dropout. To further investigate the potential impact of incomplete data, the visit-wise mean changes from baseline for completers versus dropouts are summarized in Figure 4.3. Subjects that discontinued early tended to have worse outcomes than those that completed the trial,

TABLE 4.6

Visit-Wise Raw Means in Data with Dropout

Treatment	Time	N	Mean	Median	Standard Deviation
1	1	25	−4.20	−4.0	3.66
1	2	20	−6.80	−5.5	4.63
1	3	18	−10.17	−9.0	4.88
2	1	25	−5.24	−6.0	5.49
2	2	22	−8.14	−8.0	5.27
2	3	19	−13.11	−13.0	5.44

FIGURE 4.3

Visit-wise mean changes from baseline by treatment group and time of last observation in the small example data set with dropout.

mimicking dropout for lack of efficacy. However, Treatment 2 (drug-treated) subjects that discontinued at Time 1 tended to have better outcomes than those that completed the trial, thereby potentially mimicking dropout for adverse events.

Data from the small example data sets are listed in Tables 4.7 and 4.8.

TABLE 4.7

Listing of HAMD17 Data from Small Example Data Set

Treatment		Baseline Value	Changes from Baseline					
			Complete Data			Data with Dropout		
Subject	Gender		Time 1	Time 2	Time 3	Time 1	Time 2	Time 3
1	2	F	24	−11	−16	−24	−11	.	.
2	1	F	20	−6	−8	−5	−6	.	.
3	2	F	18	−1	−1	−9	−1	−1	.
4	2	M	10	−9	−6	−9	−9	−6	−9
5	1	F	12	−6	−3	−9	−6	−3	−9
6	1	F	14	−6	−10	−10	−6	−10	−10
7	2	F	17	−7	−7	−14	−7	−7	−14
8	1	F	21	−2	−9	−9	−2	−9	−9
9	1	F	19	−9	−6	−10	−9	−6	.
10	2	F	19	−13	−12	−14	−13	−12	−14
11	2	F	20	−11	−15	−20	−11	−15	−20
12	2	F	19	−7	−15	−19	−7	.	.
13	1	M	20	−9	−12	−13	−9	−12	−13
14	1	F	19	−6	−12	−16	−6	−12	−16
15	2	F	19	−12	−15	−18	−12	−15	−18
16	1	M	19	−3	−11	−17	−3	−11	−17
17	2	F	20	−9	−13	−19	−9	−13	−19
18	1	F	23	−7	−10	−15	−7	−10	−15
19	1	M	26	−5	−5	−11	−5	−5	−11
20	2	F	19	0	−1	−8	0	−1	−8
21	2	F	24	−12	−15	−19	−12	−15	−19
22	2	M	19	0	−2	−10	0	−2	−10
23	2	F	20	−7	−8	−13	−7	−8	−13
24	1	M	20	1	−1	−6	1	−1	−6
25	1	F	22	0	−4	−9	0	−4	−9
26	2	F	23	−12	−17	−22	−12	−17	−22
27	1	M	21	−1	−2	−3	−1	−2	−3
28	1	M	21	−2	−2	−2	−2	−2	−2
29	2	F	20	−3	−8	−13	−3	−8	−13
30	1	F	19	−2	−2	0	−2	−2	.
31	2	F	13	−1	−4	−11	−1	−4	−11
32	1	M	24	−10	−14	−20	−10	−14	−20
33	2	M	18	−4	−10	−15	−4	−10	−15
34	1	M	21	−2	−1	−6	−2	−1	−6
35	2	F	20	−5	−10	−15	−5	−10	−15
36	1	M	20	−4	−4	−10	−4	.	.

(Continued)

TABLE 4.7 *(Continued)*

Listing of HAMD17 Data from Small Example Data Set

			Changes from Baseline					
Treatment		Baseline	Complete Data			Data with Dropout		
Subject	Gender	Value	Time 1	Time 2	Time 3	Time 1	Time 2	Time 3
37	2	F	20	−3	−6	−12	−3	−6	.
38	1	F	22	−3	−5	−6	−3	−5	−6
39	2	M	20	−6	−9	−13	−6	−9	−13
40	1	M	18	−5	−9	−15	−5	.	.
41	2	M	20	5	−2	−10	5	−2	−10
42	1	M	15	0	−2	−8	0	−2	−8
43	1	M	19	−3	−9	−11	−3	.	.
44	2	F	8	−6	−3	−7	−6	−3	−7
45	1	M	20	−9	−11	−9	−9	−11	−9
46	2	M	20	−6	−5	−9	−6	.	.
47	2	F	35	−8	−14	1	−8	−14	1
48	1	M	17	−10	−14	−14	−10	−14	−14
49	1	M	23	4	−4	−13	4	.	.
50	2	F	18	−1	−1	−9	−1	−1	.

TABLE 4.8

Listing of PGI Improvement from the Small
Example Data Set

Subject	Treatment	Time 1	Time 2	Time 3
1	2	3	2	2
2	1	4	4	5
3	2	4	4	4
4	2	6	2	1
5	1	2	5	4
6	1	2	2	2
7	2	2	2	2
8	1	4	2	2
9	1	2	3	2
10	2	2	2	1
11	2	3	2	2
12	2	2	2	1
13	1	3	3	2
14	1	3	1	1
15	2	3	3	2

(Continued)

TABLE 4.8 *(Continued)*

Listing of PGI Improvement from the Small
Example Data Set

Subject	Treatment	Time 1	Time 2	Time 3
16	1	3	2	2
17	2	3	2	2
18	1	3	3	2
19	1	4	4	3
20	2	4	4	3
21	2	3	3	1
22	2	4	3	2
23	2	3	3	2
24	1	4	4	2
25	1	4	3	2
26	2	2	2	1
27	1	4	4	4
28	1	4	4	4
29	2	4	3	2
30	1	4	4	4
31	2	2	2	1
32	1	2	2	1
33	2	4	3	2
34	1	4	4	3
35	2	3	2	2
36	1	3	3	2
37	2	3	3	2
38	1	3	3	4
39	2	2	2	2
40	1	2	1	1
41	2	4	3	2
42	1	4	3	2
43	1	4	4	3
44	2	1	2	1
45	1	5	3	4
46	2	3	5	3
47	2	5	7	.
48	1	3	3	3
49	1	4	3	3
50	2	4	4	4

5

Mixed-Effects Models Review

5.1 Introduction

Some readers will find the material in this chapter most useful before proceeding to subsequent chapters. Other readers may benefit more from referring to this chapter during or after digesting the contents of subsequent chapters. The intent is to provide a general review of mixed-effect models and let readers refer to it as best suited to their individual needs. As such, readers are not obligated to digest this chapter before proceeding.

Mixed-effects models provide a flexible analytic framework for clinical trial data. The term mixed model refers to the use of both fixed and random effects in the same analysis. Fixed effects have levels that are of primary interest and would be used again if the experiment were repeated. Random effects have levels that are not of primary interest, at least usually not of primary interest in clinical trials, but rather are a random selection from a larger set of levels. In the clinical trial context, subject effects are usually random effects, while treatment levels are usually fixed effects.

The use of both fixed and random effects in the same model can be thought of hierarchically, and there is a close relationship between mixed models and the class of models referred to as hierarchical linear models. The hierarchy often includes one level for subjects and another level for measurements within subjects. There can be more than two levels of the hierarchy, such as investigative sites, subjects within sites, and measurements within subjects.

Although the following example is simplistic, it provides conceptual and practical motivation for the use of mixed models for analyses of longitudinal clinical trial data. Consider a typical clinical trial scenario where the fixed effect parameters explain the average difference between treatments and the random effect parameters represent the variability among subjects (and/or sites). It is possible to fit a model with subject as a fixed effect, with for example, a unique intercept (and possibly slope) for each subject. In addition to mistreating the conceptually random subject effect as fixed, the analysis estimates one intercept parameter for each subject. Alternatively, fitting a random subject intercept requires estimating only one variance parameter that represents the spread of the random intercepts around the common intercept. Therefore, conceptual and practical motivations support use of mixed-effect models for analyses of clinical trial data.

5.2 Notation and Definitions

Laird and Ware (1982) introduced the general linear mixed-effects model to be any model that satisfies

$$Y_i = X_i\beta + Z_ib_i + \varepsilon_i \tag{5.1}$$

$$b_i \sim N(0, D)$$

$$\varepsilon_i \sim N(0, \Sigma_i)$$

$$b_1 \ldots b_{N,} \varepsilon_1 \ldots \varepsilon_N \text{ independent}$$

where Y_i is the n_i-dimensional response (column) vector for patient i; β is the p-dimensional vector of fixed effects; b_i is the q-dimensional vector of random (patient-specific) effects; X_i and Z_i are $(n_i \times p)$- and $(n_i \times q)$-dimensional matrices relating the observations to the fixed and random effects, respectively; ε_i is the n_i-dimensional vector of residuals; D is a general $(q \times q)$-dimensional covariance matrix with (i,j) element $d_{ij} = d_{ji}$; and Σ_i is a general $(n_i \times n_i)$-dimensional covariance matrix (usually the same for all *i*). It follows from this model that, marginally,

$$Y_i \sim N(X_i\beta, V)$$

$$\text{and } V = Z_iDZ_i' + \Sigma_i$$

In other words, mixed-effects models include fixed and random effects, with overall variability (V in the above equation) that can be partitioned into a part due to the random effects (Z_iDZ_i') and a part due to the errors (Σ_i). In contrast, analysis of variance models include only fixed effects (apart from the residuals).

In clinical trials, the subject-specific (random) effects are seldom the focus. Rather, the trials are typically designed to assess differences in fixed effects, most notably treatment effects. However, accounting for the random effects is needed in order to properly assess the precision of estimates and to make the most appropriate inferences regarding the fixed effects. Specifically, the difference between subjects and/or the similarity within subjects must be taken into account in order to have standard errors and confidence intervals that reflect the true uncertainty in parameter estimates.

5.3 Building and Solving Mixed Model Equations

Data from four subjects (1, 7, 9, and 14) in the small complete data set are used to illustrate the formulation of the mixed model equations. These data are listed below

Subject	Treatment	Baseline	Change from Baseline on HAMD17		
			Time1	Time2	Time3
1	2	24	−11	−16	−24
7	2	17	−7	−7	−14
9	1	19	−9	−6	−10
14	1	19	−6	−12	−16

Mechanically, mixed model equations are constructed by matrix manipulations. However, concepts underlying the manipulations are covered before illustrating the actual mechanics. The first step, whether mechanical or conceptual, is to define the linear model. Illustrations begin with a simple fixed effects model for which ordinary least squares can be applied. Subsequently, more detailed generalized least squares and mixed-effects approaches are illustrated.

5.3.1 Ordinary Least Squares

For the hand-sized example data listed above, consider a fixed effects model where only Time 3 data are used as the dependent variable, with treatment and intercept as the only fixed effects. In scalar notation

$$Y_{ij} = \mu + \beta_i + \varepsilon_{ij}$$

where μ is the population mean (intercept), β_i is the fixed effect of treatment i, and ε_{ij} is the error (residual) for subject j in treatment i.

The equations that solve for the unknown parameters (μ, β_1, and β_2) in this model can be constructed so as to minimize the error sums of squares. The sum of squared residuals for linear models is minimized by equating the means of the observed data to the associated expected values under the model.

As the simplest case, the squared sum of deviations from the mean $\Sigma(y_i - \bar{y})^2$ is smaller than the sum of squared deviations around any other provisional value, c, $\Sigma(y_i - c)^2$; hence, the least square estimate of the grand mean μ is the sample mean, $\bar{y}$. Equivalently, the estimate of grand mean can be obtained by equating the sum of observed values with the sum of expected values under the assumed model: $\Sigma y_i = \Sigma \hat{E}(Y_i) = N\hat{\mu}$.

Thus, for each effect in the model (except residual error), compute a sum such that each observation that contains the effect is included in the sum. These sums form a vector of "observations" (observed data summaries), Y. In this model, equations are needed for μ and for each treatment group, three equations total. All observations contain the effect of μ; hence, the sum for the μ effect is the sum of all observations. Likewise, the sum for each treatment group equation is the sum of all observations for the subjects in that group. The transpose of the Y vector of sums is $(-64, -26, -38)$.

The next step is to construct the ordinary least squares equations by writing the model associated with each sum in Y and equating each sum to the associated sum of the model-based predictions. The sum for the μ equation contains all four observations; therefore, the μ equation contains four μ and two β_i of one kind or another. The model and the associated equations can be written in matrix form as follows:

$$X\beta = Y$$

$$= \begin{pmatrix} 4 & 2 & 2 \\ 2 & 2 & 0 \\ 2 & 0 & 2 \end{pmatrix} \begin{pmatrix} \mu \\ \beta_1 \\ \beta_2 \end{pmatrix} = \begin{pmatrix} -64 \\ -38 \\ -26 \end{pmatrix}$$

While it is important to bear in mind the concept of equating sums to effects, the task of building the equations (coefficient matrix and right-hand side) is made much easier via the use of design (aka incidence) matrices. Incidence matrices are matrices of 0s and 1s that relate observations to the various effects. These matrices have a row for each observation and a column for each effect in the model. Whenever an observation contains an effect, a 1 is placed in the cell corresponding to the appropriate row and column, otherwise place a 0. In the example above, the X incidence matrix is

$$\begin{pmatrix} 1 & 1 & 0 \\ 1 & 1 & 0 \\ 1 & 0 & 1 \\ 1 & 0 & 1 \end{pmatrix}$$

Pre-multiplying X by its transpose (X′) creates the coefficient matrix (X′X):

$$
\begin{pmatrix} 1 & 1 & 1 & 1 \\ 1 & 1 & 0 & 0 \\ 0 & 0 & 1 & 1 \end{pmatrix}
\begin{pmatrix} 1 & 1 & 0 \\ 1 & 1 & 0 \\ 1 & 0 & 1 \\ 1 & 0 & 1 \end{pmatrix}
=
\begin{pmatrix} 4 & 2 & 2 \\ 2 & 2 & 0 \\ 2 & 0 & 2 \end{pmatrix}
$$

Pre-multiplying the vector of observations Y by X′ creates the appropriate sums:

$$
\begin{pmatrix} 1 & 1 & 1 & 1 \\ 1 & 1 & 0 & 0 \\ 0 & 0 & 1 & 0 \end{pmatrix}
\begin{pmatrix} -24 \\ -14 \\ -10 \\ -16 \end{pmatrix}
=
\begin{pmatrix} -64 \\ -38 \\ -26 \end{pmatrix}
$$

Hence, the matrix equations are now

$$(X'X)\beta = X'Y$$

And the solutions to the ordinary least square equations are

$$\beta = (X'X)^{-1}\,X'Y$$

Therefore, solving the equations requires an inverse of the coefficient matrix X′X. Unfortunately, the equations as written cannot be solved due to dependencies. That is, the two equations for the two treatments sum to the equation for μ. Therefore, the equations are not independent. The coefficient matrix is said to be singular and it cannot be inverted, nor can the equations be solved using iterative techniques.

The solution to this dilemma is to create a generalized inverse by first imposing constraints on the coefficient matrix that eliminate the dependency. For example, the coefficients for one row of the equations, which corresponds to one of the effects in β, can be set equal to zero, which eliminates the dependency of the two treatment equations summing to the μ equation. When a dependency is eliminated by using coefficients of zero for a row, zeros must also replace the original coefficients in the corresponding column for that effect.

The effects of imposing constraints, in addition to facilitating inversion of the coefficient matrix, include:

1. The expected values of solutions for fixed effects do not equal the actual fixed effect, but rather equal estimable functions of the fixed effects.

2. Solutions depend on the specific constraint(s) imposed. Different constraints for the same set of equations yield different solutions that reflect different estimable functions of the fixed effects.

3. Typically, regardless of specific constraints, the expected value of the difference in solutions reflects the difference in fixed effects. That is, the differences are estimable even if the actual effects are not.

4. Random effects solutions are unaffected by the constraints imposed on the fixed effects equations, and are said to be "translation invariant."

For the present simple example, one constraint that can be imposed is set the μ equation equal to 0, or simpler still, not include μ in the model. With this constraint the equations are:

$$\begin{pmatrix} 2 & 0 \\ 0 & 2 \end{pmatrix} \begin{pmatrix} \beta_1 \\ \beta_2 \end{pmatrix} = \begin{pmatrix} -26 \\ -38 \end{pmatrix}$$

The solutions vector β' is $(-13, -19)$, which in this simplistic example is also the simple averages for each treatment. With this constraint, the first solution represents $\mu + \beta_1$ and the second solution is $\mu + \beta_2$. The solutions in this unique example are conveniently the least square means (lsmeans) for the treatments. Typically, the estimable functions will be more complex and less convenient.

An lsmean is an estimate from a linear model, whereas a raw (arithmetic) mean is the simple average. In this simple model, the lsmeans for treatment are also the simple averages. As illustrated in later sections, the lsmeans seldom equal the raw means because the lsmeans are adjusted for other terms (covariates) in the model, thereby reflecting the independent effect of the fixed effects.

Another interesting aspect of this simple model is that changing the data for a subject in one treatment only influences the solution for that effect and the other solution is unaffected. For example, if the outcome for Subject 1 was 0 instead of 24 then $\beta' = (-13, -7)$. Later examples with more complex models will illustrate that such independence is usually not the case as estimates of fixed effects are typically correlated. That is, changing the data for a subject in treatment 1 can change the estimates of not just treatment 1 but also other effects in the model.

Another possible constraint would be to "zero out" the equation for β_2. The resulting equations with this constraint are

$$
\begin{pmatrix} 4 & 2 & 0 \\ 2 & 2 & 0 \\ 0 & 0 & 0 \end{pmatrix} \begin{pmatrix} \mu \\ \beta_1 \\ \beta_2 \end{pmatrix} = \begin{pmatrix} -64 \\ -26 \\ 0 \end{pmatrix}
$$

The solution vector $\beta' = 19, 6, 0$. The estimable functions with these solutions are that the first element $= \mu + \beta_2$ and the second element is $\beta_1 - \beta_2$.

A slightly more complex model that includes in addition to treatment the fixed covariate of baseline severity can be fit by including the actual covariate values in X. The appropriate X matrix is:

$$
X = \begin{array}{cccc} \mu & \beta_1 & \beta_2 & \beta_3 \\ \begin{pmatrix} 1 & 1 & 0 & 19 \\ 1 & 1 & 0 & 19 \\ 1 & 0 & 1 & 24 \\ 1 & 0 & 1 & 17 \end{pmatrix} \end{array}
$$

The resulting coefficient matrix (X′X) has four effects, μ, two treatment effects, and the covariate.

$$
\begin{pmatrix} 4 & 2 & 2 & 79 \\ 2 & 2 & 0 & 38 \\ 2 & 0 & 2 & 41 \\ 79 & 38 & 41 & 1587 \end{pmatrix} \begin{pmatrix} \mu \\ \beta_1 \\ \beta_2 \\ \beta_3 \end{pmatrix} = \begin{pmatrix} -64 \\ -26 \\ -38 \\ -1308 \end{pmatrix}
$$

The equation for the covariate is in the fourth row (and fourth column). The value in the first position of row 4 (79) is the sum of all baseline values, the second and third positions are sums of the baseline values in the respective treatment groups (38, 41), and the last entry (1587) is the sum of the squared baseline values. The last entry in the Y vector (–1308) is the sum of cross products. Adding this continuous covariate does not add a dependency, and (as before) only one constraint is needed to yield a coefficient matrix that can be inverted.

To fit more complex models with multiple fixed effects, the same process is used as with simple models, but the design (incidence) matrices and coefficient matrices are more extensive. Recall that the example data from four subjects includes three assessments per subject taken at 3 time points. To include time in the model, the X matrix now has 12 rows and 6 columns to associate the 12 observations with the 6 fixed effects (μ, 2 treatments, and 3 time points).

$$
X = \begin{array}{cccccc}
\mu & \beta_1 & \beta_2 & \tau_1 & \tau_2 & \tau_3 \\
\end{array}
$$

$$
X = \left(\begin{array}{cccccc}
1 & 1 & 0 & 1 & 0 & 0 \\
1 & 1 & 0 & 1 & 0 & 0 \\
1 & 1 & 0 & 0 & 1 & 0 \\
1 & 1 & 0 & 0 & 1 & 0 \\
1 & 1 & 0 & 0 & 0 & 1 \\
1 & 1 & 0 & 0 & 0 & 1 \\
1 & 0 & 1 & 1 & 0 & 0 \\
1 & 0 & 1 & 1 & 0 & 0 \\
1 & 0 & 1 & 0 & 1 & 0 \\
1 & 0 & 1 & 0 & 1 & 0 \\
1 & 0 & 1 & 0 & 0 & 1 \\
1 & 0 & 1 & 0 & 0 & 1 \\
\end{array} \right)
$$

And the coefficient matrix and right-hand sides are

$$
\left(\begin{array}{cccccc}
12 & 6 & 6 & 4 & 4 & 4 \\
6 & 6 & 0 & 2 & 2 & 2 \\
6 & 0 & 6 & 2 & 2 & 2 \\
4 & 2 & 2 & 4 & 0 & 0 \\
4 & 2 & 2 & 0 & 4 & 0 \\
4 & 2 & 2 & 0 & 0 & 4 \\
\end{array} \right)
\left(\begin{array}{c}
\mu \\
\beta_1 \\
\beta_2 \\
\tau_1 \\
\tau_2 \\
\tau_3 \\
\end{array} \right)
=
\left(\begin{array}{c}
-138 \\
-59 \\
-79 \\
-33 \\
-41 \\
-64 \\
\end{array} \right)
$$

To solve these equations, two constraints are needed; for example, the last treatment equation and the last time equation can be set to zero.

$$
\left(\begin{array}{cccccc}
12 & 6 & 0 & 4 & 4 & 0 \\
6 & 6 & 0 & 2 & 2 & 0 \\
0 & 0 & 0 & 0 & 0 & 0 \\
4 & 2 & 0 & 4 & 0 & 0 \\
4 & 2 & 0 & 0 & 4 & 0 \\
0 & 0 & 0 & 0 & 0 & 0 \\
\end{array} \right)
\left(\begin{array}{c}
\mu \\
\beta_1 \\
\beta_2 \\
\tau_1 \\
\tau_2 \\
\tau_3 \\
\end{array} \right)
=
\left(\begin{array}{c}
-138 \\
-59 \\
0 \\
-33 \\
-41 \\
0 \\
\end{array} \right)
$$

The solution vector $\beta' = 17.67, 3.33, 0, 7.75, 5.75, 0$. And the lsmeans derived from these solutions are

trt	1	-9.83
trt	2	-13.16
Time	1	-8.25
Time	2	-10.25
Time	3	-16.00

While it is easy to see that the differences in solutions for the treatment effects and the time effects match the differences in lsmeans, the estimable functions represented by each solution are more complex when more constraints are imposed.

It is often of interest to model the effects of interactions between main effects. For example, the effect of treatment may not be constant over time. The X matrix for the example data with a model that includes the effects of treatment (β_i), time (τ_j) and the treatment-by-time interaction ($\beta\tau_{ij}$) is given below.

	μ	β_1	β_2	τ_1	τ_2	τ_3	$\beta\tau_{11}$	$\beta\tau_{12}$	$\beta\tau_{13}$	$\beta\tau_{21}$	$\beta\tau_{22}$	$\beta\tau_{23}$
	1	1	0	1	0	0	1	0	0	0	0	0
	1	1	0	1	0	0	1	0	0	0	0	0
	1	1	0	0	1	0	0	1	0	0	0	0
	1	1	0	0	1	0	0	1	0	0	0	0
	1	1	0	0	0	1	0	0	1	0	0	0
X =	1	1	0	0	0	1	0	0	1	0	0	0
	1	0	1	1	0	0	1	0	0	1	0	0
	1	0	1	1	0	0	1	0	0	1	0	0
	1	0	1	0	1	0	0	0	0	0	1	0
	1	0	1	0	1	0	0	0	0	0	1	0
	1	0	1	0	0	1	0	0	0	0	0	1
	1	0	1	0	0	1	0	0	0	0	0	1

Nested effects are similar to interaction effects except that one factor of the interaction effect does not appear as a main effect. Consider again the X matrix described earlier for the model with treatment and baseline severity as fixed effects:

μ	β_1	β_2	γ
1	1	0	19
1	1	0	19
1	0	1	24
1	0	1	17

The X matrix for a model with categorical treatment, baseline severity as a covariate, and the treatment-by-baseline severity interaction is:

$$
\begin{array}{cccccc}
\mu & \beta_1 & \beta_2 & \gamma & (\beta\gamma)_1 & (\beta\gamma)_2 \\
\end{array}
$$

$$
\begin{pmatrix}
1 & 1 & 0 & 19 & 19 & 0 \\
1 & 1 & 0 & 19 & 19 & 0 \\
1 & 0 & 1 & 24 & 0 & 24 \\
1 & 0 & 1 & 17 & 0 & 17 \\
\end{pmatrix}
$$

The X matrix for a model that included treatment and baseline severity nested within treatment is:

$$
\begin{array}{ccccc}
\mu & \beta_1 & \beta_2 & (\beta\gamma)_1 & (\beta\gamma)_2 \\
\end{array}
$$

$$
\begin{pmatrix}
1 & 1 & 0 & 19 & 0 \\
1 & 1 & 0 & 19 & 0 \\
1 & 0 & 1 & 0 & 24 \\
1 & 0 & 1 & 0 & 17 \\
\end{pmatrix}
$$

As an artifact of the small example, both subjects in treatment 1 have a value of 19 for baseline severity, which creates an additional dependency making the equations unsolvable. However, in realistic scenarios where not all baseline values within a treatment were the same, the equations would be solvable and the interaction model and the nested model would yield identical fits to the data and identical treatment contrasts.

5.3.2 Generalized Least Squares

Ordinary least squares assume that observations are independent, an assumption that is not justifiable when subjects are measured repeatedly over time. Therefore, now assume that errors have a general covariance matrix, $\text{Var}[\varepsilon] = \Sigma$, such that the model becomes

$$
Y = X\beta + \varepsilon \qquad \varepsilon \sim (0, \Sigma)
$$

Generalized least squares minimizes the generalized error sum of squares

$$
\text{SSE}_g = (Y - X\beta)' \Sigma^{-1} (Y - X\beta)
$$

This leads to the generalized normal equations

$$
(X' \Sigma^{-1} X)\beta = X' \Sigma^{-1} Y
$$

and the GLS estimator

$$
\hat{\beta}_g = (X' \Sigma^{-1} X)^- X' \Sigma^{-1} Y
$$

5.3.3 Mixed-Effects Models

As noted earlier, the mixed model is written as

$$Y = X\beta + Zb + \varepsilon$$

where terms are the same as in the general linear model described above except for the addition of the known design matrix, Z, and the vector b of unknown random-effects parameters. The Z matrix can contain either continuous or dummy variables, just like X. The model assumes that b and ε are normally distributed with

$$E \begin{bmatrix} b \\ \varepsilon \end{bmatrix} = \begin{bmatrix} 0 \\ 0 \end{bmatrix}$$

$$Var \begin{bmatrix} b \\ \varepsilon \end{bmatrix} = \begin{bmatrix} G & 0 \\ 0 & R \end{bmatrix}$$

The variance of Y is $V = ZGZ' + R$, and is modeled via the random-effects design matrix Z and covariance structures G and R.

Building the coefficient matrix and right-hand side proceeds as before, albeit with more steps to incorporate both the X and Z design matrices. For simplicity, consider the example data and a model that includes only treatment and a random intercept for each subject, ignoring the correlation between the repeated observations (G and R) for now. Because the fixed effects in this model are the same as previously described, the X matrix will be the same. The Z matrix for this example is as follows:

$$\begin{pmatrix}
1 & 0 & 0 & 0 \\
1 & 0 & 0 & 0 \\
1 & 0 & 0 & 0 \\
0 & 1 & 0 & 0 \\
0 & 1 & 0 & 0 \\
0 & 1 & 0 & 0 \\
0 & 0 & 1 & 0 \\
0 & 0 & 1 & 0 \\
0 & 0 & 1 & 0 \\
0 & 0 & 0 & 1 \\
0 & 0 & 0 & 1 \\
0 & 0 & 0 & 1
\end{pmatrix}$$

The mixed model equations are

$$\begin{pmatrix} X'X & X'Z \\ Z'X & Z'Z \end{pmatrix} \begin{pmatrix} \beta \\ b \end{pmatrix} = \begin{pmatrix} X'Y \\ Z'Y \end{pmatrix}$$

which for the example data yields:

$$\begin{pmatrix} 12 & 6 & 6 & 3 & 3 & 3 & 3 \\ 6 & 6 & 0 & 0 & 0 & 3 & 3 \\ 6 & 0 & 6 & 3 & 3 & 0 & 0 \\ 3 & 0 & 3 & 0 & 3 & 0 & 0 \\ 3 & 0 & 3 & 0 & 3 & 0 & 0 \\ 3 & 3 & 0 & 0 & 0 & 3 & 0 \\ 3 & 3 & 0 & 0 & 0 & 0 & 3 \end{pmatrix} \begin{pmatrix} \mu \\ \beta_1 \\ \beta_2 \\ b_1 \\ b_2 \\ b_3 \\ b_4 \end{pmatrix} = \begin{pmatrix} -138 \\ -59 \\ -79 \\ -51 \\ -28 \\ -25 \\ -34 \end{pmatrix}$$

The mixed model equations that take into account the within-subject correlations include the G and R matrices. In practice estimates of G and R, which are denoted $\hat{G}$ and $\hat{R}$, respectively, are usually needed since the true values are not known. Estimates of β and b can be obtained from solving the following equations (Henderson 1984):

$$\begin{bmatrix} X'\hat{R}^{-1}X & X'\hat{R}^{-1}Z \\ Z'\hat{R}^{-1}X & Z'\hat{R}^{-1}Z+\hat{G}^{-1} \end{bmatrix} \begin{bmatrix} \hat{\beta} \\ \hat{b} \end{bmatrix} = \begin{bmatrix} X'\hat{R}^{-1}Y \\ Z'\hat{R}^{-1}Y \end{bmatrix}$$

The solutions can obtained as

$$\hat{\beta} = (X'\hat{V}^{-1}X)^{-}X'\hat{V}^{-1}Y$$

$$\hat{b} = \hat{G}Z'\hat{V}^{-1}(Y - X\hat{\beta})$$

If G and R are known, $\hat{\beta}$ is the best linear unbiased estimator (BLUE) of β, and $\hat{b}$ is the best linear unbiased predictor (BLUP) of b (Searle 1971; Harville 1988, 1990). In this context, "best" means minimum mean squared error.

The covariance matrix of $(\hat{\beta} - \beta, \hat{b} - b)$ is

$$C = \begin{bmatrix} X'R^{-1}X & X'R^{-1}Z \\ Z'R^{-1}X & Z'R^{-1}Z + G^{-1} \end{bmatrix}$$

Again, in practice $\hat{G}$ and $\hat{R}$ are substituted into the preceding expression to obtain

$$\hat{C} = \begin{bmatrix} X'\hat{R}^{-1}X & X'\hat{R}^{-1}Z \\ Z'\hat{R}^{-1}X & Z'\hat{R}^{-1}Z + \hat{G}^{-1} \end{bmatrix}$$

as the approximate variance-covariance matrix of $(\hat{\beta} - \beta, \hat{b} - b)$. The matrix C has as diagonal elements error variances and off-diagonals are error covariances. With estimated G and R ($\hat{G}$ and $\hat{R}$), the solutions are approximate BLUE and BLUP, which are often referred to as empirical BLUE and BLUP (EBLUE and EBLUP).

True sampling variability is underestimated by $\hat{C}$ because the uncertainty in estimating G and R is not taken into account. Inflation factors have been proposed (Prasad and Rao 1990), but they tend to be small for data sets that are fairly balanced. Another approach to accounting for the underestimation of uncertainty is approximate t and F statistics that are based on Kenward-Roger or Satterthwaite-based degrees of freedom (SAS 2013).

Returning to the example data introduced at the beginning of Section 5.3 and a model with treatment and a random intercept, now incorporating G and R, assuming values of 1 for both the random intercept and residual variances, the mixed model equations become

$$\begin{pmatrix} 12 & 6 & 6 & 3 & 3 & 3 & 3 \\ 6 & 6 & 0 & 0 & 0 & 3 & 3 \\ 6 & 0 & 6 & 3 & 3 & 0 & 0 \\ 3 & 0 & 3 & 4 & 0 & 0 & 0 \\ 3 & 0 & 3 & 0 & 4 & 0 & 0 \\ 3 & 3 & 0 & 0 & 0 & 4 & 0 \\ 3 & 3 & 0 & 0 & 0 & 0 & 4 \end{pmatrix} \begin{pmatrix} \mu \\ \beta_1 \\ \beta_2 \\ b_1 \\ b_2 \\ b_3 \\ b_4 \end{pmatrix} = \begin{pmatrix} -138 \\ -59 \\ -79 \\ -51 \\ -28 \\ -25 \\ -34 \end{pmatrix}$$

A residual variance of 1 results in no change to the X'X, X'Z, and Z'X parts of C. However, the Z'Z part of C now has 4s as non-zero values rather than 3s due to the addition of G^{-1} to that part of the coefficient matrix. If the residual variance again = 1 and the random intercept variance = 9, then the coefficient matrix and right-hand side become

$$
\begin{pmatrix}
12 & 6 & 6 & 3 & 3 & 3 & 3 \\
6 & 6 & 0 & 0 & 0 & 3 & 3 \\
6 & 0 & 6 & 3 & 3 & 0 & 0 \\
3 & 0 & 3 & 3.11 & 0 & 0 & 0 \\
3 & 0 & 3 & 0 & 3.11 & 0 & 0 \\
3 & 3 & 0 & 0 & 0 & 3.11 & 0 \\
3 & 3 & 0 & 0 & 0 & 0 & 3.11
\end{pmatrix}
\begin{pmatrix}
\mu \\
\beta_1 \\
\beta_2 \\
b_1 \\
b_2 \\
b_3 \\
b_4
\end{pmatrix}
=
\begin{pmatrix}
-138 \\
-59 \\
-79 \\
-51 \\
-28 \\
-25 \\
-34
\end{pmatrix}
$$

Note that with a larger value for intercept variance, the Z′Z part of C is augmented with smaller values.

If the residual variance = 9 and the random intercept variance = 1 then the coefficient matrix and right-hand side become

$$
\begin{pmatrix}
1.33 & 0.66 & 0.66 & 0.33 & 0.33 & 0.33 & 0.33 \\
0.66 & 0.66 & 0 & 0 & 0 & 0.33 & 0.33 \\
0.66 & 0 & 0.66 & 0.33 & 0.33 & 0 & 0 \\
0.33 & 0 & 0.33 & 1.33 & 0 & 0 & 0 \\
0.33 & 0 & 0.33 & 0 & 1.33 & 0 & 0 \\
0.33 & 0.33 & 0 & 0 & 0 & 1.33 & 0 \\
0.33 & 0.33 & 0 & 0 & 0 & 0 & 1.33
\end{pmatrix}
\begin{pmatrix}
\mu \\
\beta_1 \\
\beta_2 \\
b_1 \\
b_2 \\
b_3 \\
b_4
\end{pmatrix}
=
\begin{pmatrix}
-15.33 \\
-6.55 \\
-8.77 \\
-5.66 \\
-3.11 \\
-2.77 \\
-3.77
\end{pmatrix}
$$

Note that with a larger residual variance the values in R^{-1} are smaller; therefore, the $X'R^{-1}X$, $X'R^{-1}Z$, and $Z'R^{-1}X$ parts of C and the right-hand side $Z'R^{-1}Y$ are also smaller.

5.3.4 Inference Tests

Inferences regarding fixed- and random-effects parameters in the mixed model are obtained by testing the hypothesis

$$
H : L \begin{bmatrix} \beta \\ b \end{bmatrix} = 0
$$

where L is a contrast vector or matrix with coefficients that pull the needed elements from β and b. When L consists of a single row, a general *t* statistic is constructed as illustrated below by again using L to pull the appropriate solutions for the numerator and the appropriate variances and covariances from the coefficient matrix C for the denominator. For example, the variance of the difference between Treatment 1 and Treatment 2 is equal to the variance of Treatment 1 + the variance of Treatment 2 − 2 times the covariance between Treatments 1 and 2 (McLean and Sanders 1988; Stroup 1989). The L vector is set up to extract these elements from the coefficient matrix.

$$t = \frac{L \begin{bmatrix} \hat{\beta} \\ \hat{b} \end{bmatrix}}{\sqrt{L\hat{C}L'}}$$

Under the assumed normality of b and ε, t is in general only approximately t-distributed, and its degrees of freedom must be estimated. With $\hat{v}$ being the approximate degrees of freedom, the associated confidence interval is

$$L \begin{bmatrix} \hat{\beta} \\ \hat{b} \end{bmatrix} \pm t_{\hat{v}, \alpha/2} \sqrt{L\hat{C}L'}$$

where $t_{\hat{v}, \alpha/2}$ is the $(1-\alpha/2)100$th percentile of the $t_{\hat{v}}$ distribution. If the rank of L is greater than 1, the following general F statistic can be constructed:

$$F = \frac{\begin{bmatrix} \hat{\beta} \\ \hat{b} \end{bmatrix}' L'(L\hat{C}L')^{-1}L \begin{bmatrix} \hat{\beta} \\ \hat{b} \end{bmatrix}}{r}$$

where $r = \text{rank}(L\hat{C}L')$. Analogous to t, F in general has an approximate F distribution with r numerator degrees of freedom and $\hat{v}$ denominator degrees of freedom (SAS 2013).

5.4 Impact of Variance, Correlation, and Missing Data on Mixed Model Estimates

5.4.1 Impact of Variance and Correlation in Complete and Balanced Data

Important properties of mixed models can be illustrated by examples. For that purpose, consider the hand-sized complete data set of four subjects introduced at the beginning of Section 5.3. To these data fit a model that includes treatment, time, treatment-by-time interaction, and a random intercept for each subject. Further assume the following four combinations of values for the intercept (between subject) (σ_b^2) and residual (σ_e^2) variances:

Random Intercept Variance	Residual Variance	Total Variance
1	1	2
1	9	10
5	5	10
9	1	10

Lsmeans and standard errors for these scenarios are summarized in Table 5.1.

With complete data, the values of variance components do not influence estimates of fixed effect means. The Time 3 and treatment main effect contrast lsmeans are the same across the four combinations of variance components. However, the variance components do influence the standard errors. As expected, increasing the total variance from 2 to 10 increased the standard error of Time 3 and treatment main effect lsmeans (not shown) and of the standard error of the contrast between these lsmeans. Among the three

TABLE 5.1

Least Squares Means and Standard Errors from Mixed Model Analyses of Complete Data from the Hand-Sized Data Set

Scenario	Treatment	LSMEANS	Contrast	Contrast SE
Treatment main effect results				
$\sigma_b^2 = 1, \sigma_e^2 = 1$	1	−9.83	3.33	1.15
	2	−13.16		
$\sigma_b^2 = 9, \sigma_e^2 = 1$	1	−9.83	3.33	3.06
	2	−13.16		
$\sigma_b^2 = 5, \sigma_e^2 = 5$	1	−9.83	3.33	2.58
	2	−13.16		
$\sigma_b^2 = 1, \sigma_e^2 = 9$	1	−9.83	3.33	2.00
	2	−13.16		
Time 3 results				
$\sigma_b^2 = 1, \sigma_e^2 = 1$	1	−13.00	6.00	1.41
	2	−19.00		
$\sigma_b^2 = 9, \sigma_e^2 = 1$	1	−13.00	6.00	3.16
	2	−19.00		
$\sigma_b^2 = 5, \sigma_e^2 = 5$	1	−13.00	6.00	3.16
	2	−19.0		
$\sigma_b^2 = 1, \sigma_e^2 = 9$	1	−13.00	6.00	3.16
	2	−19.00		

scenarios where total variance = 10, that is total variance is equal, standard errors for the treatment main effect contrast increased as between-subject variance increased and residual variance decreased. In contrast, variance components did not influence standard errors of the Time 3 contrast.

The results in Table 5.1 can be explained as follows. As the between-subject variance increases, the covariance within subjects increases. That is, as the variance between subjects increases, correlation between the repeated observations on the same subjects increase and the amount of information gained from additional assessments on the same subject is decreased. Hence, standard errors for the treatment main effect are larger when the between-subject variance (and within-subject covariance) is greater. For the Time 3 contrast, a single point in time, the treatment contrast standard error is not influenced by the ratio of the variance components, only total variance. If data were unbalanced, (e.g., due to missing values) variance ratios would influence treatment contrasts at specific time points.

Generally, as the eigenvalues of G increase, G^{-1} contributes less to the equations and $\hat{b}$ is closer to what it would be if b contained fixed-effects parameters. When the eigenvalues of G decrease, G^{-1} dominates the equations and $\hat{b}$ is close to 0. For intermediate cases, G^{-1} can be viewed as shrinking the estimates of b toward 0 (Robinson 1991). This shrinkage can be seen in the estimates of the random intercepts across the varying levels of G and R. These results are summarized in Table 5.2.

The observation for Subject 1 at Time 3 (–24) was an improvement of 5 points more than the group mean. When $\sigma_b^2 = 9$ and $\sigma_e^2 = 1$ this 5-point advantage yielded an estimate for the random intercept of –3.70; that is, a result better than group average. However, when $\sigma_b^2 = 5$ and $\sigma_e^2 = 5$, the same observation yielded a random intercept estimate of –2.88, and when $\sigma_b^2 = 1$ and $\sigma_e^2 = 9$, the estimate was further shrunk to –0.96. The estimate of the intercept when $\sigma_b^2 = 5$ and $\sigma_e^2 = 5$ was the same as when $\sigma_b^2 = 1$ and $\sigma_e^2 = 1$ because the shrinkage is determined by variance ratios. A similar effect is seen in subjects who were doing worse than group mean, but of course the sign of the intercept is opposite, reflecting below-average intercepts for subjects with observations

TABLE 5.2

Estimated Intercepts and Residuals at Time 3 for Subject 1 from Mixed Model Analyses of Complete Data across Varying Values of G and R

Scenario	Observed Value	Group Mean	Estimated Intercept	Predicted Value	Residual
$\sigma_b^2 = 1, \sigma_e^2 = 1$	–24	–19	–2.88	–21.88	–2.12
$\sigma_b^2 = 9, \sigma_e^2 = 1$	–24	–19	–3.70	–22.70	–1.30
$\sigma_b^2 = 5, \sigma_e^2 = 5$	–24	–19	–2.88	–21.88	–2.12
$\sigma_b^2 = 1, \sigma_e^2 = 9$	–24	–19	–0.96	–19.96	–4.04

below average. Estimates of the intercept are again regressed toward the mean in accordance with the ratio of the variance components.

5.4.2 Impact of Variance and Correlation in Incomplete (Unbalanced) Data

Next, consider the impact of variance components in unbalanced (incomplete) data by re-examining the example data, but delete the Time 2 and Time 3 values for Subject 1 and the Time 3 value for Subject 9. Lsmeans, contrasts, and standard errors are summarized in Table 5.3. In contrast to the scenario with complete and therefore balanced data, with missing and therefore unbalanced data, variance components influenced both lsmeans and standard errors.

For the treatment main effect, increasing total variance again increased standard errors, and when σ_b^2 was a greater fraction of total variance, standard errors were larger. Changes in the lsmeans due to incomplete data were greater for the Treatment 2 main effect than the Treatment 1 main effect because more data were deleted for Treatment 2. The Time 3 contrast standard errors changed with variance components but in the opposite direction

TABLE 5.3

Least Squares Means and Standard Errors from Mixed Model Analyses of Incomplete Data from the Hand-Sized Data Set

Scenario	Treatment	LSMEANS	Contrast	Contrast SE
Treatment main effect results				
$\sigma_b^2 = 1, \sigma_e^2 = 1$	1	−10.70	0.00	1.30
	2	−10.70		
$\sigma_b^2 = 9, \sigma_e^2 = 1$	1	−10.60	0.60	3.12
	2	−11.20		
$\sigma_b^2 = 5, \sigma_e^2 = 5$	1	−10.70	0.00	2.87
	2	−10.70		
$\sigma_b^2 = 9, \sigma_e^2 = 1$	1	−10.78	−0.65	2.40
	2	−10.13		
Time 3 results				
$\sigma_b^2 = 1, \sigma_e^2 = 1$	1	−15.50	−0.50	1.91
	2	−15.00		
$\sigma_b^2 = 9, \sigma_e^2 = 1$	1	−15.29	0.51	3.42
	2	−15.80		
$\sigma_b^2 = 5, \sigma_e^2 = 5$	1	−15.50	−0.50	4.17
	2	−15.00		
$\sigma_b^2 = 1, \sigma_e^2 = 9$	1	−15.86	−1.66	4.47
	1	−14.20		

as for the treatment main effect. With a fixed total variance, as σ_b^2 increases, σ_e^2 decreases and the within-subject correlation increases. As with complete data, larger within-subject correlation resulted in smaller gain in precision from repeated observations. However, with fixed total variance, for a contrast at a single time point, as σ_b^2 increases, σ_e^2 decreases, which decreases error variance and reduces the standard error.

The shrinkage of random effect estimates can again be seen in the estimates of the random intercepts across the varying levels of σ_b^2 and σ_e^2. These results are summarized in Table 5.4 for Subject 1. The observation for Subject 1 was missing at Time 2 and Time 3. At Time 1, Subject 1's observation was 2 points better than the group mean. In contrast to the complete data, this is the only evidence about Subject 1 and it is easier to see how σ_b^2 and σ_e^2 influence estimates.

In this simple situation, the estimate of the random intercept for Subject 1 is calculated as that subject's deviation from the mean multiplied by the shrinkage factor determined by the variance components. With Subject 1, the two-point superiority in improvement resulted in an estimated intercept of -1.8 when $\sigma_b^2 = 9$, $\sigma_e^2 = 1$. The estimated intercept is 90% of the magnitude of the deviation from the group mean when the ratio of σ_b^2 to total variance $(9/(9 + 1))$ is 90%.

With $\sigma_b^2 = 5$, $\sigma_e^2 = 5$ and $\sigma_b^2 = 1$, $\sigma_e^2 = 1$, the estimated intercept was -1.0, 50% of the observed deviation from the group mean, and the ratio of σ_b^2 to total variance $= 0.5$. With $\sigma_b^2 = 1$, $\sigma_e^2 = 9$, the estimated intercept was -0.2, 1/10 the observed deviation, and the ratio of σ_b^2 to total variance $= 0.1$. If Subject 1's observation had been 2 points below the group mean, the estimated intercept would have been the same magnitude but opposite in sign ($-2 \times$ the shrinkage factor). If the observed deviation had been 4 points above average, the estimated intercept would have been calculated as four $\times$ the shrinkage factor.

These results illustrate that σ_b^2 and σ_e^2 define the regression of estimated intercept on deviation from the group mean. In this simple setting,

TABLE 5.4

Estimated Intercepts and Group Means at Time 3 for Subject 1 from Mixed Model Analyses of Incomplete Data across Varying Values of G and R

Scenario	Group Mean	Estimated Intercept	Predicted Value
$\sigma_b^2 = 1, \sigma_e^2 = 1$	-15.00	-1.00	-16.00
$\sigma_b^2 = 9, \sigma_e^2 = 1$	-15.80	-1.80	-17.60
$\sigma_b^2 = 5, \sigma_e^2 = 5$	-15.00	-1.00	-16.00
$\sigma_b^2 = 1, \sigma_e^2 = 9$	-14.20	-0.20	-14.40

when $\sigma_b^2/(\sigma_b^2 + \sigma_e^2) = 0.9$, the regression $= 0.9$, when $\sigma_b^2/(\sigma_b^2 + \sigma_e^2) = 0.5$, the regression $= 0.5$, etc. This makes intuitive sense because σ_b^2 and σ_e^2 define the intra-class correlation (a.k.a. repeatability) of the multiple observations on the same subjects. As error variance (σ_e^2) decreases, the reliability or repeatability of observations increases and the observations more closely reflect the true value; hence, a smaller shrinkage factor is applied.

The same general relationships were present in the complete data, but they were less obvious because, with three observations on each subject, the setting was that of multiple regression. With only one observation on Subject 1, the setting is simple regression and relationships are easier to see.

Although specific results are idiosyncratic to specific combinations of variance components and deviations from group means, the general idea of ratios in variance components defining the magnitude of shrinkage to estimates of random effects is common to all mixed-effect analyses. Importantly, change to random effect estimates due to changes in variance components in unbalanced data also influence estimates of fixed effects.

5.5 Methods of Estimation

5.5.1 Inferential Frameworks

Three general frameworks for inference are frequentist, Bayesian, and likelihood-based. With frequentist inference conclusions are drawn from significance tests, or results are expressed in terms of sample-derived confidence intervals. With Bayesian inference results are expressed in terms of probability distributions for the parameters being estimated. Likelihood-based inference arises from the assertion that all the information in samples is contained in probability distributions—called likelihood functions. The extent to which the evidence supports one parameter value or hypothesis against another is therefore equal to the ratio of their likelihoods. From these likelihoods (probabilities), confidence intervals and hypothesis tests can be constructed.

Obviously, method of inference and method of estimation are linked. Subsequent sections in this chapter briefly review common methods of estimation: least squares and generalized estimating equations (GEE), and takes a more in-depth look at maximum likelihood-based estimation.

5.5.2 Least Squares

A standard reference for least squares estimation is Snedecor and Cochran (1980). Least squares minimizes $(Y-X\beta)'(Y-X\beta)$, that is, minimizes squared deviations. The mechanics of least squares estimation for fixed effects was illustrated in Section 5.3.1. The following section provides additional detail.

Fisher (1925) introduced the method for estimating variance components by equating sum of squares to their expected values. Possibly the most important paper in least squares estimation for unbalanced data is Henderson (1953). The three methods presented in that paper, later known as Henderson's methods, were the standard estimation methods for linear mixed-effect models until fast computers became available.

In simple regression, the method of least squares determines the best fit line to the data by minimizing the error sums of squares. The degree to which the data points are scattered around the line determines how well the model "fits" the data. The more tightly clustered the points are around the line, the better the fit to the data. Best fit can be determined for any finite linear combination of specified functions and is not limited to regression settings. That is, any number of categorical and continuous independent variables can be fit via least squares.

Least squares has been used broadly across many fields of research because it is a flexible method that can be applied to simple data structures using simple models, or can be adapted to complex situations with complex models. A simple data structure could have, for example, one observation on the outcome variable per subject. More complex data structures arise when the outcome variable is measured repeatedly on each subject (or experimental unit). Least squares can be adapted to these more complex data structures. As illustrated in Sections 5.3.1 and 5.3.2, least squares can be subdivided into two categories: ordinary least squares for simple data structures and generalized least squares to accommodate correlated data.

An important attribute of least squares estimation and the associated frequentist inference is that missing data are only ignorable if arising from a missing completely at random (MCAR) mechanism. Important missing data concepts are covered in Section III, including the benefits of ignorability. See in particular Chapters 12 and 13. For now, it is sufficient to know that methods such as least squares that require MCAR for ignorability are less well-suited to longitudinal clinical trial data than methods that require the less restrictive assumption of missing at random (MAR).

5.5.3 Generalized Estimating Equations

A standard reference for generalized estimating equations (GEE) is Liang and Zeger (1986). Intuitively, GEE allows for correlation between repeated measurements on the same subjects without explicitly defining a model for the origin of the dependency. As a consequence, GEE is less sensitive to parametric assumptions than maximum likelihood, and is computationally more efficient. Some connections can be drawn between the origins of GEE and maximum likelihood. However, GEE is a non-likelihood based method, and hence frequentist, and similar to least squares. The very restrictive assumption of an MCAR missing data mechanism is required for ignorabily of missing data in GEE.

In GEE, estimates arise as generalizations of both quasi-likelihood and generalized linear models from univariate to multivariate outcomes. It is a viable approach for conducting inference on parameters that can be expressed via the first moments of some underlying multivariate distributions (e.g., treatment contrast in repeated measures analysis), especially in situations when specification of the entire multivariate distribution may be challenging. For example, GEE can be useful for analysis of non-normally distributed (e.g., binary) correlated data when maximum likelihood methods either do not exist or are hard to implement. See Chapter 10 for additional details on analyses of categorical data.

The attractiveness of GEE is in that it does not require modeling within-subject correlation structures. Even if the structure is incorrectly specified (e.g., assumed to be independent), the point estimates of parameters are consistent and the correct standard errors can be computed by using the robust sandwich estimator that is based on residuals from the fitted model. However, the relaxed distributional assumptions and non-reliance on correlation structure comes at the price of generally decreased statistical efficiency. That is, all else equal, parameter estimates from GEE will have greater standard errors than corresponding maximum likelihood estimates.

GEE obtains estimates as solutions of estimating equations that have the following form.

$$s(\beta) = \sum_{i=1}^{N} D_i^T V_i^{-1} \left(Y_i - \mu_i(\beta) \right) = 0$$

Here, the summation is over N patients, μ_i is a vector of expected marginal means for the ith subject (i.e., the set of n_i visit-wise marginal means μ_{ij} for the ith subject with evaluations at visits $j = 1,...,n_i$) that are expressed in terms of linear combination $X_{ij}^T\beta$ through an appropriate link function. For example, when modeling binary data using the logit link, the marginal means are probabilities of the event of interest that are related to a linear predictor $l_{ij} = X_{ij}^T\beta$ via an inverse logit transformation $Pr(Y_{ij}=1) = \mu_{ij}=1/(1+\exp(-l_{ij}))$. The linear combination l_{ij} is the product of row-vector X_{ij}^T in the $N \times p$ design matrix X_i and the p-dimensional vector of parameters β (e.g., associated with treatment variable, baseline severity score).

The $n_i \times p$ matrix D_i contains partial derivatives of μ_i with respect to parameters β and the $n_i \times n_i$ matrix V_i is essentially a "working model" for the covariance of Y_i that is decomposed into a so-called working correlation matrix $R(\alpha)$ (where α is the vector of estimated parameters) that is pre- and post-multiplied by the square root of diagonal matrix A_i with marginal variances.

$$V_i = \phi A_i^{\frac{1}{2}} R(\alpha) A_i^{\frac{1}{2}}$$

Note that the GEE actually contains p equations. In the simplest case of a univariate normal regression, these specialize to p "normal equations" that are obtained by differentiating the log-likelihood (or least squares) with respect to p parameters in β.

5.5.4 Maximum Likelihood

Maximum likelihood (ML) estimation for normal distribution variance component models was considered by Crump (1947). The landmark papers on ML estimation include Hartley and Rao (1967), in which the first asymptotic results for the maximum likelihood estimators (MLE) were established. Restricted maximum likelihood was introduced by Thompson (1962) and later extended by Patterson and Thompson (1971). Harville (1977) presented a comprehensive review of maximum likelihood and restricted maximum likelihood estimation in linear mixed-effects models and is a standard reference, along with papers by Laird and Ware (1982), and Jennrich and Schluchter (1986).

Loosely speaking, a likelihood function is the probability distribution function associated with the parameter(s) being estimated from the observed data sample. Parameter values are set such that the observed data sample is most likely to be generated from the underlying probability distribution. In maximum likelihood estimation, the value of a parameter that maximizes the likelihood function is chosen as the estimate for that parameter. For example, the appropriate likelihood function for a continuous variable may be the normal probability distribution, which includes parameters for the mean and variance. A key implication is that parameters for the mean and variance need to be estimated. When extending this to repeated measures taken in a longitudinal clinical trial, parameters for mean, variance, and covariance (correlation) need to be estimated.

With likelihood-based estimation and inference (as well as with Bayesian inference), missing data can be ignored if it arises from either an MCAR or MAR mechanism. This is an extremely important advantage for longitudinal clinical trial data analyses over least squares and GEE that require the more restrictive assumption of MCAR for ignorability. (See Section III, especially Chapter 12 and 13, for additional details.)

Use of least squares does not mean the errors (residuals from the model) will be small, only that no other estimates will yield smaller errors.

And ML does not guarantee the parameter estimates have a high likelihood of being the true value, only that there is no other value of the parameter that has a greater likelihood, given the data. Under certain conditions, ML and least squares yield the same results.

Restricted maximum likelihood estimates (RMLE) of the variance-covariance components are usually preferred to MLE in linear mixed-effects models because RMLEs take into account the estimation of the fixed effects when calculating the degrees of freedom associated with the variance-components estimates, while MLEs do not.

Maximum likelihood and restricted maximum likelihood estimates of G and R can be obtained by constructing appropriate objective functions and maximizing that function over the unknown parameters. The corresponding log-likelihood functions are as follows:

$$\text{ML:} \quad l(G, R) = -\frac{1}{2}\log|V| - \frac{1}{2}r'V^{-1}r - \frac{n}{2}\log(2\pi)$$

$$\text{REML:} \quad l_R(G, R) = -\frac{1}{2}\log|V| - \frac{1}{2}\log|X'V^{-1}X| - \frac{1}{2}r'V^{-1}r - \frac{n-p}{2}\log(2\pi)\}$$

where $r = Y - X(X'V^{-1}X)^{-}X'V^{-1}Y$ and p is the rank of X.

In practice, commercial software packages minimize −2 times these functions by using a ridge-stabilized Newton–Raphson algorithm, which is generally preferred over the expectation-maximum algorithm (Lindstrom and Bates 1988). One advantage of using the Newton–Raphson algorithm is that the second derivative matrix of the objective function evaluated at the optima (H) is available upon completion.

The asymptotic theory of maximum likelihood shows that H^{-1} is an estimate of the asymptotic variance-covariance matrix of the estimated parameters of G and R. Therefore, tests and confidence intervals based on asymptotic normality can be obtained. However, these tests can be unreliable in small samples, especially for parameters such as variance components that have sampling distributions that tend to be skewed to the right (SAS 2013). See Verbeke and Molenberghs (2000) for additional details on estimation and testing of variance components in likelihood-based models.

5.6 Marginal, Conditional, and Joint Inference

Within each inferential framework/method of estimation, it is also important to consider whether marginal, conditional, or joint inference is most relevant for the clinical question at hand.

To illustrate the conceptual distinctions between marginal, conditional, and joint inference, consider the following example regarding the probability of developing a certain disease. Assume that D is a discrete random variable with a value of 1 for subjects with the disease and 0 for those who do not have the disease. Further assume that R is a discrete random variable with a value of 1 for subjects with known risk factors for the disease and 0 for those who do not have risk factors. Further assume that the probabilities of D depend on R. That is, $P(D = 1)$ and $P(D = 0)$ vary depending on whether R is 0 or 1. With $R = 1$, $P(D = 1)$ is greater than if $R = 0$. Hypothetical probabilities for the example are listed below.

	R = 0	R = 1	Marginal Probability
D = 0 (healthy)	0.70	0.10	0.80
D = 1 (disease)	0.10	0.10	0.20
Total	0.80	0.20	1.0

Finding the probability for specific pairs of outcomes, D and R, requires knowledge of the joint probability distribution. An example would be the probability of a subject having $D = 1$ and $R = 0$. That is, what is the probability of having the disease and no risk factors, which in this example is 0.10 (10%).

An example of marginal inference from these data would be questions about the probability of D without regard for R. That is, what is the probability of having the disease without regard for whether or not risk factors are present? The marginal $P(D = 1)$ can be found by summing the joint probabilities for $D = 1$ across levels of R. In the example, the marginal $P(D = 1) = 0.10 + 0.10 = 0.20$. The marginal $P(D = 0)$ can be found similarly by summing across levels of R where $D = 0$ (0.80 in the example). Thus the marginal probability of having the disease = 20% and the marginal probability of not having the disease = 80%.

An example of conditional inference from these data would be questions about the probability of having the disease conditional on having (or not having) risk factors. The conditional probability of having disease in subjects with risk factors is based on only those subjects with $R = 1$. Hence, the probability $D = 1$ given $R = 1$ (which can be denoted as $P(D = 1|\ R = 1) = 0.10/(0.10 + 0.10) = 50\%$. Similarly, the probability of having the disease in subjects with no risk factors is $P\ (D = 1|R = 0)$, which is calculated as $0.10/(0.70 + 0.10) = 12.5\%$.

None of these three inferential frameworks (joint, marginal, and conditional) is inherently more relevant than the others; each can be the most relevant or not relevant depending on the question being addressed. The distinction between marginal and conditional inference is relevant in longitudinal trials of medical interventions, but perhaps not as straightforward as in the previous simplistic example.

This topic is most often considered with regard to random effects, such as subject.

The marginal and conditional means in the linear mixed model are $E[Y] = X\beta$ and $E[Y|b] = X\beta + Zb$, respectively. Therefore, the marginal and conditional residuals are $Y - X\beta$ and $Y - X\beta - Zb$, respectively. Recall that random effects are constrained to have mean $= 0$. Therefore, in normally distributed data with a linear model $X\beta = X\beta + Zb$. That is, with regard to fixed effects contrasts, there is no difference between the marginal and the conditional result. However, for data that are not normally distributed, this will not be the case.

Another way to conceptualize the distinction is that marginal inference involves the estimate of the average response in the population of subjects whereas conditional inference involves the estimates of response for the average subject (the subject for which $b = 0$). In normally distributed data, the average response and the response of the average subject are identical. In nonnormal data, they are not identical. However, the important issues are not so much numeric equality or inequality, but rather which estimate is best to address the question at hand.

Section II

Modeling the Observed Data

Given the variety of scenarios that may be encountered in longitudinal clinical trials, no universally best model or modeling approach exists. This implies that the analysis must be tailored to the situation at hand. To an extent, characteristics of the data are driven by the design of the study. And, an appropriate analysis therefore follows logically from the design—and the estimand. The analyst must therefore understand how data characteristics and estimands influence choice of analysis. In Section II, each chapter addresses a common modeling consideration for the analysis of longitudinal clinical trial data. Chapter 6 discusses various choices for the dependent variable. Chapter 7 covers approaches to modeling mean trends over time. Chapter 8 covers common methods to account for correlation between repeated measurements. Chapter 9 covers considerations for whether covariates should be included and, if so, how best to include them. Chapter 10 covers categorical data. Chapter 11 covers model checking and validation.

6

Choice of Dependent Variable and Statistical Test

6.1 Introduction

A logical place to begin in developing analyses for longitudinal clinical trial data is to determine the dependent (i.e., response or outcome) variable and upon what basis it will be evaluated. These may seem like obvious decisions dictated by the design of the trial and historical precedent. However, a number of subtleties apply and these factors reinforce the need for the iterative study development process detailed in Chapter 2. Specifically, the trial design informs the analysis, but analytic consequences also need to inform the design.

Of course, the distribution of the outcome variable influences the method of analysis. Statistical methods for a wide array of distributions are well known. In many longitudinal clinical trials the primary analysis is based on a continuously distributed variable. Continuous outcome variables can be analyzed as: the actual outcomes collected, change from baseline, percent change from baseline, or a dichotomized version of the outcome indicating whether or not some relevant threshold in the actual score, change, or percent change is achieved.

In addition, the statistical test used to evaluate these various versions of the outcome variable could be based on a contrast at a single, landmark time point, or based on multiple time points, such as a slopes analysis, treatment main effect or treatment-by-time interaction. Convention may guide the analyst to choices for the primary analysis. Nevertheless, consequences of the conventional choice should be understood. Secondary analyses of alternative choices or an alternative choice may be needed as the primary analysis.

6.2 Statistical Test—Cross-Sectional and Longitudinal Contrasts

In clinical trials, it is common to base the primary analysis on a contrast at a landmark time point. Such contrasts are often referred to as cross-sectional contrasts because the focus is on a "cross section in time." However, other "longitudinal contrasts" that involve multiple time points, for example, the entire longitudinal profile, are often worth considering for the primary analysis or secondary analysis.

An important distinction must be made for cross-sectional contrasts. Historically, cross-sectional contrasts have often been based upon just the data at the landmark time point. However, it is possible to construct the same cross-sectional contrast from the longitudinal sequence of data. Single-point-in-time analyses were likely motivated by simplicity and ease of computation in an era when computational efficiency was a legitimate concern. However, with advancements in hardware and software, such compromises are no longer needed.

Incorporating all repeated measures from a subject into an analysis rather than including just a single outcome per subject opens many possibilities for analyses. Perhaps the most important benefit from longitudinal analyses, regardless of whether or not focus is on a landmark time point, is in accounting for missing data. With repeated measurements, the correlation between outcomes within subjects can be exploited under certain conditions to provide safeguards against potential bias from missing data. Missing data is a nuanced and detailed discussion that is covered in detail in Section III of this book. The important point here is that longitudinal data require a longitudinal analysis, even when focus is on a single point in time. Therefore, the emphasis throughout this book is on longitudinal analysis, with illustrations of how contrasts can be constructed if focus is on a single point in time.

The following examples in Figures 6.1 through 6.3 illustrate some of the key considerations in choosing between test statistics that involve a single landmark time point versus test statistics that include data from all time points.

Figure 6.1 illustrates a significant treatment-by-time interaction wherein the difference between treatments varies over time. The two groups are equal at endpoint, but the effect evolved more slowly in one group. Such a scenario reinforces the need to understand the longitudinal profiles that lead to the endpoint results.

Figure 6.2 illustrates a significant treatment main effect, with a rapidly evolving treatment effect that is sustained until endpoint. The consistency of the time trends suggests the treatment main effect, which includes data from all time points, could be a useful primary analysis. The treatment main effect is in essence an average effect over all visits and can be interpreted similarly to an area under the curve analysis.

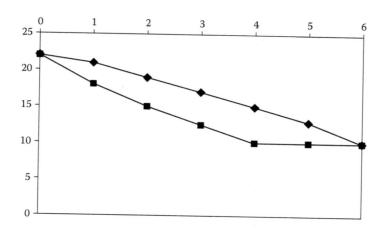

FIGURE 6.1
Illustration of a significant treatment-by-time interaction with a transitory benefit in one arm.

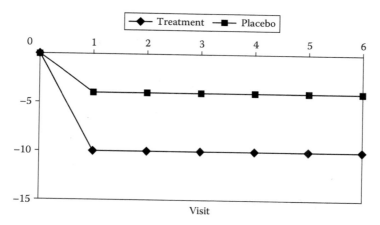

FIGURE 6.2
Illustration of a significant treatment main effect.

Figure 6.3 illustrates a significant treatment-by-time interaction where the treatment effect increases over time. The treatment contrast at endpoint is usually of particular interest in such scenarios. However, in certain situations similar to this example, focus may be on the rate of change over time, that is, time is fit as a continuous effect (see Chapter 8 for further examples).

In situations with more than two treatment arms, additional options for primary test statistics exist. For example, a global F test might be used at a landmark time point to assess if any differences exist between treatments at that visit. Or, if treatment main effects are relevant, a global F test for the treatment main effect can be used that includes data from all visits in all arms.

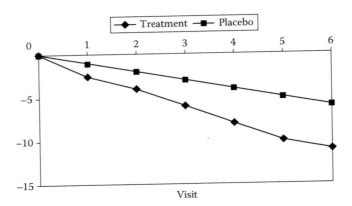

FIGURE 6.3
Illustration of a significant treatment-by-time interaction with an increasing treatment differ-ence over time.

6.3 Form of Dependent Variable (Actual Value, Change, or Percent Change)

Clinical relevance is an important factor in the choice of how a continuous outcome is expressed. In some scenarios, the outcomes are well-understood at face value and the actual values may be favored for the dependent variable. Consider blood pressure, a well-understood, objective measure for which the actual outcomes are meaningful and could be used in the primary analysis. However, medical interventions are hoped to elicit change in a condition. Therefore, even if the actual outcome is meaningful and well-understood, change from baseline may be the more intuitive and preferred outcome.

For other outcomes, the actual values may not be readily meaningful or widely understood. Take, for example, the psoriasis area and severity index (PASI) (Langley et al. 2004). The PASI combines the amount of skin covered by the psoriatic plaques (area) and the severity (thickness, redness, etc.) of the plaques into a single number that can range from 0 to 72. Experienced research-ers understand PASI scores, but the broader dermatology community may lack context and find such values difficult to interpret. Similarly, if the actual values have limited meaning, then change scores may also be difficult to interpret. Therefore, psoriasis clinical trials typically use percent change from baseline because relative changes are easier for broader audiences to appreciate.

However, the analytic consequences of the choices need to be considered. Perhaps foremost among these analytic consequences is the distribution of the dependent variable. To illustrate key points, consider the histograms of all post-baseline values for actual HAMD17 total scores, change from base-line, and percent change from baseline obtained from the small complete data set that are depicted in Figures 6.4 through 6.6.

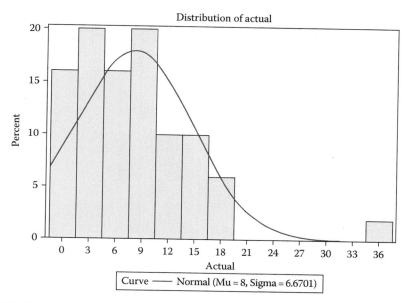

FIGURE 6.4
Distribution of actual scores in the small complete data set.

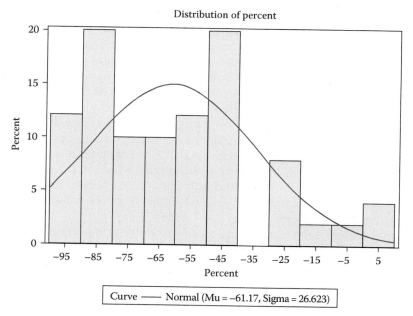

FIGURE 6.5
Distribution of percent changes from baseline in the small complete data set.

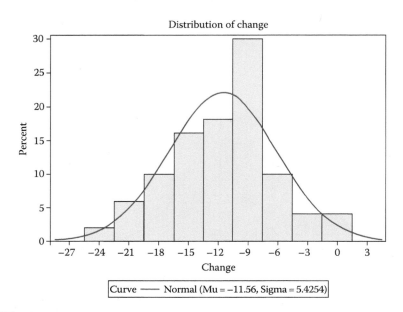

FIGURE 6.6
Distribution of changes from baseline in the small complete data set.

The actual values and the percent changes have truncated distributions, bounded by 0 for actual values and –100% for percent change. Actual scores and percent changes also have skewed distributions, with actual scores having an extreme outlier value. In contrast, changes from baseline are not truncated and are more symmetrically distributed. Of course, this is only one example and situations vary. However, whenever an appreciable portion of subjects have a score of 0, and accordingly –100 percent change, truncation and its impact should be considered.

To that end, nonnormality of the outcome variable is not the key issue. Normality of the residuals is the key distributional assumption. However, residuals are more likely to be nonnormal as the distribution of the outcome variable departs further from normality. As will be seen in Chapter 9, under certain formulations of a longitudinal analysis (including baseline score for the outcome variable as a covariate) treatment contrasts based on actual change and change from baseline will be identical.

Considerations for percent change are particularly important when there is no minimum requirement for baseline severity, as would be the case for many secondary outcomes. To illustrate, consider the hypothetical data in Table 6.1 for a 100 mm visual analog scale for pain. Subjects rate pain by marking a spot in the line describing their pain (current pain, pain during the assessment interval, etc.). Zero denotes no pain and 100 denotes the worst possible pain.

TABLE 6.1

Hypothetical Data Illustrating Actual Outcomes, Change from Baseline, and Percent Change from Baseline

Subject	Treatment	Baseline	Endpoint	Change	Percent Change
1	1	60	30	−30	−50%
2	1	1	10	9	900%
3	2	20	10	−10	−50%
4	2	80	30	−50	−62%
Mean	1		20	−10.5	425%
Mean	2		20	−30	−56%

TABLE 6.2

Hypothetical Data Illustrating Dichotomization of a Continuous Endpoint

Subject	Treatment	Percent Change	Response Status
1	1	−70%	Yes
2	1	+20%	No
3	2	−49%	No
4	2	−50%	Yes

Based on the unadjusted (raw) means, mean endpoint scores are equal for Treatments 1 and 2 (20 for each treatment). The mean change from baseline is nearly threefold greater for Treatment 2 (30 versus −10.5). The mean percent change from baseline for Treatment 1 is strongly influenced by Subject 2, who had minimal pain at baseline and a small increase at endpoint. The low baseline severity results in an extreme outlier value for percent change. While this hypothetical example is purposefully extreme, it illustrates how percent change can create outlier values and nonnormal distributions, especially when analyzing a variable with no minimum requirement for baseline severity.

In situations where percent change is customary, an alternative may be to conduct the analyses based on changes from baseline and then convert the mean changes into *percent mean change*, rather than using percent change as the dependent variable to assess *mean percent change*. In the example above, the percent mean changes for Treatments 1 and 2 are approximately −34% (mean change of −10.5 divided by baseline mean of 30.5) and −60% (mean change of −30 divided by baseline mean of 50), respectively.

Dichotomization of continuous outcomes into binary outcomes of whether or not a certain threshold of response was met causes a loss of information. To illustrate, consider the hypothetical data in Table 6.2. Assume that a 50% improvement from baseline is used as the cut off to define responder status.

The percent changes for Subjects 2 and 3 are very different (20% worsening vs. 49% improvement), but both are classified as nonresponders. The percent changes for Subjects 3 and 4 are essentially identical, but Subject 3 is a nonresponder and Subject 4 is a responder. Both treatment groups have a 50% responder rate, whereas the mean percent change is approximately twofold greater for Treatment 2.

In situations where responder rate is a common outcome, it may be useful to consider some form of mean change analysis to assess if a treatment signal exists and then use the dichotomized responder status to describe the clinical relevance of a signal, if one is found based on the mean change analysis.

6.4 Summary

Cross-sectional contrasts have often been based upon just the data at the landmark time point. However, it is possible to construct the same cross-sectional contrast from the longitudinal sequence of data. Using longitudinal analyses rather than cross-sectional analyses opens many possibilities for tailoring the analysis to the situation at hand. Actual change from baseline will usually have better distributional properties than percent changes, especially when there is no baseline minimum requirement for the dependent variable.

7

Modeling Covariance (Correlation)

7.1 Introduction

Clinical trials often assess subjects repeatedly over time. Correlations between repeated measurements *within* the same subjects often arise from between-subject variability and adjacency in time or location of evaluations. Therefore, independence of observations cannot be assumed in longitudinal trials. Failure to properly account for the association between observations can result in biased point estimates and standard errors that do not properly reflect the uncertainty in the data.

Between-subject variability (i.e., heterogeneity between individual profiles) may arise from inherent, subject-specific factors, such as genotype. Additional association may arise from unaccounted for fixed effects, such as age or gender, which like genotype influence every observation and therefore create association between repeated observations. Further association may arise due to time course (i.e., serial) correlation, which exists when observations closer to each other in time (or location) are more similar than observations further apart in time (or location).

Correlation *between* subjects is generally less of a concern in longitudinal clinical trials than correlations within subjects. Sources of correlation between subjects may include genetic or environmental factors. Generally, the frequency of relatives in a clinical trial is so low that genetic correlation can be ignored. The most common environmental source of correlation is that observations on subjects at the same investigative site (location) may be more similar to each other than to the sample as a whole.

Random measurement errors contribute to variability. In the longitudinal setting it is particularly important to consider the potential for error variance to increase or decrease over time (Mallinckrodt et al. 2003). Measurement errors tend to weaken the association between the measurements.

Longitudinal analyses can account for the correlation between observations as functions of the random effects, the residual effects, or both. Appropriate means of accounting for correlations between observations begins with considering the sources of covariation. The relative importance of the various sources of (co)variance can be useful in guiding modeling choices for specific circumstances.

For example, in analyses of objective physical measures such as blood pressure or laboratory values, subject-specific factors may have the greatest contribution to within-subject correlations. Fixed effects that are not included in the analysis (e.g., subject's age or gender) may also give rise to a compound symmetric error structure because, like random effects, these fixed effects may have the same effect on each observation. Detailed descriptions for a wide array of correlation structures are available (SAS 2013).

In analyses of subjective ratings, such as the Hamilton Depression Rating Scale (Hamilton 1960), serial correlation that decays with increasing distance in time (such as in an autoregressive structure) may also be important.

In clinical trials where the focus is primarily on the fixed effects, it may be equally appropriate, and more straightforward, to omit explicit modeling of the subject-specific effects and model them as part of the within-subject error (residual) correlation structure. In such cases, the subject-specific effects and serial correlations combine, with or without changes in error variance over time, to yield what is often an unstructured correlation pattern for the within-subject (residual) errors.

In certain settings the number of parameters that must be estimated for an unstructured covariance matrix can be prohibitive. However, many clinical trials have observations taken on the primary outcome measure at a relatively small number of time points. These measurement times are typically fixed, with narrow intervals. Thus measurements may be taken perhaps once per week, with the Week 1 observation mandated to take place between days 5 and 9, the Week 2 observation between days 12 and 16, and so on.

Therefore, unstructured modeling of residual correlation is a popular approach in clinical trials, especially confirmatory trials, because fewer restrictions/assumptions are imposed on the pattern of correlations over time. However, this should not be confused with an assumption-free approach. For example, unstructured modeling of within-subject correlation may still require assumptions, such as the same correlation structure applies to each treatment group. Of course, this restriction can be relaxed by specifying separate structures for each treatment group. However, separate structures for each group may trigger the issue of having to estimate a prohibitively large number of parameters relative to the number of subjects.

7.2 Assessing Model Fit

Given the importance of appropriately modeling the covariance between repeated measures, and the variety of approaches that can be used, it is important to assess the fit of a prespecified model and to compare the fit of alternative models.

With likelihood-based estimation the objective function can be used to assess model fit and to compare the fit of candidate models. If one model is a submodel of another, likelihood ratio tests can be used to assess if the more general model provides superior fit. The likelihood ratio test is constructed by computing −2 times the difference between the log likelihoods of the candidate models. This statistic is then compared to the χ^2 distribution with degrees of freedom equal to the difference in the number of parameters for the two models.

For models that are not submodels of each other, various information criteria can be used to determine which model provides the best fit. The Akaike (AIC) and Bayesian (BIC) information criteria are two common approaches (Hurvich and Tsai 1989). These criteria are essentially log likelihood values adjusted (penalized) for the number of parameters estimated, and can thus be used to compare different models. The criteria are set up such that the model with the smaller value is preferred.

7.3 Modeling Covariance as a Function of Random Effects

Two common means of modeling within-subject correlation include fitting a random intercept or the random coefficient regression approach that fits a random intercept and random effect(s) for time. Random coefficient regression is covered in Section 8.3. Code fragments for fitting a random intercept model in SAS and R for the small complete data set are listed in Section 7.8 (Code Fragment 7.1). Results from fitting a random intercept model are summarized in Table 7.1.

The between-subject variance (random intercept) was 15.08 and the residual variance was 8.11, resulting in within-subject correlations of approximately 0.65 [15.08/(15.08 + 8.11)]. This formulation of the mixed model assumes constant variance over time. Therefore, the within-treatment standard errors and the standard errors of the contrasts between treatments do not change over time. At Time 3 the between-treatment contrast was 3.39 and the SE was 1.36.

The correlation between observations on different subjects at the same investigative site could be modeled by adding a random intercept for site to the model above.

TABLE 7.1

Results from Fitting a Random Intercept Model to the Small Complete Data Set

Visit-wise Least Square Means			
Treatment	Time	LSMEAN	Standard Error
1	1	−4.120	0.9641
1	2	−6.70	0.9641
1	3	−9.86	0.9641
2	1	−5.31	0.9641
2	2	−8.69	0.9641
2	3	−13.25	0.9641

Visit-wise Contrasts			
Time	Difference LSMEAN	Standard Error	P
1	1.19	1.36	0.3860
2	1.99	1.36	0.1487
3	3.39	1.36	0.0151

Random intercept variance = 15.08

Residual variance = 8.11

−2 res log likelihood = 823.2

AIC = 827.2

7.4 Modeling Covariance as a Function of Residual Effects

Subject-specific effects and serial correlation or other sources of correlation can be modeled simultaneously. However, if the subject-specific effects are not of direct interest, a simpler formulation of the model can be implemented in which the random effects are not explicitly modeled, but rather are included as part of the error correlation matrix, leading to what could be described as a multivariate normal model. Under certain model specifications discussed in Section 7.5, fitting versus not fitting a random intercept in addition to fitting a residual correlation structure has no effect on treatment contrasts.

Modeling the random effects as part of the within-subject error correlation structure is the feature that distinguishes the so-called MMRM (mixed model for repeated measures) analysis from other implementations of mixed-effects models (Mallinckrodt 2013).

Many residual covariance structures can be implemented for analyses. Some example structures are described below and subsequently used in analyses of the small example data set. The compound symmetric (CS) structure has constant variance and constant covariance across all assessments. The heterogeneous compound symmetric (CSH) structure has a different variance for each assessment time and it uses the square roots of these parameters in the off-diagonal entries. The heterogeneous Toeplitz (TOEPH) structure has a different variance for each assessment time and uses the same correlation value whenever the degree of adjacency is the same (correlation between Time 1 and 2 is the same as between Times 2 and 3). An unstructured covariance matrix is completely unstructured, with different variances at each visit and different covariances for each combination of visits.

Each of the selected structures is described in further detail in Figure 7.1. Those descriptions use four assessment times even though the example data set has only three assessment times. Adding a fourth assessment time makes it easier to appreciate how the structures differ.

Code fragments for fitting the selected residual covariance structures in SAS and R for the small complete data set are listed in Section 7.8 (Code Fragment 7.2). Estimated covariance matrices from fitting these structures are summarized in Table 7.2.

With a compound symmetric structure the within-subject covariance is equal to the between-subject variance when fitting a random intercept model and the total variance is equal for the two models. When adding heterogeneous variance over time to the compound symmetric structure variance estimates increase over time, especially at Time 3. Compound symmetric models fit a single correlation parameter for all combinations of visits. Therefore, when variance increases over time the covariance must increase for observations further apart in time to maintain equal correlation.

Covariance estimates from the unstructured model and the TOEPH model were similar, with variances increasing over time and covariance decreasing for observations further apart in time. Given only three assessment times, the number of parameters estimated for the various structures did not differ

$$
\begin{bmatrix}
\sigma^2+\sigma_1 & \sigma_1 & \sigma_1 & \sigma_1 \\
\sigma_1 & \sigma^2+\sigma_1 & \sigma_1 & \sigma_1 \\
\sigma_1 & \sigma_1 & \sigma^2+\sigma_1 & \sigma_1 \\
\sigma_1 & \sigma_1 & \sigma_1 & \sigma^2+\sigma_1
\end{bmatrix}
\quad
\begin{bmatrix}
\sigma_1^2 & \sigma_1\sigma_2\rho & \sigma_1\sigma_3\rho & \sigma_1\sigma_4\rho \\
\sigma_2\sigma_1\rho & \sigma_2^2 & \sigma_2\sigma_3\rho & \sigma_2\sigma_4\rho \\
\sigma_3\sigma_1\rho & \sigma_3\sigma_2\rho & \sigma_3^2 & \sigma_3\sigma_4\rho \\
\sigma_4\sigma_1\rho & \sigma_4\sigma_2\rho & \sigma_4\sigma_3\rho & \sigma_4^2
\end{bmatrix}
$$
$$\text{(a)} \qquad\qquad \text{(b)}$$

$$
\begin{bmatrix}
\sigma_1^2 & \sigma_1\sigma_2\rho_1 & \sigma_1\sigma_3\rho_2 & \sigma_1\sigma_4\rho_3 \\
\sigma_2\sigma_1\rho_1 & \sigma_2^2 & \sigma_2\sigma_3\rho_1 & \sigma_2\sigma_4\rho_2 \\
\sigma_3\sigma_1\rho_2 & \sigma_3\sigma_2\rho_1 & \sigma_3^2 & \sigma_3\sigma_4\rho_1 \\
\sigma_4\sigma_1\rho_3 & \sigma_4\sigma_2\rho_2 & \sigma_4\sigma_3\rho_1 & \sigma_4^2
\end{bmatrix}
\quad
\begin{bmatrix}
\sigma_1^2 & \sigma_{21} & \sigma_{31} & \sigma_{41} \\
\sigma_{21} & \sigma_2^2 & \sigma_{32} & \sigma_{42} \\
\sigma_{31} & \sigma_{32} & \sigma_3^2 & \sigma_{43} \\
\sigma_{41} & \sigma_{42} & \sigma_{43} & \sigma_4^2
\end{bmatrix}
$$
$$\text{(c)} \qquad\qquad \text{(d)}$$

FIGURE 7.1
Description of selected covariance structures for data with four assessment times: (a) compound symmetry, (b) heterogeneous CS, (c) heterogeneous Toeplitz, and (d) unstructured.

TABLE 7.2

Residual (Co)variances and Correlations from Selected Models

				Covariances		
Time	1	2	3	1	2	3
	Compound Symmetric (CS)			*CS with Heterogeneous Variance*		
1	23.19	15.08	15.08	21.28	13.62	16.24
2	15.08	23.19	15.08	13.62	20.08	15.77
3	15.08	15.08	23.19	16.24	15.77	28.54
	Unstructured			*Toeplitz with Heterogeneous Variance*		
1	20.61	15.30	12.28	20.59	15.28	12.28
2	15.30	21.36	17.67	15.28	21.36	17.70
3	12.28	17.67	27.61	12.28	17.70	27.64
				Correlations		
Time	1	2	3	1	2	3
	Compound Symmetric (CS)			*CS with Heterogeneous Variance*		
1	1.00	0.65	0.65	1.00	0.66	0.66
2	0.65	1.00	0.65	0.66	1.00	0.66
3	0.65	0.65	1.00	0.66	0.66	1.00
	Unstructured			*Toeplitz with Heterogeneous Variance*		
1	1.00	0.73	0.51	1.00	0.73	0.51
2	0.73	1.00	0.72	0.73	1.00	0.73
3	0.51	0.72	1.00	0.51	0.73	1.00

TABLE 7.3

Treatment Contrasts, Standard Errors, P Values, and Model Fit Criteria from Selected Residual Correlations Structures

Structure	AIC	Time 3 Contrast	Standard Error	P
CSH	828	3.391	1.514	0.0299
TOEPH	820	3.391	1.490	0.0272
UN	823	3.391	1.489	0.0274
UN GROUP = TRT	831	3.381	1.490	0.0279

Note: CSH = compound symmetric with heterogeneous variance, TOEPH = toeplitz with heterogeneous variance, UN = unstructured, GROUP = TRT indicates separate structures were fit for each treatment group.

as much as would be the case with more assessment times. Therefore, results from the different covariance structures were more similar than would be the case with more assessment times.

Treatment contrasts, standard errors, P values and model fit criteria for fitting selected residual correlation structures are summarized in Table 7.3.

The treatment contrasts from models that fit a single covariance structure for all subjects were identical. This would not be expected to happen if some data were missing or the data were otherwise unbalanced. Fitting separate structures by treatment had a small effect on the contrast. Standard errors and P values varied slightly across the various models. The best fit came from the TOEPH model. Although the unstructured covariance model yielded nearly identical results to the TOEPH model, the TOEPH yielded the best fit based on Akaike's information criteria because it estimated fewer parameters.

A banded correlation structure may be useful in scenarios where fitting an unstructured correlation matrix is desired but problematic due to the number of parameters to be estimated. In a banded unstructured covariance matrix, not all covariance parameters are estimated. Instead, only those covariance terms within the specified degree of adjacency (number of bands) are fit and all other covariance terms are set to zero. For example, in a study with 10 post-baseline visits, if an unstructured matrix with 3 bands is fit, then for any time point only those assessments within 3 visits of the reference visit are fit, with all other covariances assumed to $= 0$. With 10 post-baseline assessments, a fully unstructured approach requires estimation of $10(10 + 1)/2 = 55$ variance and covariance parameters. Banding can therefore dramatically reduce the number of parameters to be fit, but imposes restrictions on how rapidly the correlations decay.

A vast array of residual correlation structures may be fit, far too many to fully consider here. See, for example, the SAS PROC Mixed documentation (SAS 2013) for full descriptions of the structures that can be fit within that software. While choice of covariance structure is in general an important issue, for clinical trials an unstructured approach, either overall or separate structures for each treatment, is generally preferred and almost always feasible given the number of observations relative to the number of parameters to be estimated.

7.5 Modeling Covariance as a Function of Random and Residual Effects

Code fragments for fitting a random intercept and residual correlations in SAS and R for the small complete data set are listed in Section 7.8 (Code Fragment 7.3).

Results from fitting a random intercept and an unstructured residual covariance structure is summarized below. Standard errors, treatment contrasts, and P values were identical for models with unstructured residual covariance structures that fit and did not fit a random intercept for subject.

In actual practice, a model with unstructured covariance and random effects should not be fit because this results in overspecified models. Specifically, if an unstructured covariance is fit, there is nothing left for random effects to explain about the within-subject correlations.

An unstructured covariance was used here in conjunction with a random intercept to illustrate the very point that random effects can be accounted for via residual within-subject correlations and that there is nothing left in addition to be explained by the random intercept. Note that the model fit in SAS as specified in code fragment 7.3 yields the following warning: "NOTE: Convergence criteria met but final hessian is not positive definite." Results from fitting versus not fitting a random intercept will not be identical if a residual structure other than unstructured is fit, but usually results are similar.

Even when interest centers on the fixed effects, it is still useful to understand the random effects. Variance and covariance parameters from the model fitting a random intercept and an unstructured residual covariance structure are summarized in Table 7.4. Adding the random intercept variance to each element of the residual covariance matrix in Table 7.4 reproduces the unstructured covariance matrix in Table 7.3 that was estimated from the model that did not fit the random intercept. The random intercept accounts for most of the total variance at Time 1 and Time 2, and over half the total variance at Time 3. The random intercept accounts for virtually all of the within-subject covariance.

As further noted in Chapter 8, a variety of means can be used to model correlations as a function of the random effects, and as noted above, many possibilities exist for modeling correlations as a function of the residual effects. In principle, most of the approaches can be combined in order to model correlations as functions of random and residual effects. However, model complexity should be considered and it is seldom necessary to fit both a complex random effects and residual effects modeling of correlation; usually, at least one of the two will involve a simple structure and require only one or a few parameters to be estimated.

TABLE 7.4

Variance and Covariance Parameters from
the Model Fitting a Random Intercept and an
Unstructured Residual Covariance Structure

Intercept Variance 16.06

| | **Residual Covariance** | | |
Time	1	2	3
1	4.56	−0.75	−3.77
2	−0.75	5.30	1.61
3	−3.78	1.61	11.56

7.6 Modeling Separate Covariance Structures for Groups

In Section 7.3, results from separate residual correlation structures by treatment group were included. In this example, there was little difference in results from fitting separate structures by treatment versus a single, common structure for both treatments. However, in many realistic scenarios it is necessary to at least consider the possibility that correlation structures differ for certain groups of patients. In principle, this is an extension of a *t*-test with heterogeneous variance to the repeated measures setting.

Code fragments for fitting separate random intercepts (Code Fragment 7.4) and separate residual correlations (Code Fragment 7.5) by treatment group in SAS and R for the small complete data set are listed in Section 7.8. Results in Table 7.3 showed that in these examples, fitting separate residual correlation structures by treatment had little effect on results. However, in other scenarios, especially those with unbalanced data and/or missing data, choice of correlation structure is likely to have a greater impact. Therefore, consideration of separate structures for groups is important. Separate correlation structures based on demographic or illness characteristics can also be considered.

7.7 Study Design Considerations

Although understanding the relative magnitude of, for example, a random intercept variance and residual (co)variances is not necessary to interpret fixed effects results, the variance components have implications for study design and power. Refer to the examples in Section 5.4 where given a fixed total variance, the ratio of between-subject variance to within-subject variance influenced standard errors, with the direction (increase or decrease) of effect varying depending on what parameter was being estimated.

Therefore, in powering and designing studies, it is not sufficient to consider only the total variance, rather the between-subject variance and within-subject variance both need to be considered. Historical data can be mined to determine plausible variances for the study under development. Simulations can be used to assess how differing combinations of between- and within-subject variance influence power for specific parameters.

7.8 Code Fragments

CODE FRAGMENT 7.1   SAS and R Code for Fitting a Random Intercept Model

SAS code

```
PROC MIXED DATA=ONE;
 CLASS SUBJECT TRT TIME;
 MODEL CHANGE = BASVAL TRT TIME BASVAL*TIME TRT*TIME /
   DDFM=KR;
 RANDOM INT / SUBJECT=SUBJECT*;
 LSMEANS TRT*TIME/DIFFS;
RUN;
```

R code[†]

```
# using lme function from nlme package
require(nlme)

# setting the time and treatment variables as factors
# (corresponds to the use of CLASS statement in SAS
   procedures
# Note: unlike SAS, R is case-sensitive and variable names
# should be written exactly
# as they are imported in R data frame from a csv file
complete$TIME <-as.factor(complete$TIME)
complete$trt <-as.factor(complete$trt)

# specifying random intercept model in nlme
fitmle<-lme(change ~ basval +trt+ TIME + basval*TIME+
   trt*TIME, data = complete, random = ~ 1 |subject)

# displaying model fit summary
summary(fitmle)

#displaying variance components
VarCorr(fitmle)

# evaluating treatment least square means and contrast at
   specific visit
require(contrast)
```

---

* In the data set, the patient identification variable is named "subject." If that variable were named ID, then the statement would read RANDOM INT / SUBJECT=ID;

† Obtaining P-values using the Kenward–Roger approximation in R to match results from SAS requires first fitting a random effects model using the lme4 package and then computing KR degrees of freedom using another package (pbkrtest).

```
# least squares means
contrast(fitmle ,a = list(trt = "1", basval=
   mean(complete$basval), TIME = "3"),
       type = "individual")
contrast(fitmle ,a = list(trt = "2", basval=
   mean(complete$basval), TIME = "3"),
       type = "individual")

contrast(fitmle ,a = list(trt = "1", basval=
   mean(complete$basval), TIME = "3"),
                 b = list(trt = "2", basval=
                    mean(complete$basval), TIME = "3"),
       type = "individual")

# Computing p-value based on KR df can be done using lme4
   and pbkrtest packages.
require(lme4)
require(pbkrtest)

# setting the reference (base) level for time and treatment
   variables as the last level
contrasts(complete$TIME) <- contr.treatment(3, base = 3)
contrasts(complete$trt) <- contr.treatment(2, base = 2)

# runs a random effect model using lmer procedure from lme4
   package
lmerfit<-lmer(change ~ basval +trt+ TIME + basval*TIME+
   trt*TIME+(1|subject), data = complete, REML = TRUE)
sumlmer<-summary(lmerfit)

# displays estimated variance components
sumlmer$varcor

# displays estimated coefficients; since we set reference
   levels for trt and time at the last visit the coefficient
   for variable trt estimates treatment effect at the last
   visit.
coefs<-data.frame(coef(sumlmer))
coefs

# obtaining Kenward-Roger degrees of freedom for treatment
   contrast at time 3 using pbkrtest package
trt.df.KR <-get_Lb_ddf(lmerfit, c(0,0,1,0,0,0,0,0,0))
trt.df.KR

# computing p-value from t-distribution with KR degrees of
   freedom
trt.p.KR <- round(2 * (1 - pt(abs(coefs["trt1","t.value"]),
   trt.df.KR)),5)
trt.p.KR.
```

CODE FRAGMENT 7.2   SAS and R Code
for Fitting Residual Correlations

SAS code

```
PROC MIXED DATA=ONE;
 CLASS SUBJECT TRT TIME;
 MODEL CHANGE = BASVAL TRT TIME BASVAL*TIME TRT*TIME /
    DDFM=KR;
 REPEATED TIME / SUBJECT=SUBJECT TYPE =XX;*
 LSMEANS TRT*TIME/DIFFS;
RUN;
```

R code

```
require(nlme)

fitmodel <- gls(change ~ basval +trt+ TIME + basval*TIME+
   trt*TIME, data = complete,
      weights = varFunc(form= ~ 1 | TIME),
      correlation= corStruct(form=~ 1| subject))
```

Notes

```
corStruct is specific error correlation structure,
e.g. corAR1, corCompSymm, corSymm (see R help for
corClasses{nlme}), specifying weights via varFunc
allows for various error covariance structures, for
example, combining varFunc =varIdent with
correlation = corCompSymm fits a model with
heterogeneous compound symmetry (see help for varFunc{nlme}
```

```
To evaluate treatment contrasts at time x, one can use the
contrast function from the contrast package as shown in
code fragment 7.3.
```

CODE FRAGMENT 7.3   SAS and R Code for Fitting
a Random Intercept and Residual Correlations

SAS code

```
PROC MIXED DATA=ONE;
 CLASS SUBJECT TRT TIME;
 MODEL CHANGE = BASVAL TRT TIME BASVAL*TIME TRT*TIME /
    DDFM=KR;
```

---

* TYPE = XX indicates entries for this option determine the correlation structure that is fit,
e.g., UN, AR(1), ARH(1)

```
RANDOM INT / SUBJECT=SUBJECT;
REPEATED TIME / SUBJECT=SUBJECT TYPE =XX;
LSMEANS TRT*TIME/DIFFS;
ODS OUTPUT DIFFS=_DIFFS (where=(TIME= _TIME))
LSMEANS=_LSMEANS;
RUN;
```

Type = XX indicates entries for this

R code

```
fitLME.erun.rint <- lme(change ~ basval +trt+ TIME +
  basval*TIME+ trt*TIME, data = complete, random = ~ 1
 |subject, weights = varIdent(form= ~ 1 | TIME),
correlation=corSymm(form=~ 1| subject))

summary(fitLME.erun.rint)

# treatment contrasts can be evaluated using the contrast
  package (see Code Fragment 7.5)
```

**CODE FRAGMENT 7.4   SAS Code for Fitting
Separate Random Intercepts by Treatment**

```
ODS LISTING CLOSE;
PROC MIXED DATA=ONE;
 CLASS SUBJECT TRT TIME;
 MODEL CHANGE=BASVAL TRT TIME BASVAL*TIME TRT*TIME /
   DDFM=KR;
 RANDOM INT / SUBJECT=SUBJECT GROUP=TRT G GCORR;
 LSMEANS TRT*TIME/DIFFS;
 ODS OUTPUT DIFFS=_DIFFS LSMEANS=_LSMEANS G=_G;
RUN;
```

**CODE FRAGMENT 7.5   SAS Code for Fitting Separate
Residual Correlation Structures by Treatment**

```
PROC MIXED DATA=ONE
 CLASS SUBJECT TRT TIME;
 MODEL CHANGE =BASVAL TRT TIME BASVAL*TIME TRT*TIME /
   DDFM=KR;
 REPEATED TIME / SUBJECT=SUBJECT TYPE=UN Group=TRT;
 LSMEANS TRT*TIME/DIFFS;
 ODS OUTPUT DIFFS=_DIFFS LSMEANS=_LSMEANS R=_R
   RCORR=_RCORR;
RUN;
```

7.9 Summary

The association between repeated measurements on the same subjects can be modeled as a function of the random effects, the residual effects, or both. No approach is universally better than another. The analysis must be tailored to the situation at hand.

In clinical trials, the random effects are seldom of direct interest and the number of assessment times relative to the number of subjects is often fairly small. Such situations are amenable to unstructured modeling of within-subject covariance (residual errors). Unstructured modeling places few restrictions (assumptions) on the model and is often a preferred modeling approach, especially in large, confirmatory trials.

The number of parameters for unstructured modeling of correlations is equal to $n(n + 1)/2$, where n is the number of assessment times. However, it is unlikely that the number of covariance parameters to be estimated is prohibitively large in clinical trial settings unless separate unstructured matrices are fit for multiple groups (e.g., treatment arms) within the same data set.

Model fitting criteria can be used to pick the best fitting model after data become available. Alternatively, an unstructured (or other appropriate) approach can be prespecified and alternative structures tested for better fit.

8

Modeling Means Over Time

8.1 Introduction

In longitudinal clinical trials, means can vary over time due to, among other things, study effects and the natural evolution of the disease. Even when focus is on a single landmark time point (e.g., endpoint visit), properly understanding and modeling the time trends is important.

In mixed-effects models, time can be modeled in either a structured or unstructured manner. In unstructured modeling of time, the time variable is considered a categorical (i.e., class) effect. The fixed effect solutions in such a mixed model represent the unique effects of each assessment time and have t-1 degrees of freedom for t time points. In structured modeling of time, the time variable is treated as a continuous independent variable (covariate) as is typically done in regression and covariate analyses. Therefore, structured models for time can use fewer degrees of freedom and be more powerful than unstructured approaches, provided that the functional form of the time trend is correctly specified. In structured approaches the time variable can be considered strictly a fixed effect, strictly a random effect or have both fixed and random components. Models with time as a random effect are commonly referred to as random coefficients regression models (SAS 2013).

Although the longitudinal pattern of treatment effects is usually of interest, the functional form of the mean responses over time may be difficult to anticipate. In particular, linear time trends may not adequately describe the mean responses. Nonlinear trends may arise from inherent characteristics of the particular disease and the drug under study, and/or from trial design features. For example, if titration dosing is used with initial dosing at a subtherapeutic level to reduce adverse events, there may be a lag period with little or no improvement. Conversely, if a drug has rapid onset of a fully therapeutic effect, the beneficial effects may increase rapidly across early assessments and then level off thereafter. In such cases, parsimonious approaches to modeling means over time may lead to inaccurate results and more general unstructured models may be preferred (Mallinckrodt et al. 2003). Therefore, in many scenarios, an unstructured modeling of means over assessment times requires fewer assumptions, does not require estimation of an inordinate number of parameters, and can be depended upon to yield a useful result (Mallinckrodt et al. 2003).

Figure 8.1 illustrates linear time trends for means superimposed on top of unstructured time trends. In this example, the treatment group differences at the endpoint (Time 8) visit appear relatively equal for the unstructured and linear approaches. However, the linear model underestimates within-group changes at early visits and overestimates within-group changes at later visits.

Figure 8.2 illustrates the same unstructured time trends for treatment means with linear plus quadratic trends for means by treatment superimposed. The two models yield similar within-group changes and between-group contrasts at each time point.

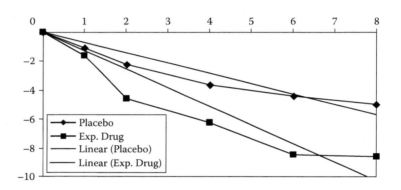

FIGURE 8.1
Unstructured modeling of time compared with linear trends.

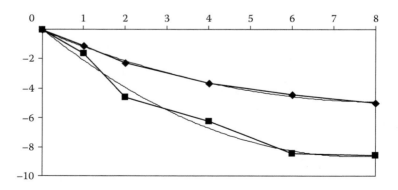

FIGURE 8.2
Unstructured modeling of time compared with linear plus quadratic trends.

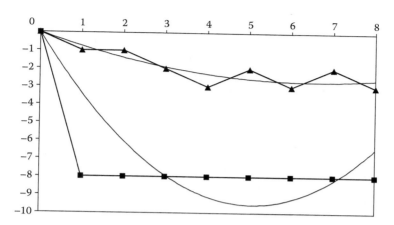

FIGURE 8.3
Unstructured modeling of time compared with linear plus quadratic trends in a scenario with a rapidly evolving treatment effect.

Figure 8.3 illustrates a scenario where one treatment has a rapid and sustained effect and the other treatment has a smaller effect that evolves more slowly over time. The linear plus quadratic model provides good fit to the treatment arm with smaller changes. Compared to the unstructured model, the linear plus quadratic model smoothed the somewhat erratic and seemingly random mean changes around the overall trend. However, the linear plus quadratic model provides poor fit to the arm with a rapid and sustained effect.

The examples are not intended to be a full exploration of modeling alternatives. Rather, the intent is merely to show that in some cases structured time models adequately describe mean trends over time and in other situations they don't.

Another aspect of mean trends over time that must be considered is with regard to the other covariates included in the analysis and their interaction with time. For example, the effect of baseline severity may be an important covariate because subjects' responses may depend on their condition at the start of the trial. It is usually preferable to allow a full interaction of covariates with time because, if not, a restriction is imposed that the dependence of response on the covariate is the same at all assessment times (Mallickrodt et al. 2008, 2014).

Alternatively, both the baseline and post-baseline measures can be treated as response variables (Liang and Zeger 2000). This topic is covered in detail in Chapter 9. For other covariates, it may be appropriate not to include interaction with time because the effects are constant; but such decisions need to be justified a priori (Mallinckrodt et al. 2008).

TABLE 8.1

Results from the Unstructured Time Model in SAS PROC MIXED

Treatment	TIME	Estimate	Standard Error	LSMEAN Difference	P
1	1	−4.12	0.91	1.19	0.360
2	1	−5.31	0.91		
1	2	−6.70	0.93	1.99	0.135
2	2	−8.69	0.93		
1	3	−9.86	1.05	3.39	0.0274
2	3	−13.25	1.05		

Residual covariance matrix

1	20.61	15.30	12.28
2	15.30	21.36	17.67
3	12.28	17.67	27.61

Note: P values for treatment main effect, the main effect of time, and treatment-by-time interaction were 0.073, 0.001, and 0.287, respectively. The values for − 2 x residual log likelihood and AIC were 810.4 and 822.4, respectively.

8.2 Unstructured Modeling of Means Over Time

Code fragments for fitting an unstructured model for means over time in SAS and R for the small complete data set are listed in Section 8.4 (Code Fragment 8.1). Key aspects of this code include specifying time as a class effect and fitting the treatment-by-time interaction along with all other two-way interactions of covariates with time. Unstructured modeling of means over time was used throughout Chapter 7 when considering approaches to model correlations between repeated measurements.

Results from the unstructured means model in SAS PROC MIXED are summarized in Table 8.1. Both the treatment (2) and control group (1) had significant mean improvement over time (P = 0.001). The mean difference between treatments increased over time, reaching statistical significance (P < 0.05) at the endpoint visit (Time 3). The treatment main effect approached significance (P < 0.10).

8.3 Structured Modeling of Means Over Time

8.3.1 Time as a Fixed Effect

Code fragments for fitting time as a linear fixed effect in SAS and R for the small complete data set are listed in Section 8.4 (Code Fragment 8.2).

Key aspects of this code include specifying time as a continuous effect (time not included in class statement), thereby using a single degree of freedom each for time and the treatment-by-time interaction. The endpoint contrast is obtained by comparing treatment lsmeans at the value of 3 for time.

Results from fitting time as a linear fixed effect are summarized in Table 8.2. Results did not differ remarkably from fitting time as unstructured in this example. However, the model fit was slightly worse for the linear fixed effect analysis.

Code fragments for fitting time as linear plus quadratic fixed effects in SAS and R for the small complete data set are listed in Section 8.4 (Code Fragment 8.3). In this approach, as in the unstructured model, time and the treatment-by-time interaction both use two degrees of freedom. In fact, the two approaches are equivalent and yield identical results. Fitting time as unstructured is equivalent to fitting a t-1 degree polynomial. Therefore, with 3 time points, a model with linear and quadratic terms for time is equivalent to the unstructured model. Of course, a linear plus quadratic model would not be equivalent to unstructured with more than 3 time points.

8.3.2 Time as a Random Effect—Random Coefficients Regression

Code fragments for SAS and R implementations of a random coefficients regression model with random terms for intercept and slope (i.e., time is a linear random effect) are listed in Section 8.4 (Code Fragment 8.4). Key aspects of this code include specifying time as a continuous fixed effect (continuous variable TIME not included in class statement) and as a random effect, along with intercept. The Type = option in the random statement allows for correlation between the random terms. As in the fixed

TABLE 8.2

Results from Fitting Time as a Linear Fixed Effect in SAS PROC MIXED

Treatment	TIME	Estimate	Standard Error	LSMEAN Difference	P
1	1	−4.07	0.92	1.14	0.389
2	1	−5.21	0.92		
1	2	−6.91	0.86	2.21	0.076
2	2	−9.13	0.86		
1	3	−9.76	1.06	3.28	0.034
2	3	−13.05	1.06		

Note: P values for treatment main effect, the main effect of time, and treatment-by-time interaction were 0.076, 0.003, and 0.133, respectively. The values for $-2 \times$ residual log likelihood and AIC were 819.5 and 831.5, respectively.

TABLE 8.3

Results from Fitting a Random Coefficient Regression Model with
Intercept and Time as Random Effects in SAS PROC MIXED

Treatment	TIME	Estimate	Standard Error	LSMEAN Difference	P
1	1	− 4.03	0.91	1.09	0.401
2	1	− 5.12	0.91		
1	2	− 6.90	0.84	2.19	0.073
2	2	− 9.09	0.8		
1	3	− 9.77	1.04	3.29	0.030
2	3	− 13.06	1.04		

Estimated G Matrix

	Intercept	Time	Residual
Intercept	24.14	− 0.528	
Time	− 0.528	3.54	
Residual			4.75

Note: P values for treatment main effect, the main effect of time, and treatment-by-time interaction were 0.073, 0.001, and 0.117, respectively. The
values for −2 x residual log likelihood and AIC were 820.1 and 828.1,
respectively.

effects model, the endpoint contrast is obtained by comparing treatment
lsmeans at the value of 3 for time.

Results from fitting the random coefficient regression model with intercept
and time as random effects are summarized in Table 8.3. Results did not differ remarkably from fitting time as unstructured or as a linear fixed effect in
this example.

A quadratic term for time could be added to the random statement.
However, in such models it may be useful to center the time variable (subtract the mean time from each value for time) and to use a time scale that
is not overly granular. For example, fitting time in years may be preferable to fitting time in days because the latter is likely to yield smaller variance, which could cause convergence problems or result in a nonpositive
definite hessian matrix. It may also be useful to transform time variables
into orthogonal polynomials, especially for fitting higher-order (e.g., cubic)
terms.

It is possible to capture additional correlation between repeated measurements in a random coefficients regression analysis via a residual correlation structure. However, guarding against overspecification of models
is important. For example, fitting random intercepts and slopes plus an
unstructured error covariance specifies too many parameters for the variance function, and a more parsimonious error covariance structure is
needed.

8.4 Code Fragments

CODE FRAGMENT 8.1   SAS and R Code for
Fitting an Unstructured Time Model

SAS code

```
PROC MIXED DATA=ONE;
 CLASS SUBJECT TRT TIME;
 MODEL CHANGE = BASVAL TRT TIME BASVAL*TIME TRT*TIME /
   DDFM=KR;
 REPEATED TIME / SUBJECT=SUBJECT TYPE =UN R;
 LSMEANS TRT*TIME/DIFFS;
 ODS OUTPUT DIFFS=_DIFFS (where=(TIME= _TIME)) LSMEANS=_
   LSMEANS ;RUN;
```

R code

```
fitgls.erun <- gls(change ~ basval +trt+ TIME +
            basval*TIME+ trt*TIME, data = complete,
            weights = varIdent(form= ~ 1 | TIME),
            correlation=corSymm(form=~ 1| subject))

summary(fitgls.erun)

# computing error variance-covariance matrix
getVarCov(fitgls.erun)

# evaluating least squares means at time 3
contrast(fitgls.erun ,a = list(trt = "1",
            basval= mean(complete$basval), TIME = "3"),
            type = "individual")
contrast(fitgls.erun ,a = list(trt = "2",
            basval= mean(complete$basval), TIME = "3"),
            type = "individual")

# evaluating treatment contrast at time 3
contrast(fitgls.erun ,a = list(trt = "1", basval=
            mean(complete$basval), TIME = "3"),
            b = list(trt = "2", basval=
            mean(complete$basval), TIME = "3"),
            type = "individual")
```

**CODE FRAGMENT 8.2   SAS and R Code for
Fitting Time as a Linear Fixed Effect**

SAS code

TIME2 is continuous time variable assuming values 1, 2, 3. Variable TIME
is also needed as a CLASS variable because it is used in REPEATED
statement.

```
PROC MIXED DATA=ONE;
CLASS SUBJECT TRT TIME;
MODEL CHANGE =BASVAL TRT TIME2 BASVAL*TIME2 TRT*TIME2 /
  DDFM=KR;
REPEATED TIME/SUBJECT=SUBJECT TYPE=UN R RCORR;
LSMEANS TRT / at TIME2 = 1 DIFFS;
LSMEANS TRT / at TIME2 = 2 DIFFS;
LSMEANS TRT / at TIME2 = 3 DIFFS;
ODS OUTPUT DIFFS=_DIFFS (where=(TIME= _TIME))
  LSMEANS=_LSMEANS;
RUN;
```

R code

```
# using continuous time, creating timec variable
complete$timec<-as.numeric(complete$TIME)

fitgls.cont.time <- gls(change ~ basval +trt+ timec +
             basval*timec+ trt*timec, data = complete,
             weights = varIdent(form= ~ 1 | timec),
             correlation=corSymm(form=~ 1| subject))

# note since timec is continuous variable, it is set at
  numerical value=3, not a character value ="3"
contrast(fitgls.cont.time ,a = list(trt = "1",
             basval= mean(complete$basval), timec = 3),
             b = list(trt = "2", basval=
             mean(complete$basval), timec = 3),
             type = "individual")
```

CODE FRAGMENT 8.3   SAS and R Code for Fitting
Time as Linear + Quadratic Fixed Effects

SAS code

TIME2 is continuous time variable assuming values 1, 2, 3.

```
PROC MIXED DATA=ONE;
 CLASS SUBJECT TRT;
 MODEL CHANGE =BASVAL TRT TIME2 BASVAL*TIME2 TRT*TIME2
   TIME2*TIME2 TRT*TIME2*TIME2 BASVAL*TIME2*TIME2 /
   DDFM=KR;
 REPEATED TIME/SUBJECT=SUBJECT TYPE=UN R RCORR;
 LSMEANS TRT/ at TIME2= 1 DIFFS;
 LSMEANS TRT/ at TIME2= 2 DIFFS;
 LSMEANS TRT/ at TIME2= 3 DIFFS;
 ODS OUTPUT DIFFS=_DIFFS (where=(TIME= _TIME))
   LSMEANS=_LSMEANS;
RUN;
```

R Code

```
# creating additional variable, time squared
complete$tsq<-complete$timec^2

fitgls.cont.time2 <- gls(change ~ basval +trt+ timec +
              basval*timec+ trt*timec+tsq+trt*tsq+
              basval*tsq, data = complete, weights =
              varIdent(form= ~ 1 | timec),
              correlation=corSymm(form=~ 1| subject))

summary(fitgls.cont.time2)

# evaluating treatment contrast at time=3
# need to specify squared time tsq in the contrast at fixed
  value
contrast(fitgls.cont.time2, a = list(trt = "1",
              basval = mean(complete$basval), timec = 3,
              tsq = 9), b = list(trt = "2", basval=
              mean(complete$basval), timec = 3, tsq=9),
              type = "individual")
```

**CODE FRAGMENT 8.4   SAS and R Code for
Fitting a Random Coefficient Regression Model
with Intercept and Time as Random Effects**

SAS Code

```
PROC MIXED DATA=ONE;
 CLASS SUBJECT TRT;
 MODEL CHANGE =BASVAL TRT TIME BASVAL*TIME TRT*TIME /
   DDFM=KR;
 RANDOM INT TIME / SUBJECT=SUBJECT TYPE=UN G GCORR;
 LSMEANS TRT/ at TIME= 1 DIFFS;
 LSMEANS TRT/ at TIME= 2 DIFFS;
 LSMEANS TRT/ at TIME= 3 DIFFS;
 ODS OUTPUT DIFFS=_DIFFS LSMEANS=_LSMEANS;
RUN;
```

R Code

```
fitLME.rint.time <- lme(change ~ basval +trt+ timec +
              basval*timec+ trt*timec, data =complete,
              random = ~ 1+timec |subject)

summary(fitLME.rint.time)
getVarCov(fitLME.rint.time)

# lsmeans at timec=3
contrast(fitLME.rint.time ,a = list(trt = "1", basval=
                   mean(complete$basval), timec = 3)
                   type = "individual")
contrast(fitLME.rint.time ,a = list(trt = "2", basval=
                   mean(complete$basval), timec = 3)
                   type = "individual")

# treatment contrast at timec=3
contrast(fitLME.rint.time ,a = list(trt = "1", basval=
                   mean(complete$basval), timec = 3),
                   b = list(trt = "2", basval=
                   mean(complete$basval), timec = 3),
                   type = "individual")
```

8.5 Summary

Although the longitudinal pattern of mean treatment effects is usually of interest, the functional form of the response profiles may be difficult to anticipate. Structured (parsimonious) approaches to modeling means over time may be more powerful if appropriate, but may not fit the data adequately, leading to inaccurate results.

Clinical trials typically have a set number of assessment times that are fixed within narrow intervals. The number of assessment times relative to the number of patients is typically small. The number of parameters to describe the means over time from an unstructured model increase linearly with the number of assessment times. These attributes suggest that unstructured modeling of mean trends over time is often possible. This is important, especially in confirmatory studies, because an unstructured model for the means requires no assumption about the time trend and models with fewer assumptions are preferred.

In many situations, an unstructured model for the mean trends over time can be prespecified because the number of parameters to be estimated relative to the number of observations is small. If the anticipated data structure is not expected to be amenable to unstructured modeling, likelihood ratio tests can be used to pick the best fitting model after data become available.

9

Accounting for Covariates

9.1 Introduction

Covariates are commonly included in analyses of longitudinal clinical trials. In Section 8.1, it was noted that it is usually preferable, or at least it should be considered, to allow a full interaction of covariates with time. Fitting covariate-by-time interactions avoids imposing restrictions that the dependence of response on the covariates is the same at all assessment times. Therefore, throughout this chapter, examples will be used that include not only the covariate but also the covariate interaction with time.

Covariates are often included in longitudinal analyses to account for the variability due to these effects, thereby yielding more precise estimates of treatment effects. This can be particularly important when values of continuous covariates or levels of categorical covariates are not balanced across treatments.

Covariate-by-treatment interactions, commonly called subgroup analyses when the covariate is a categorical effect, are included in longitudinal analyses to assess the consistency of treatment effects across levels of the covariate. Consistency of treatment effect across subgroups indicates that the average treatment effect is in general applicable regardless of the specific characteristic described by the covariate. Substantial heterogeneity in treatment effect may indicate that treatment benefit pertains only to a subset of the population. However, apparent heterogeneity in the observed treatment effect across subgroups can arise due to chance as a result of partitioning the population into several subgroups. Furthermore, clinical trials are generally not powered for detecting heterogeneity in treatment effects, thus statistical tests may miss detection of existing heterogeneity due to low power (Alosh et al. 2015). This chapter emphasizes how to fit covariates and the consequences of so doing. It does not cover model building approaches to decide which covariates to include. For more details on model building, see Verbeke and Molenberghs (2000).

The impact of baseline severity on outcomes is an important consideration in longitudinal clinical trials. Baseline severity is a special case of covariate adjustment because it can be taken into account either through covariate adjustment or by including baseline as part of the response vector. Both approaches, along with their respective strengths, limitations, and considerations, will be illustrated.

This chapter begins with an illustration of including a continuous covariate for baseline severity. Other continuous covariates can be fit in the same manner as illustrated for baseline severity. Subsequent sections illustrate how baseline severity can be accounted for as a response variable, how to account for categorical covariates, and covariate-by-treatment interactions. Covariates and model development can be an important consideration in the handling of missing data. See Chapter 12 and Chapter 15 for more details on the role of covariates with regard to handling missing data.

9.2 Continuous Covariates

9.2.1 Baseline Severity as a Covariate

The small complete data set is used to illustrate key concepts in fitting covariates. Code Fragment 9.1 in Section 9.5 provides details on fitting a model with baseline severity as a covariate in SAS and R.

To illustrate covariate adjustment, consider the results in Table 9.1 from likelihood-based analyses. Two models were used. The "simple" model included only treatment, time, and the treatment-by-time interaction. The "baseline" or ANCOVA model included those same effects plus baseline and baseline-by-time interaction as specified in Code Fragment 9.1. In the simple model, because the data were completely balanced (same number of observations for each treatment-by-time combination) the lsmeans for the treatment-by-time interaction effects are equal to their

TABLE 9.1

Results from Analyses of Small Complete Data Set with and without Baseline Severity as a Covariate

Treatment	Time	Simple Model		Model Including Baseline	
		LSMEAN	SE	LSMEAN	SE
1	1	−4.20	0.94	−4.13	0.91
2	1	−5.24	0.94	−5.32	0.91
1	2	−6.80	0.97	−6.70	0.93
2	2	−8.60	0.97	−8.70	0.93
1	3	−9.88	1.04	−9.86	1.05
2	3	−13.24	1.04	−13.26	1.05
Endpoint Contrast		3.36	1.47 (p = 0.0270)	3.39	1.49 (p = 0.0274)

corresponding raw means. In the model with baseline and baseline-by-time interaction, the lsmeans do not equal the raw means, thereby reflecting the influence of correcting for differences between treatments in baseline values.

Recall from Table 4.3 that the mean baseline values were 19.80 and 19.32 for Treatments 1 and 2, respectively. Given this similarity of baseline means, differences in treatment contrasts between models fitting versus not fitting baseline severity are expected to be small. With greater imbalance between baseline means, the greater the potential for covariate adjusted results to differ from unadjusted results.

The relationship between baseline and change was such that for each 1 point increase in baseline severity, change (improvement) from baseline increased on average approximately 0.06 points. Therefore, correcting for the approximately 0.50 point greater mean baseline in Treatment 1 (by including baseline as a covariate) increased the difference between treatments in change at Time 3 by about 0.03 (0.50 mean difference in baseline × the 0.06 change in response per unit change in baseline severity).

To further clarify how including baseline as a covariate influenced results, consider the observed and predicted values for selected subjects summarized in Table 9.2. In the simple model, each subject's predicted value equals the corresponding lsmean for the treatment-by-time combination. That is, the model contained only group effects; no information unique to individual subjects was in the model. Therefore, individuals' predictions were entirely derived from the group means. Including baseline as a covariate introduced information specific to individual subjects, and the predicted values for each subject were based on a combination of group means and individual subject data (baseline values). Lower baseline values

TABLE 9.2

Predicted Values for Selected Subjects from Analyses of Complete Data with a Simple Model and a Model that Included Baseline Values as a Covariate

Subject	Model[a]	Treatment	Time	Baseline	Actual Change	Predicted Change
1	Simple	2	3	24	− 24	−13.24
	Baseline					−13.54
2	Simple	1	3	20	− 5	−9.88
	Baseline					−9.89
4	Simple	2	3	10	− 9	−13.24
	Baseline					−12.64
5	Simple	1	3	12	− 9	−9.88
	Baseline					−9.37

[a] Simple model: Change = trt time trt*time. Baseline model added basval and basval*time.

were predictive of smaller improvements and higher baseline values were predictive of greater improvements.

The mean baseline value was 19.56 (approximately 20). The baseline value for Subject 1 was 24, approximately 4 points higher than the baseline mean; the baseline values for Subjects 4 and 5 were 10 and 12, respectively, considerably below the mean. Therefore, when including baseline as a covariate, the predicted improvement for Subject 1 was greater than the corresponding treatment group mean. Similarly, when including baseline as a covariate, the predicted improvements for Subjects 4 and 5 were smaller than the corresponding group means. Subject 2 had a baseline value of 20, close to the overall mean; therefore, the predicted values from the models including versus not including baseline were nearly identical.

By default, lsmeans are typically estimated based on the mean value of continuous covariates. However, it is also useful to look at results when values other than the mean are used. [See the "AT" option in the lsmean statement of SAS PROC MIXED (SAS 2013) for implementation]. Treatment lsmeans and contrasts based on baseline severity of 15 and 25 are summarized in Table 9.3. The treatment contrasts, standard errors, and P values are the same across baseline severities of 15, 25, or the default, which is the mean value of 19.56. Within-group means, however, are influenced by the baseline value, consistent with the regression coefficient for change on baseline severity, which in this case is approximately 0.06. Therefore, conditioning on a baseline value of 15 resulted in lsmeans approximately 0.60 lower than when conditioning on a baseline value of 25.

9.2.2 Baseline Severity as a Response

Although fitting baseline severity as a covariate is a common approach, it is not the only option. Baseline severity is a special case of covariate adjustment because baseline severity can be considered a response at Time 0 and therefore may also be accounted for through including baseline outcomes as part of the response vector (Liang and Zeger 2000). This subsection details two methods that include baseline as a response, the so-called LDA (longitudinal data analysis) and the cLDA (constrained longitudinal data analysis)

TABLE 9.3

Least Squares Means and Treatment Contrasts Conditioning on Various Levels of Baseline Severity

Baseline	TRT	LSMEAN	LSMEAN Difference	Standard Error	P Value
15	1	−9.57			
	2	−12.96	3.39	1.49	0.0274
25	1	−10.21			
	2	−13.60	3.39	1.49	0.0274

(Liu et al. 2009). The constraint in cLDA is that the baseline values are equal in the intervention groups.

Code fragments are listed in Section 9.5 to implement LDA and cLDA models in SAS and R (Code Fragments 9.2 and 9.3, respectively). For these analyses, data are arranged so that there are four responses per subject, with baseline being the Time = 0 response. For the cLDA analysis, additional steps are required to create the time-specific treatment indicators tt0-tt3. These dummy variables are components of the treatment-by-time interaction: ttk=I(TIMEk*TRT) for k=1,2,3, where I(.) is the indicator function, returning 1 when the argument is TRUE and 0 if FALSE. The model is fit with time as a class variable (to estimate time-specific least squares means at Time=1, 2, 3) and the three dummy variables tt1, tt2, tt3 that capture treatment-specific least-squares means at time=1, 2, 3.

The tt0 variable and the I(Time=0)*Treatment interaction term are not fit in the model in order to implement the constraint of equal baseline means. The two treatments in essence have a common set of baselines, hence equal baselines, as would be expected on average from randomization; Table 9.4 lists data for selected subjects as prepared for LDA and cLDA.

TABLE 9.4

Data for LDA and cLDA Analyses

Subject	TRT	TIME	Y			
Data for LDA						
16	1	0	19			
16	1	1	16			
16	1	2	8			
16	1	3	2			
17	2	0	20			
17	2	1	9			
17	2	2	5			
17	2	3	1			

Subject	TIME	Y	TT0	TT1	TT2	TT3
Data for cLDA						
16	0	19	0	0	0	0
16	1	16	0	0	0	0
16	2	8	0	0	0	0
16	3	2	0	0	0	0
17	0	20	1	0	0	0
17	1	9	0	1	0	0
17	2	5	0	0	1	0
17	3	1	0	0	0	1

Note: The tt0 variable is not fit in the model in order to constrain lsmean by omitting the (Time=0)*TRT interaction term.

Endpoint contrasts from the various methods of accounting for baseline severity in the small complete data set are summarized in Table 9.5 and residual variances and correlations are summarized in Table 9.6. The endpoint (Time 3) contrast from the cLDA and ANCOVA models were identical. This will only be the case in complete data. Standard errors and P values were similar across methods, as were correlations between the residuals. However, residual variances were greater for the LDA and cLDA models.

Although results from the ANCOVA, LDA, and cLDA methods tend to be similar in many situations, circumstances exist when important differences are likely. To illustrate, data from the small complete data set were

TABLE 9.5

Endpoint Contrasts from Various Methods of Accounting for Baseline Severity in the Small, Complete Data Set

Method	LSMEAN Difference	Standard Error	P
ANCOVA	3.391	1.489	0.0274
LDA	3.360	1.473	0.0270
cLDA	3.391	1.501	0.0284

TABLE 9.6

Residual Variances and Correlations from Various Methods of Accounting for Baseline Severity in the Small, Complete Data Set

Time	0	1	2	3
Baseline as Covariate (ANCOVA)				
1		20.612	0.729	0.515
2			21.358	0.724
3				27.614
LDA				
0	16.613	0.529	0.473	0.591
1		28.038	0.796	0.665
2			26.938	0.797
3				41.577
cLDA				
0	16.333	0.526	0.470	0.588
1		27.906	0.795	0.663
2			26.836	0.796
3				41.331

altered in the following ways. In alteration 1, the *baseline values* for Subjects 1 to 15 were deleted. In alteration 2, no baseline values were deleted but *all post-baseline data* for Subjects 1 to 15 were deleted. Endpoint contrasts from the three methods of handling baseline severity (ANCOVA, LDA, cLDA) are summarized in Table 9.7 for alteration 1 and in Table 9.8 for alteration 2.

For the ANCOVA method, results were identical from the two alterations, with the treatment contrast smaller than in the complete data. That is, when fitting baseline as a covariate, deleting 15 baseline values had the same impact as deleting all the post-baseline data for those 15 subjects—because observations with missing covariates are not used in the analysis. However, in the LDA and cLDA analyses where baseline is considered a response, deleting 15 baseline values left 185 of the 200 values to be used in the analysis, and all post-baseline observations are used. Therefore, missing baseline values had a smaller effect on the LDA and cLDA analyses than on the ANCOVA analyses.

For alteration 2, deleting all the post-baseline data for Subjects 1 to 15, results were similar across methods.

9.2.3 Choosing the Best Approach

In the ANCOVA model where baseline is accounted for as a covariate, baseline is considered a fixed effect. In the LDA and cLDA models where baseline

TABLE 9.7

Endpoint Contrasts from Various Methods of Accounting for Baseline Severity in the Small, Complete Data Set with 15 Baseline Values Deleted

Method	LSMEAN Difference	Standard Error	P Value	Number of Observations	
				Used	Not Used
ANCOVA	2.239	1.846	0.234	155	45
LDA	3.125	1.619	0.060	185	15
cLDA	3.323	1.613	0.045	185	15

TABLE 9.8

Endpoint Contrasts from Various Methods of Accounting for Baseline Severity in the Small, Complete Data Set with All Post Baseline Values Deleted for 15 Subjects

Method	LSMEAN Difference	Standard Error	P Value	Number of Observations	
				Used	Not Used
ANCOVA	2.239	1.846	0.234	155	45
LDA	2.264	1.828	0.224	155	45
cLDA	2.239	1.862	0.238	155	45

is considered a response, it is a random effect. The ANCOVA model tends to be the easier and the more common approach. In the ANCOVA model, F tests for the treatment main effect and treatment-by-time interaction are more meaningful than in the LDA or cLDA approaches. Treatment main effects in LDA and cLDA are diluted because at Time 0 (baseline) there is no difference between treatments. This zero difference at Time 0 can also inflate the treatment-by-time interaction term in LDA and cLDA.

However, when an appreciable number of baseline observations are missing, or when an appreciable number of subjects have a baseline but no post-baseline values, the LDA or cLDA approaches can have advantages, and it is important for analysts to understand the strengths and limitations of various approaches to account for baseline severity.

If baseline severity is considered a fixed effect, then the ANCOVA model is appropriate. This model addresses the conditional question of the treatment effect in subjects with the baseline values fixed as in the current clinical trial. If baseline severity is considered a random effect, then the LDA and cLDA models are appropriate. By considering baseline severity as a random effect, inference can be extended to the general population of subjects from which the sample was drawn.

9.3 Modeling Categorical Covariates

Categorical covariates are fit in longitudinal models similar to continuous covariates, except the covariate is considered a class effect. Code fragments are listed in Section 9.5 to fit gender as a categorical variable in the small complete data set using SAS and R (Code Fragment 9.4). As with continuous covariates, adding just the main effect of the covariate assumes a constant covariate effect at all assessments. Therefore, it is often useful to fit the interaction of the categorical covariate with time, and that is the approach taken in this section. However, if the categorical covariate has many levels, especially when combined with numerous assessment times, fitting the covariate-by-time interaction can require estimating too many parameters unless the sample size is large. In practice, this consideration most often comes into play for fitting investigative site and its interaction with time.

Results from fitting a model with gender and gender-by-time interaction are compared to results from the simple model that included only treatment, time, and the treatment-by-time interaction in Table 9.9. As illustrated in Section 9.2 for continuous covariates, because the data were completely balanced (same number of observations for each treatment-by-time combination), the lsmeans for the treatment-by-time interaction effects in the simple model are equal to their corresponding raw means. In the model with gender and gender-by-time interaction, the lsmeans for each treatment-by-time

TABLE 9.9

Results from Analyses of Small Complete Data Set with and without Gender as a Covariate

Treatment	Time	Simple Model		Model Including Gender	
		LSMEAN	SE	LSMEAN	SE
1	1	−4.20	0.94	−4.53	0.90
2	1	−5.24	0.94	−4.39	0.96
1	2	−6.80	0.97	−6.98	0.98
2	2	−8.60	0.97	−8.14	1.04
1	3	−9.88	1.04	−9.91	1.06
2	3	−13.24	1.04	−13.15	1.13
Endpoint Contrast		3.36	1.47 (p = 0.0270)	3.24	1.60 (p = 0.049)

combination do not equal the raw means, thereby reflecting covariate adjustments for gender.

Treatment 1 included 40% females and 60% males, whereas Treatment 2 had 76% females and 24% males. Females tended to have greater changes from baseline than males. Therefore, the covariate-adjusted analyses correct for the overrepresentation of females—subjects with more favorable outcomes—in Treatment 2, resulting in smaller mean changes for Treatment 2 and smaller differences between treatments than in the unadjusted analyses.

9.4 Covariate-by-Treatment Interactions

Sections 9.2 and 9.3 discussed models with continuous and categorical covariates. In longitudinal clinical trials, it can also be useful to understand if the effects of the covariate differed by treatment group; that is, to assess subgroup-by-treatment interactions. A full discussion of model development and testing is beyond our present scope. The intent here is to illustrate an implementation of such models and to consider what the results imply.

9.4.1 Continuous Covariates

Code fragments are listed in Section 9.5 to implement models with baseline severity-by-treatment interactions in SAS and R (Code Fragment 9.5). Results from models using the default approach that conditions on the mean baseline value are compared to results when conditioning on baseline values of 15 and 25 in Table 9.10. Increasing baseline from 15 to 25 increased the lsmean for Treatment 1 by 1.40, whereas the increase for Treatment 2 was only 0.35, reflecting heterogeneity in the regression of change on baseline

TABLE 9.10

Least Square Means at Time 3 Conditioning on
Various Levels of Baseline Severity in Models Including
Baseline-by-Treatment Interaction

Baseline	Treatment	Time 3 LSMEAN	LSMEAN Difference	Standard Error
Mean	1	−9.85		
	2	−13.25	3.40	1.50
15	1	−9.20		
	2	−13.08	3.88	2.46
25	1	−10.60		
	2	−13.43	2.83	2.69

across treatments. Therefore, the net impact of adding the various interaction terms to account for differential baseline effects across treatments was greater treatment differences at lower baseline severity.

As in simpler regression settings, moving further away from mean levels of an independent variable increased uncertainty. Therefore, the standard error of the treatment contrast was smaller when assessed at the mean level of baseline severity.

9.4.2 Categorical Covariates

Code fragments are listed in Section 9.5 to implement models with gender-by-treatment interaction in SAS and R (Code Fragment 9.6). Lsmeans for the three-way gender-by-treatment-by-time interaction and the two-way treatment-by-time interaction are summarized in Table 9.11. From the three-way interaction, the difference between treatments at Time 3 was approximately 5 in females and 0.5 in males. The two-way interaction lsmeans reflect the equal weighting given to each gender and the lsmean is the average of the corresponding gender-specific lsmeans from the three-way interaction. For example, the treatment difference at Time 3 = 2.75, which is the average of the 5 point treatment contrast in females and the 0.5 point treatment contrast in males.

Recall that in the simple model that included only treatment, time and treatment-by-time interaction, the difference between treatments was 3.36. Therefore, when correcting for the imbalance in the number of subjects by gender in each treatment via including gender and gender-by-time interactions, the treatment difference was 3.24. When including the gender-by-treatment interaction terms to further account for a differential treatment effect by gender, the treatment effect was further reduced to 2.75.

Code fragment 9.5 includes as part of the SAS code an option in the lsmeans statement "SLICE=GENDER*TIME". The slice option is a convenient way to partition interactions into component parts. Specifying slices

TABLE 9.11

Least Square Means at Time 3 by Gender and Treatment

Treatment	Gender	N	LSMEAN	LSMEAN Difference
Gender-by-Treatment lsmeans at Time 3				
1	F	10	−8.90	5.04
2	F	19	−13.94	
1	M	15	−10.53	
2	M	6	−11.00	0.47
Treatment lsmeans at Time 3				
1		25	−9.72	
2		25	−12.47	2.75

TABLE 9.12

Significance Tests Based on the Slices Option in SAS

Treatment Contrast		
Time	Gender	P
1	F	0.220
1	M	0.096
2	F	0.169
2	M	0.648
3	F	0.017
3	M	0.854

for gender by time yields significance tests for treatment contrasts for each gender-by-time combination.

Because this example has two treatment arms, the P values are essentially *t*-tests, but with three or more groups these would be *F*-tests. Similar tests could be achieved via contrast statements. However, correctly coding the series of three-way interaction contrasts is far more tedious than simply specifying the slices option. Results from the slices option are summarized in Table 9.12.

The slice option allows partitioning of a three-way interaction into its component two-way interactions and to assess a main effect for each level of the other two factors, as was done in assessing treatment differences for each gender-by-time combination. For example, the slice option could be used to assess gender differences for each treatment-by-time combination (slice=trt*time); the two-way treatment-by-time interaction for each gender (slice=gender); the gender-by-treatment interaction for each time (slice=time), or the gender-by-time interaction for each treatment (slice=treatment).

9.4.3 Observed versus Balanced Margins

Further consideration of the results in the previous section illustrates an important point for categorical subgroup-by-treatment interactions. Treatment 1 had 40% females and Treatment 2 had 76% females. By default, when the three-way gender-by-treatment-by-time interaction is fit, lsmeans for treatment-by-time reflect equal weighting by gender—the results expected if there were 50% males and 50% females in each treatment.

It is important to consider if the question being addressed by the analysis is best approached with lsmeans reflecting these so-called balanced margins (equal weightings). When subjects are randomized to treatment, gender representation in each treatment is expected to be equal. If by chance that is not the case, covariate adjustment can help restore analytically the balance that did not materialize via design. However, randomization is expected to yield equal (similar) representation of gender in each treatment, but not equal representation of gender within each group. For example, if 2/3 of the clinical trial population is female, randomization is expected to yield approximately 2/3 females in each treatment group. However, by default lsmeans are based on complete balance such that lsmeans reflect 50% females and 50% males in each treatment group.

If the population from which a clinical trial sample is drawn is not approximately 50/50 male/female, then default lsmeans assuming balance in number by gender within treatment would not be appropriate. It is possible to use software options to obtain lsmeans that reflect the margins observed in the actual sample, or user-specified margins. [See, for example, the observed margins option for the lsmean statement in SAS PROC MIXED (SAS 2013).] This feature allows an interaction to be fit without forcing the use of balanced margins.

9.5 Code Fragments

CODE FRAGMENT 9.1   SAS and R Code for
Fitting Baseline Severity as a Covariate

SAS Code

```
PROC MIXED DATA=All;
  CLASS SUBJECT TRT TIME;
  MODEL Y = BASVAL TRT TIME BASVAL*TIME TRT*TIME/ DDFM=KR;
  REPEATED TIME / SUB=SUBJECT TYPE=UN R RCORR;
  LSMEANS TRT*TIME /DIFFS;
RUN;
```

R Code

```
fitgls.bas <- gls(Y ~ basval +trt+ TIME + basval*TIME,
  data = complete,
      weights = varIdent(form= ~ 1 | TIME),
      correlation= corSymm(form=~ 1| subject))
```

CODE FRAGMENT 9.2   SAS and R Code for Fitting an LDA Model

SAS Code

```
PROC MIXED DATA=RESPONSE;
 CLASS SUBJECT TRT TIME;
 MODEL Y = TRT TIME TRT*TIME / DDFM=KR;
 REPEATED TIME / SUB=SUBJECT TYPE=UN R RCORR;
 ESTIMATE' ' trt*time -1 0 0  1
                       1 0 0 -1;
 RUN;
```

R Code

```
# setting reference for TIME and trt factors at the last
level
contrasts(response$TIME) <- contr.treatment(4, base = 4)
contrasts(response$trt) <- contr.treatment(2, base = 2)

fitgls.resp <- gls(Y ~ trt+ TIME + trt*TIME,
  data = response,
      weights = varIdent(form= ~ 1 | TIME),
      correlation= corSymm(form=~ 1| subject))

# with the parameterization of factors used the difference
between treatment effects at TIME 3
# and at baseline time is the -1* [coefficient at
interaction effect trt1:TIME1]
```

CODE FRAGMENT 9.3   SAS and R Code for Fitting a cLDA Model

SAS Code

```
PROC MIXED DATA=cLDA;
Class SUBJECT TRT TIME;
MODEL Y = TIME TT1 TT2 TT3 / DDFM=KR;
REPEATED TIME / SUBJECT=SUBJECT TYPE=UN R RCORR;
ESTIMATE 'endpoint diff (trt-pbo)' TT3 -1 /cl;
ESTIMATE 'trt main effect' tt1 -1 tt2 -1 tt3 -1;
CONTRAST 'trt*time interaction' tt1 1 tt2 0 tt3 -1,
                                tt1 0 tt2 1 tt3 -1;
RUN;
```

R Code

```
fitgls.cLDA <- gls(Y ~ TIME + tt1+tt2+tt3, data = cLDA,
       weights = varIdent(form= ~ 1 | TIME),
       correlation= corSymm(form=~ 1| subject))

# evaluating treatment contrast at TIME=3
contrast(fitgls.cLDA, a = list(TIME = "3", tt1=0,tt2=0,
        tt3=-1), b = list(TIME = "3", tt1=0,tt2=0, tt3=0),
        type = "individual")

# evaluating the overall treatment effect
contrast(fitgls.cLDA, a = list(TIME = "3", tt1=-1, tt2=-1,
        tt3=-1), b = list(TIME = "3", tt1=0, tt2=0,tt3=0),
        type = "average")
```

Note: contrast package does not allow evaluation of contrasts with DF>1)

CODE FRAGMENT 9.4   SAS and R Code for
Fitting Gender as a Categorical Covariate

SAS Code

```
PROC MIXED DATA=ONE;
CLASS SUBJECT TRT TIME GENDER;
MODEL CHANGE = GENDER TRT TIME GENDER*TIME TRT*TIME/DDFM=KR
OUTP=Cov;
REPEATED TIME/SUBJECT=SUBJECT TYPE=UN R RCORR;
LSMEANS TRT*TIME/DIFFS;
ODS OUTPUT DIFFS=_DIFFS (where=(TIME= _TIME)) LSMEANS=_
  LSMEANS ;
RUN;
```

R Code

```
complete$GENDER <- as.factor(complete$GENDER)

fitgls.gender <- gls(change ~ GENDER +trt+ TIME +
  GENDER*TIME+ trt*TIME, data =complete, weights =
  varIdent(form= ~ 1 | TIME), correlation= corSymm(form=~ 1|
  subject))

# treatment effect at TIME=3 (note since gender by treatment
     interaction is not fit in the # model, GENDER can be
     fixed at any level in the call to contrast function

cont <- contrast(fitgls.gender,a = list(trt = "1",
        TIME = "3", GENDER=c("F")), b = list(trt = "2",
        TIME = "3", GENDER=c("F")), type = "individual")
```

CODE FRAGMENT 9.5   SAS and R Code for Fitting Baseline as a Covariate and its Interaction with Treatment

SAS Code

```
PROC MIXED DATA=ALL ;
 CLASS SUBJECT TRT TIME;
 MODEL CHANGE =BASVAL TRT TIME BASVAL*TIME TRT*TIME
               BASVAL*TRT
 BASVAL*TRT*TIME/DDFM=KR;
 REPEATED TIME/SUBJECT=SUBJECT TYPE=UN R RCORR;
 LSMEANS TRT*TIME/DIFFS;
 LSMEANS TRT*TIME/DIFFS at BASVAL=15;
 LSMEANS TRT*TIME/DIFFS at BASVAL=25;
 ODS OUTPUT DIFFS=_DIFFS (where=(TIME= _TIME)) LSMEANS=_
   LSMEANS ;
RUN;
```

R Code

```
fitgls.base <- gls(change ~ basval +trt+ TIME + basval*TIME+
  trt*TIME+basval*trt+basval*trt*TIME, data = complete,
  weights = varIdent(form= ~ 1 | TIME),
  correlation=corSymm(form=~ 1| subject))

# evaluating treatment contrast at TIME=3 and baseline
    value =25
cont <- contrast(fitgls.base, a = list(trt = "1",
        TIME = "3", basval=25), b = list(trt = "2",
        TIME = "3",basval=25), type = "individual")
```

CODE FRAGMENT 9.6   SAS and R Code for Fitting Gender as a Categorical Covariate and its Interaction with Treatment

SAS Code

```
PROC MIXED DATA=ALL;
 CLASS SUBJECT TRT TIME GENDER;
 MODEL CHANGE =GENDER TRT TIME GENDER*TIME TRT*TIME
               GENDER*TRT
 GENDER*TRT*TIME/DDFM=KR;
 REPEATED TIME/SUBJECT=SUBJECT TYPE=UN R RCORR;
 LSMEANS GENDER*TRT*TIME/DIFFS SLICE=GENDER*TIME;
 LSMEANS TRT*TIME/DIFFS;
 ODS OUTPUT DIFFS=_DIFFS (where=(TIME= _TIME))
   LSMEANS=_LSMEANS;
RUN;
```

R Code

```
# fitting in "gender-by-treatment" interactions
fitgls.gender <- gls(change ~ GENDER +trt+ TIME +
             GENDER*TIME+ trt*TIME+GENDER*trt+GENDER*trt*
             TIME, data = complete,
             weights = varIdent(form= ~ 1 | TIME),
             correlation=corSymm(form=~ 1| subject))

# least squares means by gender for trt=1, TIME=3
contrast(fitgls.gender, a = list(trt = "1", TIME = "3",
        GENDER=c("F","M")), type = "individual")

# treatment contrast at TIME=3, for Gender="F"
contrast(fitgls.gender, a = list(trt = "1",
TIME = "3", GENDER=c("F")), b = list(trt = "2",
TIME = "3",GENDER=c("F")), type = "individual")

# treatment contrast (averaged across gender groups)
cont <- contrast(fitgls.gender, a = list(trt = "1",
        TIME = "3", GENDER=c("F","M")), b = list(trt = "2",
        TIME = "3",GENDER=c("F","M")), type = "average")
```

9.6 Summary

In the ANCOVA model where baseline is accounted for as a covariate, baseline is considered a fixed effect. In the LDA and cLDA models where baseline is considered a response, it is a random effect. The ANCOVA model tends to be the easier and the more common approach. However, when an appreciable number of baseline observations are missing, or when an appreciable number of subjects have a baseline but no post-baseline values, the LDA or cLDA approaches can have advantages.

Fitting just the main effect of the covariate assumes a constant effect at all assessments. This assumption may not be justifiable. Therefore, it is often useful to fit the interaction of covariates with time.

In longitudinal clinical trials, it can also be useful to understand if the effects of the covariate differed by treatment group; that is, to assess subgroup-by-treatment interactions. It is important to consider for categorical covariates, especially when fitting covariate-by-treatment interactions, whether focus should be on the observed versus balanced margins. When fitting a continuous covariate, especially when fitting the covariate-by-treatment interaction, it may be useful to assess treatment contrasts at values of the covariate other than the default of using the mean value.

10

Categorical Data

10.1 Introduction

A comprehensive review of categorical data analyses can be found in Agresti (2002). McCullagh and Nelder (1989) provide specific focus on generalized linear models, which are used extensively in categorical data analyses. This chapter provides an overview of longitudinal categorical analyses.

Many of the principles guiding analyses of continuous outcomes also apply to categorical outcomes. For example, considerations regarding modeling means over time and correlations between repeated measurements are essentially the same as previously outlined for continuous outcomes (see Chapters 7 and 8). Additional similarities include the ability to formulate a longitudinal categorical analysis with treatment contrasts that exactly match the results from an analysis of the endpoint time only. However, analyses of categorical endpoints entail additional complexity compared with continuous endpoints that are typically modeled using linear models with Gaussian error distributions. This additional complexity stems from the (typically) nonlinear relationship between the dependent variable and independent variables and from the nonnormal distribution of errors.

Conceptually, accommodating these aspects is as simple as specifying an appropriate link function to account for nonlinearity and an appropriate distribution for the errors. However, these accommodations necessitate additional computational complexity and intensity, which in turn limits flexibility in implementing analyses.

Moreover, unlike the "linear normal" modeling of continuous outcomes where a single result has both a marginal and a hierarchical (random effects) interpretation, the parameters estimated from marginal and random-effects models with categorical data, and more broadly for any generalized linear mixed model with a nonidentity link function, describe different effects and have different interpretations (Jansen et al. 2006). Therefore, the choice between marginal and random-effect models should ideally be driven by the scientific goals, but the computational complexity and availability of software tools are also a consideration.

Conceptually, the distinction between marginal and random effects models is that marginal models estimate the average response in the population, whereas random effects models estimate responses for the average subject (the subject for which b = 0). In linear mixed-effects models with normally distributed data, the average response and the response of the average subject are the same because the random effects cancel out when taking expectation over the outcome variable. This is due to the additivity of linear models with an identity link and also random effects having a mean and expected value = 0. Hence, fixed effect parameters estimated from a linear mixed-effects model in Gaussian data have both a marginal and hierarchical interpretation. In nonnormal data these two targets of inference are not identical because the function connecting outcome variables and covariates is not linear.

A similar consideration for categorical data analyses is with regard to inclusion of covariates. When a covariate is included, the resultant estimates and inferences are conditional on the covariate. By default, analyses are typically adjusted to the mean value of the covariate. When the association between the response and the covariate is linear, as in Gaussian data, the population average response and the response of the average subject with the mean covariate value are the same. Therefore, in Gaussian data, including versus not including covariates does not influence the target of inference; but in non-Gaussian data, including versus not including the covariate does influence the target of inference because the population average is not equal to the expected value for the subject with the average covariate value. The technical details in the next section help to further clarify these issues.

10.2 Technical Details

10.2.1 Modeling Approaches

Three common modeling approaches to longitudinal categorical data include marginal, random effects, and conditional models.

A marginal model for nonnormally distributed data can be written as

$$h\left(E\left(Y_{ij} \mid X\right)\right) = x'_{ij}\beta$$

where $h(.)$ is a link function that creates a linear association between the mean of Y_{ij} (outcome measured on subject i on jth occurrence) and associated covariate vector x_{ij}.

In marginal models, marginal distributions are used to describe the outcome vector Y, given a set of X predictor variables. The correlation among the components of Y (e.g., repeated measurements on subjects) and fixed effects parameters can be estimated via fully parametric approaches such as likelihood-based analyses, or by working assumptions in the semiparametric GEE framework (Molenberghs and Kenward 2007).

In random-effect models the predictor variables in X are supplemented with a vector of random effects:

$$h\left(E\left(Y_{ij} \mid X, b_i\right)\right) = x'_{ij}\beta + z'_{ij}b_i$$

This model has been termed a generalized linear mixed-effect model. It is generalized in the sense that the link function generalized the linear mixed-effects model to a more general class, allowing for nonnormal (e.g., count or binary) data.

In a random-effects model, the fixed effects estimates are conditional upon the random-effects vector. In principle, it is possible to model correlations among components in Y as a function of both random effects and residual correlation. However, in most applications, the computational complexity necessitates assuming that conditional upon the random effects the components of Y are independent. The linear mixed model for continuous data is a special case of this model with an identity link function. The random effects b_i are, as in general linear models for continuous data, assumed to be sampled from a (multivariate) normal distribution with mean 0 and covariance matrix D. With a logit link and normally distributed random effects, the familiar logistic-linear generalized linear mixed-effects model (GLMM) follows (Molenberghs and Kenward 2007).

In conditional models, the distribution of the components of Y are conditional on X and conditional on (a subset of) the other components of Y. In the example below, outcomes are conditional on the previous outcomes:

$$h\left(E\left(Y_{ij} \mid Y_{i,j-1,...,} Y_{i1}, x_{ij}\right)\right) = x'_{ij}\beta + \alpha Y_{i,j-1}$$

That is, rather than add random effects, expectations are based on previous outcomes. In clinical trials, interest is often on an overall, or population average treatment effect, not on a treatment effect associated with specific outcome histories. Therefore, conditional models will not be further considered here.

As noted above, linear mixed model analyses exploit the elegant properties of the multivariate normal distribution, resulting in fixed effect parameters having both a marginal and hierarchical (random effects model) interpretation. Given this connection, it is easy to appreciate why the linear mixed model provides a unifying framework for analyses of Gaussian data. However, the connection between the model families does not exist when outcomes are nonnormal (Jansen et al. 2006). Therefore, analysts need different tools for marginal and random-effects analyses of categorical data. However, as described in the next section, computational considerations restrict implementation of analyses, especially likelihood-based analyses.

10.2.2 Estimation

In a generalized linear model (GLM), the log likelihood is well-defined and an objective function for estimation of the parameters is straightforward to construct. In a GLMM, categorical data pose increased complexity over continuous data. These complexities hinder construction of objective functions. Even if the objective function is feasible mathematically, it still can be out of reach computationally (SAS 2013). These complexities and restrictions have led to the development of a number of estimation methods. Many of these methods are based on either approximating the objective function or approximating the model.

Integral approximation methods approximate the log likelihood of the GLMM and submit the approximated function to numerical optimization. The advantage of integral approximation methods is that an actual objective function is optimized. This facilitates likelihood ratio tests among nested models and likelihood-based fit statistics. A significant disadvantage of integral approximation methods for typical clinical trial scenarios is the inability to accommodate residual covariance structures. Hence, the within-subject correlations must be modeled as a function of only random effects. The number of random effects must be small for integral approximation methods to be practically feasible (SAS 2013).

Algorithms to approximate the model can be expressed in terms of Taylor series (linearization) and are hence also known as linearization methods. They employ expansions to approximate the model based on pseudo data with fewer nonlinear components (SAS 2013). For example, one approach is based on a decomposition of the data into the mean and an appropriate error term. All methods in this class differ in the order of the Taylor approximation and/or the point around which the approximation is expanded. More specifically, one approach uses the decomposition

$$Y_{ij} = \mu_{ij} + \varepsilon_{ij} = h^{-1}\left(x'_{ij}\beta + z'_{ij}b_i\right) + \varepsilon_{ij}$$

where h^{-1} is the inverse link function and the error terms have the appropriate distribution (Molenberghs and Kenward 2007).

Several approximations of this model can be considered. The basic idea is to create the so-called pseudo data Y_i^* to which a general linear model can then be fit. Results from this model are then used to update the pseudo data and the linear model is refit to the updated pseudo data. This doubly iterative procedure continues until the desired level of convergence is met (Molenberghs and Verbeke 2005; Molenberghs and Kenward 2007). A specific example is the so-called pseudo-likelihood approach where

$$Y_i^* \equiv W_i^{-1}\left(Y_i - \mu_{ij}\right) + X_i\beta + Z_ib_i \approx X_i\beta + Z_ib_i + \varepsilon_i^*$$

with W_i being a diagonal matrix with entries equal to $v(\mu_{ij})$, and with $\varepsilon * I$ equal to $W_i^{-1}\varepsilon_i$, which still has mean zero. This model is essentially a linear mixed model for the pseudo data (Molenberghs and Kenward 2007).

Advantages of linearization-based methods include a relatively simple form of the linearized model that can be fit based on only the mean and variance in the linearized form. Models for which the joint distribution of outcome variables (repeated measurements) is difficult—or impossible—to ascertain can be fit with linearization-based approaches. Models with correlated errors and a large number of random effects are well-suited to linearization methods. The disadvantages of linearization approaches include the absence of a true objective function for the overall optimization process and potentially biased estimates, especially for binary data when the number of observations per subject is small (SAS 2013).

Generalized estimating equations can circumvent the computational complexity of likelihood-based analyses of categorical data, and is therefore a viable alternative whenever interest is restricted to the mean parameters (treatment difference, time evolutions, effect of baseline covariates, etc.). As introduced in Chapter 5, generalized estimating equations are rooted in the quasi-likelihood ideas expressed by McCullagh and Nelder (1989). Modeling is restricted to the correct specification of the marginal mean function, together with the so-called working assumptions about the correlation structure among the repeated measures.

10.3 Examples

10.3.1 Binary Longitudinal Data

To illustrate analyses of a longitudinal binary outcome, the continuous HAMD17 outcomes from the small example data set were dichotomized as is often done in depression clinical trials based on whether or not improvement from baseline was $\geq 50\%$, the so-called responder rate analysis. The percentage of responders by treatment and time are summarized below.

Treatment	Time	Percent Responders
1	1	8
2	1	24
1	2	32
2	2	44
1	3	56
2	3	88

The model for binary data can be very similar to that used for the corresponding continuous endpoint. Fixed effects include treatment, time, treatment-by-time interaction, along with the continuous HAMD17 score as baseline covariate and its interaction with time. For hierarchical inference that require explicit fitting of random subject effects, likelihood-based estimation would typically be used. For the present purpose marginal inference is preferred. Therefore, estimation can be either likelihood-based or via generalized estimating equations.

Code fragment 10.1 lists code to fit a pseudo likelihood-based marginal model using SAS. Code fragment 10.2 lists code to fit the same marginal model using generalized estimating equations. Results are summarized in Tables 10.1 and 10.2, respectively. These summaries focus on visit-wise contrasts. As with continuous data, emphasis can also be on the fixed effect parameter estimates, but are not discussed here. Also note that an unstructured correlation matrix was fit in both the pseudo likelihood and GEE analyses. Although fitting of alternative correlation structures is not discussed here, many of the same principles and approaches apply as in continuous data.

TABLE 10.1

Pseudo Likelihood-Based Results for Binary Data from the Small Example Data Set

| Treatment | Time | Logit Scale | | Percent Scale[a] | | P Value |
		Estimate	SE	Estimate	SE	
1	1	−2.511	0.738	0.075	0.051	0.166
2	1	−1.282	0.493	0.217	0.083	
1	2	−0.732	0.439	0.325	0.096	0.458
2	2	−0.279	0.414	0.431	0.101	
1	3	0.392	0.425	0.597	0.102	0.023
2	3	2.240	0.683	0.904	0.059	

[a] Results on the percent scale are obtained by using the inverse link function.

TABLE 10.2

Generalized Estimating Equation-Based Results for Binary Data from the Small Example Data Set

| Treatment | Time | Logit Scale | | Percent Scale[a] | | P Value |
		Estimate	SE	Estimate	SE	
1	1	−2.518	0.706	0.075	0.048	0.194
2	1	−1.293	0.577	0.215	0.097	
1	2	−0.729	0.423	0.325	0.093	0.456
2	2	−0.292	0.409	0.428	0.100	
1	3	0.386	0.406	0.595	0.097	0.020
2	3	2.206	0.671	0.901	0.059	

[a] Results on the percent scale are obtained by using the inverse link function.

Results from the pseudo likelihood and GEE approaches were similar, both yielding significant treatment contrasts at Time 3, as was seen for the continuous HAMD scores in previous Chapters. At Time 3, response rates from both analyses were approximately 90% for Treatment 2 and 60% for Treatment 1, reflecting slight differences from the observed percentages due to the adjustment for baseline score.

Dichotomization of continuous outcomes results in a loss of information. However, this will not always translate into "less significant" treatment contrasts. Treatment differences for the dichotomized outcome depend on the distribution of the continuous data relative to the cut point chosen for dichotomization. It is possible that the cut off for dichotomization is chosen at a point that is achieved by many subjects in one group but not another, despite relatively small differences in means. This can happen because of greater variance in one group or as an artifact of chance, especially in a small sample such as this example where results from the dichotomized outcome were actually more significant than from the continuous outcome. The P value for the treatment contrast at Time 3 from continuous data was 0.027 (see Table 7.3), versus 0.023 from pseudo likelihood and 0.020 from GEE analyses of the dichotomized (categorical) data.

10.3.2 Ordinal Model for Multinomial Data

Analyses of the PGI improvement (patient global impression) is used to further illustrate categorical analyses of longitudinal data. The PGI is an ordinal variable with scores that can range from 1 (very much improved) to 7 (very much worse), with 4 meaning no change (see Chapter 4). The frequency of responses in the 5, 6 and 7 categories were rare. Therefore, all scores greater than 4 were recoded as 4 for these analyses.

Code fragment 10.3 lists SAS code to fit a marginal, ordinal model for these multinomial data using GEE. The only differences from Code Fragment 10.2 that was for a binary outcome is use of a cumulative logit link and multinomial error distribution rather than a logit link and a binomial error distribution.

Although software tools generally accommodate a wide variety of correlation structures that can be fit to categorical data, for multinomial data typically independence must be assumed. This strong limitation can be addressed by using empirical standard errors based on the sandwich estimator. Results are summarized in Table 10.3.

First, focus on results at Time 3. The results in Table 10.3 as obtained in default output reflect accumulations over categories. Probabilities for individual categories can be obtained by subtracting adjacent categories. For example, the estimated probabilities for category 3 are $0.501 - 0.209 = 0.292$ for Treatment 1 and $0.174 - 0.053 = 0.121$ for Treatment 2. Estimated probabilities for category 1 (very much improved) = $1 - \text{prob 2 or worse}$, which is 0.079 for Treatment 1 and 0.291 for Treatment 2. Both treatments had estimated probabilities for category 2 of approximately 0.4.

TABLE 10.3

Generalized Estimating Equation-Based Results of Ordinal
Data from the Small Example Data Set

| Time | Category | Estimated Probabilities | | P Value[a] |
		Treatment 1	Treatment 2	
1	4 or worse	0.522	0.378	
	3 or worse	0.806	0.697	
	2 or worse	0.980	0.964	0.262
2	4 or worse	0.386	0.235	
	3 or worse	0.705	0.539	
	2 or worse	0.965	0.931	0.151
3	4 or worse	0.209	0.053	
	3 or worse	0.501	0.174	
	2 or worse	0.921	0.709	0.014

[a] Results on the original percentage scale are obtained by using the inverse link function.

Therefore, Treatment 1 had greater estimated probabilities in categories 3 and 4 (worse outcomes) and Treatment 2 had a greater estimated probability for category 1. The significant P value (0.014) reflects the differences between treatments across all categories. Similar trends were seen at Time 1 and Time 2; however, as in continuous and binary analyses, improvements and differences between treatments at earlier times were less than at endpoint.

10.4 Code Fragments

CODE FRAGMENT 10.1   SAS Code for a Pseudo Likelihood-Based Analysis of Binary Data from the Small Example Data Set

```
PROC GLIMMIX DATA=ONE PLOTS=ALL METHOD=RMPL;
  NLOPTIONS MAXITER=50 TECHNIQUE=NEWRAP;
  CLASS SUBJECT TRT TIME GENDER ;
  MODEL RESP = BASVAL TRT TIME BASVAL*TIME TRT*TIME /
    DIST=BINOMIAL LINK=LOGIT;
  RANDOM TIME / SUBJECT=SUBJECT RESIDUAL TYPE=UN V VCORR;
  LSMEANS TRT*TIME / diffs ILink;
  ODS OUTPUT LSMEANS=_LSMEANS DIFFS=_DIFFS V=_V VCORR=_VCORR;
RUN;
```

CODE FRAGMENT 10.2 SAS Code for a Generalized Estimating Equation-Based Analysis of Binary Data from the Small Example Data Set

```
PROC GENMOD DATA =ONE DESCENDING;
 CLASS TRT TIME SUBJECT;
 MODEL RESP=BASVAL TRT TIME BASVAL*TIME TRT*TIME
 /LINK=LOGIT DIST=BINOMIAL;
 REPEATED SUBJECT=SUBJECT / TYPE=UN;
 LSMEANS TRT*TIME / DIFFS ILINK;
 ODS OUTPUT LSMEANS=_LSMEANSG;
 ODS OUTPUT DIFFS=_DIFFSG;
RUN;
```

CODE FRAGMENT 10.3 SAS Code for a Generalized Estimating Equation-Based Analysis of Multinomial Data from the Small Example Data Set

```
PROC GENMOD DATA=ONE DESCENDING;
 CLASS TRT TIME SUBJECT;
 MODEL PGI= TRT TIME TRT*TIME / LINK = CLOGIT DIST=MULT;
 REPEATED SUBJECT=SUBJECT / TYPE=IND;
 LSMEANS TRT*TIME / DIFFS ILINK;
RUN;
```

10.5 Summary

Many of the modeling considerations and principles regarding longitudinal analysis of continuous outcomes also apply to categorical outcomes. However, one key difference is with regard to inference. Fixed effect parameters estimated from a linear mixed-effects model in Gaussian data have both a marginal and hierarchical interpretation. In nonnormal data, these are different targets of inference because the link between the mean of the outcome variable and the covariates is not identity. Therefore, separate models are needed for marginal and hierarchical inference in categorical data.

Incorporating an appropriate link function to account for nonlinearity and an appropriate distribution for the errors in categorical data increases computational complexity. This complexity limits the implementation of certain models, especially for likelihood-based estimation. Therefore, generalized estimating equation-based analyses can be particularly useful in categorical data.

11

Model Checking and Verification

11.1 Introduction

Important assumptions required for valid regression-type analyses of continuous outcomes include linearity, normality, and independence (Wonnacott and Winacott 1981). The first assumption is about the true form of the mean function and the last two assumptions are with regard to the error term. Errors (i.e., residuals) are the difference between observed and predicted values. Several options to account for correlation between repeated observations on the same subjects in mixed-effect model analyses were presented in Chapter 7. Options to account for nonlinearity were presented in Chapter 10.

An inherent challenge in model checking—evaluating the mean structure and the errors—is that they are conditional on one another. Therefore, checking assumptions is typically an iterative process that entails refitting the model. For example, the errors may have some type of skewed distribution due to an incorrect mean model. After altering the mean model and refitting the model, the residuals can be rechecked.

11.2 Residual Diagnostics

Outliers are anomalous values in the data that may have a strong influence on the fitted model, resulting in a worse fit for the majority of the data. Outliers typically increase the residual variance, thereby widening confidence intervals and reducing power. Outliers may be due to errors in data collection and recording. These errors can be corrected. Examples include recording weight in pounds rather than kilograms, recording systolic blood pressure as diastolic blood pressure, etc. Therefore, checking for outliers can be a useful part of establishing the integrity of a database.

Outliers not due to correctable errors may result from several causes. For example, if important fixed effects are not included in the model, then sampling is in essence from a mixture distribution. Apparent outliers may also result from sampling from a nonnormal distribution. Or a few outliers may exist because these values are unusual simply due to chance.

Outliers may be detected in simple scatterplots of the data. However, more sophisticated approaches can be useful. Boxplots and the so-called Q–Q or normal probability plots for the residuals may be useful. Signs of nonnormality include skewed (lack of symmetry), light-tailed, or heavy-tailed distributions. Although specific tests for normality exist, these tests may lack power in small data sets, and in large data sets statistically significant departures from normality may have a trivial impact. Therefore, the important issue to address is whether outliers had an important effect on results, not whether outliers or nonnormality existed.

Some general considerations for residual diagnostics include:

- If the residuals are from a normal distribution, normal probability plots should approximate a straight line, and boxplots should be symmetric, with the median and mean close together in the middle of the box.
- If the normal probability plot is generally a straight line with a few points lying off that line, those points are likely outliers.
- If both ends of the normality plot bend above the straight line, the distribution from which the data were sampled may be skewed to the right.
- If both ends of the normality plot bend below the straight line, the distribution from which the data were sampled may be skewed to the left.
- If the right (upper) end of the normality plot bends below the straight line while the left (lower) end bends above that line (an S curve), the distribution from which the data were sampled may be light-tailed.
- If the right (upper) end of the normality plot bends above the straight line while the left (lower) end bends below it, the distribution from which the data were sampled may be heavy-tailed.

Several types of residuals can be calculated. A raw residual is simply the difference between the observed and predicted value. A studentized residual is the raw residual divided by the standard deviation in residuals. A Pearson residual is the raw residual divided by the standard deviation in the observed values.

11.3 Influence Diagnostics

The general idea of quantifying the influence of one or more observations relies on computing parameter estimates based on all data points, removing the case(s) in question from the data, refitting the model, and computing statistics based on the change between the full-data and reduced-data estimations.

Influence statistics can be grouped by their primary target of estimation.

- Restricted likelihood distance is a measure of general change; that is, change in the overall objective function.
- The influence on parameter estimates, such as treatment effects or other fixed effects can be assessed using Cook's D.
- Influence on fitted and predicted values can be assessed using the PRESS residual and PRESS statistic.
- Influence on precision of estimates can be evaluated using the CovRatio and CovTrace tests.

Additional details on these quantities and how they are calculated in mixed-effect models can be obtained in the SAS documentation for PROC MIXED (SAS 2013). An example of how the measures can be used in practice is provided in Section 11.5 using the small example data set.

11.4 Checking Covariate Assumptions

In a simple regression setting, if the assumption of equal variance across values of the dependent variable is correct, the plot of the observed Y values against X should suggest a band across the graph with roughly equal vertical width for all values of X. A pattern to the scatterplot with greater vertical spread at either the right or left end suggests that the variance in the values increases in the direction with greatest vertical spread. In such cases, a transformation of the Y values might be useful.

11.5 Example

A code fragment to implement residual and influence diagnostics in SAS is listed below. Results from the small example data set follow the code fragment.

CODE FRAGMENT 11.1   SAS Code for Implementing Residual and Influence Diagnostics

```
ODS GRAPHICS ON;
PROC MIXED DATA=ONE plot=all;
  CLASS TRT TIME GENDER SUBJECT;
  MODEL CHANGE= TRT TIME BASVAL TRT*TIME BASVAL*TIME /
  INFLUENCE(EFFECT=SUBJECT ITER=5 estimates);
  REPEATED TIME / SUBJECT=SUBJECT TYPE=UN;
  ODS OUTPUT INFLUENCE=INFLUENCE;
RUN;
ODS GRAPHICS OFF;
```

Studentized residuals are plotted in Figure 11.1. The normal probability plot (lower left panel) shows both ends bending above the straight line, suggesting the distribution is skewed to the right. This skewness is also suggested by the plot of the studentized residuals (upper right panel). Pearson residuals (not shown) indicated the same pattern.

Residual plots by treatment, time and treatment-by-time are depicted in Figures 11.2, 11.3, and 11.4, respectively. These plots reinforce the suggestion of some skewness to the distribution of residuals.

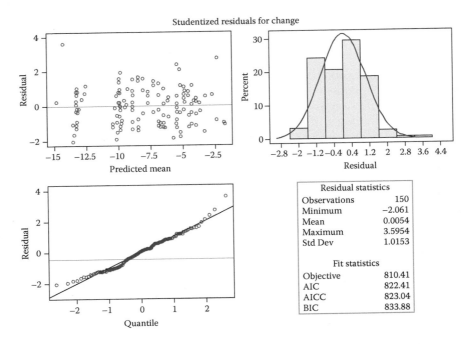

FIGURE 11.1
Residual diagnostics based on studentized residuals from the small example data set.

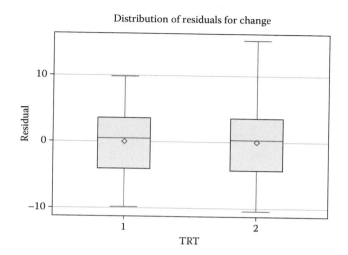

FIGURE 11.2
Distribution of residuals by treatment group from the small example data set.

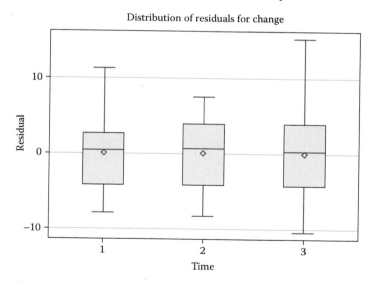

FIGURE 11.3
Distribution of residuals by time from the small example data set.

Restricted likelihood distances are plotted in Figure 11.5. Subject 47 had by far the greatest influence on the overall fit to the model, with Subject 4 standing out to a lesser degree.

To better understand how these influential subjects affected results, influence statistics for fixed effects and covariance parameters are plotted in Figure 11.6. Subjects 4 and especially 47 were appreciably more

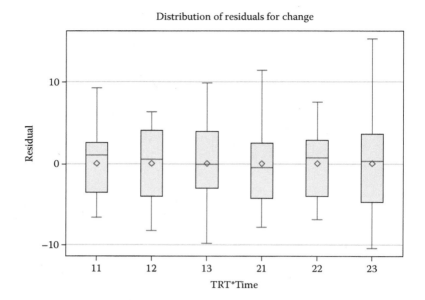

FIGURE 11.4
Distribution of residuals by treatment group and time from the small example data set.

FIGURE 11.5
Plot of restricted likelihood distances by subject from the small example data set.

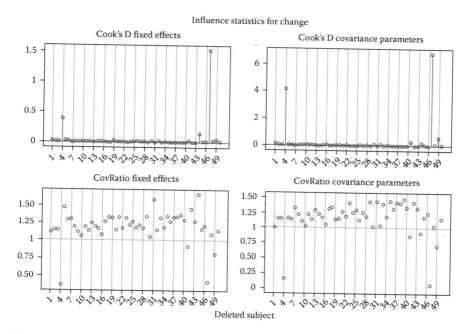

FIGURE 11.6
Influence statistics for fixed effects and covariance parameters from the small example data set.

TABLE 11.1

Comparisons of Endpoint Contrasts from All Data and Data
with Influential Subjects Excluded

Data	Endpoint Treatment Contrast	Standard Error	P Value
All data	3.39	1.49	0.0274
Excluding Subject 4	3.54	1.51	0.0234
Excluding Subject 47	4.55	1.31	0.0011

influential than other subjects for fixed effects, covariance parameters, and for precision in those estimates.

Influence statistics for individual fixed effect parameters are also produced by the code in Code Fragment 11.1. However, plots are not shown here. Subject 47 had a large influence on almost every parameter. The influence of Subject 4 was less consistent. Influence statistics for individual covariance parameters are also produced by the code in Code Fragment 11.1. However, plots are not shown here. Deleting Subject 47 reduced variance at Times 2 and 3, and deleting Subject 4 reduced variance at Time 1.

Treatment lsmeans after deleting Subject 47 and Subject 4 are compared to results from including all Subjects in Table 11.1. Excluding Subject 4 slightly increased the treatment contrast, had little effect on the standard error, and resulted in a small decrease to the P value. Deleting Subject 47 resulted in a large increase in the treatment contrast and a decrease in the standard error. Therefore, the T statistic when excluding Subject 47 was much larger and the P value much smaller compared with results from including all subjects.

If these were real data, the consequences of excluding Subject 47 would warrant additional investigation from a clinical perspective. In general, final inferences from confirmatory trials are based on results from including all randomized subjects. However, if this was an early phase or otherwise nonconfirmatory study, clinical considerations could warrant basing conclusions on data with Subject 47 excluded. Regardless of the scenario, it is important to know about influential subjects and how they influenced results.

The additional investigations might focus on subject history or other demographic or illness characteristics to verify whether the subject was indeed appropriate for inclusion in the study. If nothing anomalous was discovered, the subject may simply seem unusual because the data set was small and in a larger data set other subjects more similar to Subject 47 may be present.

For this example, results were statistically significant with or without Subject 47 included. Therefore, the anomalous profile of Subject 47 did not alter conclusions about the existence of a treatment effect. However, the difference in magnitude of the treatment effect could still be a consideration.

11.6 Summary

Outliers are anomalous values in the data that may have a strong influence on the fitted model, resulting in a worse fit for the majority of the data. The important issue to address is whether outliers had an important effect on results, not whether outliers or nonnormality existed.

Checking for patterns of residuals, such as associations between residuals and covariates, helps ascertain whether or not the mean function is appropriately specified; that is, are all the important effects fitted and is the modeled form of the association (linear etc.) correct? This emphasizes the iterative nature of model checking in that after identifying such patterns the model would be modified and refit, and the residuals reevaluated.

Another important aspect of model checking is to assess the influence of clusters of observations on model fit. In clinical trials, the clusters of interest usually include subject and investigative site. The general idea of quantifying the influence of clusters relies on computing parameter estimates based on all data points, removing the cases in question from the data, refitting the model, and computing statistics based on the change between the full-data and reduced-data estimations. Again, the main idea is not so much whether or not influential clusters existed, but rather to understand what impact the most influential clusters had on results.

Section III

Methods for Dealing with Missing Data

Missing data is an incessant problem in longitudinal clinical trials. The fundamental problem caused by missing data is that the balance provided by randomization is lost if, as is usually the case, the subjects who discontinue differ with regard to the outcome of interest from those who complete the study. This imbalance can lead to biases in the comparison of the treatment groups.

Fortunately, missing data has been an active area of research, with many advances in statistical theory and in our ability to implement the theory. Section III focuses on statistical methods for dealing with incomplete data. However, missing data is a cross-functional problem that is best dealt with by preventing missing data. Therefore, other aspects of missing data, including trial design and conduct to minimize missing data, were covered in Section I.

The focus in this section is to introduce various methods and their general attributes. How to use these various methods in developing a comprehensive analysis plan is covered in Section IV.

12

Overview of Missing Data

12.1 Introduction

Missing data in longitudinal clinical trials is a complex and wide-ranging topic, in part because missing data may arise in many ways. Intermittent missing data occurs when subjects miss scheduled assessments but attend subsequent visits. Dropout (withdrawal, attrition) is when subjects miss all subsequent assessments after a certain visit. Intermittent missing data are generally less problematic than withdrawal/attrition because, having observed data bracketing the unobserved value makes it easier to verify assumptions about the missing data compared to when no subsequent values are observed.

In addition, values may be missing because a subject is lost to follow-up, with nothing known about treatment or measurements past the point of dropout. Alternatively, a subject may withdraw from the initially randomized study medication and be given an alternative (rescue) treatment, but with no further measurements taken. Or, follow-up measurements may continue after initiation of the rescue treatment. All these and other scenarios may happen within a single trial, with differing implications for analyses (Mallinckrodt and Kenward 2009).

Importantly, missing data may need to be handled differently for different estimands. In addition, the consequences of missing values are situation-dependent. For example, in a clinical trial for rheumatoid arthritis, if a subject is lost to follow-up halfway through the trial, some of the information needed to understand how well the drug worked for that subject is indeed missing. On the other hand, if the subject discontinued for lack of efficacy, it is known the drug was, at least in a global sense, not effective for that subject and no information is missing for that subject relative to global effectiveness. However, other information regarding safety or secondary aspects of efficacy may be hindered by the incompleteness of the data.

The following hypothetical data illustrates the ambiguity missing data can cause. Assume that Treatment 1 is an investigational medicine and Treatment 2 is the standard of care. Results for each subject are categorized as success or failure and the outcomes are summarized in Table 12.1.

TABLE 12.1

Hypothetical Trial Results (Number of
Subjects by Outcome Category)

	Treatment 1	Treatment 2
Success	35	40
Failure	35	50
Missing	30	10
Total	100	100

Success rates based on the observed data are 50% (35/70) for Treatment 1 and 44% (40/90) for Treatment 2 (for ease of illustration, significance testing is ignored). Therefore, if it is assumed that presence or absence of the observations was not related to the outcome, then the observed percentages reflect what would have been observed if data were complete, and Treatment 1 would appear to have the greater success rate. In contrast, if it is assumed that all subjects with unknown outcomes were failures, then the success rate would be greater for Treatment 2 (35% vs. 40%).

These results illustrate how missing outcomes can undermine the clarity and robustness of trial conclusions. According to one assumption the success rate for Treatment 1 was greater, but under another assumption Treatment 2 was better. Drawing the proper inference depends on which assumption was most appropriate. However, assumptions about missing data cannot be evaluated from the available data because the data about which the missing data assumptions are made are missing (Verbeke and Molenberghs 2000).

Despite the presence of missing data, a clinical trial may still be valid provided the statistical methods used are sensible (www.ich.org/cache/compo/276–254-1.html). Carpenter and Kenward (2007) define a sensible analysis as one where:

1. The variation between the intervention effect estimated from the trial and that in the population is random. In other words, trial results are not systematically biased.

2. As the sample size increases, the variation between the intervention effect estimated from the trial and that in the population gets smaller and smaller. In other words, as the size of the trial increases, the estimated intervention effect hones in on the true value in the population. Such estimates are called consistent in statistical terminology.

3. The estimate of the variability between the trial intervention effect and the true effect in the population (i.e., the standard error) correctly reflects the uncertainty in the data.

If these conditions hold, then valid inference can be drawn despite the missing data. However, the analyses required to meet these conditions may be different from the analyses that satisfy these conditions when no data are missing. Regardless, whenever data intended to be collected are missing, information is lost and estimates are less precise than if data were complete (Mallinckrodt 2013).

When drawing inference from incomplete data, it is important to recognize that the potential bias from missing data can either mask or exaggerate the true difference between treatments (Mallinckrodt et al. 2008; NRC 2010). Moreover, the direction of bias has different implications in different scenarios. For example, underestimating treatment differences in efficacy is bias *against* an experimental treatment that is superior to control, but is bias *in favor* of an experimental treatment that is inferior to control. This situation has particularly important inferential implications in noninferiority testing.

Underestimating treatment differences in safety is bias in favor of an experimental treatment that is less safe than control, but is bias against the experimental drug that is safer than control.

12.2 Missing Data Mechanisms

In order to understand the potential impact of missing data and to choose an appropriate analytic approach for a particular situation, the stochastic process(es) (i.e., mechanisms) leading to the missingness must be considered. The following taxonomy of missing data mechanisms is now well-established in the statistical literature (Little and Rubin 2002).

Data are missing completely at random (MCAR) if, conditional upon the covariates (e.g., treatment group, baseline severity, investigative site) in the analysis, the probability of missingness does not depend on either the observed or unobserved outcomes of the variable being analyzed.

Data are missing at random (MAR) if, conditional upon the covariates in the analysis and the observed outcomes of the variable being analyzed, the probability of missingness does not depend on the unobserved outcomes of the variable being analyzed.

Data are missing not at random (MNAR) if, conditional upon the covariates in the analysis model and the observed outcomes of the variable being analyzed, the probability of missingness does depend on the unobserved outcomes of the variable being analyzed. Another way to think about MNAR is that if, conditional on observed outcomes, the statistical behavior (means, variances, etc.) of the unobserved data is equal to the behavior had the data been observed, then the missingness is MAR; if not, then MNAR.

With MCAR, the outcome variable is not related to the probability of dropout (after taking into account covariates). In MAR, the observed values of the outcome variable are related to the probability of dropout, but the unobserved outcomes are not (after taking into account covariates and observed outcome). In MNAR the unobserved outcomes are related to the probability of dropout even after the observed outcomes and covariates have been taken into account.

The practical implications of the distinction between MAR and MNAR is best appreciated by example. Consider a clinical trial where subjects are assessed every 4 weeks for 24 weeks, and a subject had clinically meaningful improvement during the first 12 weeks. Subsequent to the Week-12 assessment the subject had a marked worsening and dropped out. If the subject was lost to follow-up and there was no Week-16 observation to reflect the worsened condition, the missingness was MNAR. If the Week-16 observation was obtained before the subject dropped out, it is possible the missingness was MAR (provided the outcomes were incorporated in the analysis model). Note that this example illustrates what happens on average under the two mechanisms. With the stochastic nature of the missingness processes, it is impossible to claim with certainty whether missingness for a particular subject was driven by an MAR or MNAR mechanism.

Mallinckrodt et al. (2008) summarized several key points that arise from the precise definitions of the missingness mechanisms given above. First, given that the definitions are all conditional on the model, characterization of the missingness mechanism does not rest on the data alone; it involves both the data and the model used to analyze them. Consequently, missingness that might be MNAR given one model could be MAR or MCAR given another. In addition, since the relationship between the dependent variable and missingness is a key factor in the missingness mechanism, the mechanism may vary from one outcome to another within the same data set.

Moreover, when dropout rates differ by treatment group, it would be incorrect to conclude on these grounds alone that the missingness mechanism was MNAR and that analyses assuming MCAR or MAR were invalid. If dropout depended only on treatment, and treatment was included in the model, the mechanism giving rise to the dropout was MCAR. This is one example of what some have termed covariate-dependent MCAR (Little 1995; O'Kelly and Ratitch 2014). The distinction between covariate-dependent MCAR and MCAR applies to all covariates, not just treatment.

Given that the missingness mechanism can vary from one outcome to another in the same study, and may depend on the model and method, statements about the missingness mechanism without reference to the model and the variable being analyzed are problematic to interpret. This situational dependence also means that broad statements regarding missingness, and validity of particular analytic methods across specific disease states are unwarranted (Mallinckrodt 2013).

Moreover, terms such as ignorable missingness can also be problematic to interpret. For example, in the case of likelihood-based estimation, if the parameters defining the measurement process (i.e., governing the distribution of both observed and missing outcomes) are independent of the parameters defining the missingness process (this condition sometimes is referred to as the separability or distinctness condition), the missingness is ignorable if it arises from an MCAR or MAR mechanism but is nonignorable if it arises from an MNAR process (Verbeke and Molenberghs 2000).

In this context, ignorable means the missing-data mechanism need not be modeled because unbiased estimates of the parameters governing the measurement process can be obtained from the maximum likelihood analysis of observed data. However, if other forms of estimation are used, missing data may be ignorable only if arising from an MCAR mechanism. Hence, if missing data are described as ignorable or nonignorable, this must be done with reference to both the estimation method and the analytic model (Mallinckrodt 2013).

Informative censoring is yet another term used to describe the attributes of missing data. Censoring is best understood in the context of survival analyses. If the response variable was time to an event, subjects not followed long enough for the event to occur have their event times censored at the time of last assessment. It is often assumed in survival time analyses that what caused a subject to be censored is independent of what would cause her/ him to have an event. This assumption is often taken after conditioning on available baseline covariates or strata, such as in a Cox proportional hazards regression model. If the outcome is related to the likelihood of censoring, conditional on available covariates, informative censoring is said to have been present. For example, if subjects discontinue because of poor response to treatment but did not yet have the event of interest, the censoring times indirectly reflect bad outcomes. Thus, the censoring is said to be informative. Analogously, the censoring can be said to be not at random because the statistical behavior or distribution of event times for censored patients is not equal to that of uncensored patients.

However, an important consideration differentiates informative censoring in the survival time setting from the repeated measures setting. In survival time settings, typically there is one observation of the analyzed outcome (event time) per subject; no intermediate observations exist. In longitudinal settings with repeated measures, most subjects will have at least partially observed sequences. With repeated measurements, for censoring (dropout) to be informative, this must be in addition to what is known from the observed outcomes. With no intermediate observations included in the model in the survival time setting, it is more likely censoring would be informative than in an otherwise similar scenario where analyses can condition on the intermediate observations. Simply put, MAR (noninformative censoring) is more likely valid with intermediate observations in a repeated measures setting. In survival time settings, these intermediate observations are often not included in analysis.

Throughout the remainder of this book, missing data are described via the mechanism giving rise to the missingness (Mallinckrodt 2013).

12.3 Dealing with Missing Data

12.3.1 Introduction

Dealing with missing data is of course in part an analytic problem. However, the best way to deal with missing data is to prevent it (NRC 2010; Fleming 2011; Mallinckrodt 2013; O'Kelly and Ratitch 2014). A comprehensive approach to the prevention and treatment of missing data involves three pillars: (1) setting clear objectives and defining the causal estimands; (2) minimizing the amount of missing data; and, (3) defining an appropriate primary analysis supported by plausible sensitivity analyses (Mallinckrodt et al. 2014).

Minimizing missing data was covered in Chapter 3. Objectives and estimands were discussed in Chapter 2. Recall that some estimands can be formulated such that early discontinuation from treatment or initiation of recuse treatment are considered an outcome and do not result in missing data, whereas for other estimands discontinuation or rescue result in missing data. This chapter and Part III of the book focuses on the second situation. The remainder of this chapter introduces key concepts in analysis of incomplete data. Details on specific analyses are covered in subsequent chapters.

12.3.2 Analytic Approaches

Missing data can be dealt with by:

1. Ad hoc (single) imputation approaches (e.g., imputation with last observed values)
2. Ignoring the missing data
3. Accounting for the missing data via principled approaches to imputation, likelihood-based analyses, or weighting the observed values to adjust for the probability of dropout
4. Jointly modeling the outcome variable and the missingness process

Until recently, guidelines for the analysis of clinical trial data provided only limited advice on how to handle missing data, and analytic approaches tended to be simple and ad hoc (Molenberghs and Kenward 2007). Simple and ad hoc methods became popular during a time of limited computing power because they restored the intended balance to the data, allowing implementation of the simple analyses for complete data. However, with the seminal work on analysis of incomplete data by Rubin (1976), including the now common taxonomy of missingness mechanisms, attention began to shift to accounting for the potential bias from missing data.

Nevertheless, widespread use of simple methods for dealing with missing data set historical precedent that fostered their continued acceptance even after alternative methods were well known. In regulatory settings, methods like baseline observation carried forward (BOCF) and last observation carried forward (LOCF) remained popular choices for the primary analysis long after more principled alternatives could be easily implemented with commercial software (Mallinckrodt 2013).

In addition to historical precedent, continued acceptance of LOCF and BOCF despite strong evidence of their shortcomings was also fostered by the belief that these methods led to conservative estimates of treatment effects. Conservative in this context means not favoring the treatment; that is, underestimating the advantage of treatment over control. Hence, even though it became well known that imputing missing data via LOCF or BOCF yielded biased estimates of treatment effects, that bias was considered appropriate for confirmatory clinical trials of medical interventions because the bias was thought to provide protection against erroneous approval of ineffective interventions (Kenward and Molenberghs 2009).

However, as detailed in Chapter 13, the conditions under which LOCF and BOCF yield conservative estimates and maintain control of Type I error rates are not straightforward and cannot be assured at the start of the trial. Not surprisingly, LOCF and BOCF are now generally not seen as suitable for use as a primary analysis (Molenberghs and Kenward 2007; Mallinckrodt et al. 2008; NRC 2010; O'Kelly and Ratitch 2014).

For an analysis to yield unbiased results when ignoring missing data, the missingness must typically arise from an MCAR mechanism. One notable exception to the requirement of MCAR for ignorability is direct likelihood analyses, which can be valid under the far less restrictive assumption of MAR. Part II of this book described many aspects of direct likelihood analyses. Chapter 14 provides further detail on how likelihood-based analyses can ignore missing data that arise from an MCAR or MAR mechanism.

Multiple imputation has several variations, but the key idea is to impute the missing values using a likelihood-based model, combine the actually observed and imputed values to create a complete data set, analyze the now complete data, and repeat the process multiple times. Results are combined across data sets for final inference in a manner that takes into account the uncertainty due to missing data. More details on multiple imputation are provided in Chapter 15.

Inverse probability weighting is another MAR approach wherein a specific model is used to estimate the probability of dropout given the observed data. The inverse of these probabilities are applied to the observed data to create a pseudo-sample reflecting what would have been observed if no data were missing. Chapter 16 includes additional theoretical details and specifics on implementing inverse probability weighting.

Jointly modeling the outcome of interest and the dropout process typically involves MNAR analyses. Chapter 18 includes additional theoretical details and some implementation specifics on MNAR methods.

The analytic conundrum missing data pose is that MCAR is usually not a reasonable assumption, MAR may be reasonable but there is no way to know for certain, and there is no way to be certain that an MNAR method and model is appropriate (Mallinckrodt 2013). A sensible compromise between blindly shifting to MNAR models and ignoring them altogether is to use MNAR methods in sensitivity analyses (Molenberghs and Kenward 2007; Mallinckrodt et al. 2008). Indeed, broad consensus has emerged indicating that the primary analyses of longitudinal clinical trials should often be based on methods that assume MAR, and that robustness of the MAR result should be assessed using sensitivity analyses (Verbeke and Molenberghs 2000; Molenberghs and Kenward 2007; Mallinckrodt et al. 2008; Siddiqui et al. 2009; NRC 2010; Mallinckrodt et al. 2014).

12.3.3 Sensitivity Analyses

Sensitivity analyses can be a single analysis or a series of analyses with differing assumptions. The aim is that by comparing results across sensitivity analyses it becomes apparent how much inferences rely on the assumptions (NRC 2010; Phillips et al. 2016). In longitudinal clinical trials, sensitivity analyses typically focus on inferences regarding the treatment effects. Therefore, a primary aim of sensitivity analyses is to assess how treatment effects vary depending on assumptions about the missing data.

Sensitivity analyses in principle can be used for any analytic assumption. However, it is useful to distinguish between testable and nontestable assumptions. Assumptions regarding covariance between repeated measurements, mean trends over time, distribution of residuals, etc. can be tested from the observed data. In contrast, the fundamental sensitivity task for missing data will often center on the distinction between MAR and MNAR mechanisms; however, a formal data-based distinction between MAR and MNAR is not possible because each MNAR model fit to a set of observed data can be reproduced exactly by an MAR counterpart (Molenberghs and Kenward 2007). Of course, such a pair of models will produce different predictions of the unobserved outcomes, given the observed outcomes.

That is, it is not possible to distinguish MAR versus MNAR in practice (NRC 2010; Mallinckrodt et al. 2014). Therefore, the aim of sensitivity analyses for missing data is typically to evaluate the degree to which inferences are influenced by departures from MAR. Departure from MAR is typically quantified via one or several sensitivity parameters. Unlike parameters that can be estimated from observed data, there is no information in the observed data about the missing data sensitivity parameters. Therefore, the sensitivity parameters are typically chosen by the analyst in order to create a relevant departure from MAR from which results can be compared to the MAR result (Carpenter et al. 2013).

It is important to keep missing data sensitivity analyses within the overall context of assessing uncertainty in clinical trial results. This uncertainty arises from different sources: (1) inherent imprecision in parameters of the model estimated from a finite sample; (2) model selection (e.g., for the mean and covariance functions); and, (3) the level of uncertainty due to incompleteness. Sources 1 and 2 can be assessed from the observed data. What sets missing data apart is that uncertainty from incompleteness cannot be objectively evaluated from observed data. Hence, the need for missing data sensitivity analyses (Molenberghs and Kenward 2007).

12.3.4 Inclusive and Restrictive Modeling Approaches

Collins et al. (2001) describe restrictive and inclusive modeling philosophies. Restrictive models typically include only the design factors of the experiment, and perhaps one or a few covariates. Inclusive models include, in addition to the design factors, auxiliary variables whose purpose is to improve the performance of the missing data procedure.

Recalling the specific definition of MAR provides rationale for inclusive modeling. Data are MAR if, conditional upon the variables in the model, missingness does not depend on the unobserved outcomes of the variable being analyzed. Therefore, if additional variables are added to the model that explains missingness, MAR can be valid; whereas if the additional variables are not included, the missing data would be MNAR.

Ancillary variables can be included in likelihood-based analyses by either adding the ancillary variable as a covariate or as an additional response to create a multivariate analysis. However, the complexity of multivariate analyses and the features of most commercial software make it easier to use ancillary variables via MI. With separate steps for imputation and analysis, post-baseline, time-varying covariates—possibly influenced by treatment—can be included in the imputation step of MI to account for missingness but then not included in the analysis step to avoid confounding with the treatment effects, as might be the case in a likelihood-based analysis.

12.4 Summary

Missing data is an incessant and complex problem in longitudinal clinical trials. Dealing with missing data is in part an analytic problem. However, the best way to deal with missing data is to prevent it. A comprehensive approach to the prevention and treatment of missing data involves setting clear objectives and defining the causal estimands, minimizing missing data, and having an appropriate primary analysis supported by plausible sensitivity analyses.

The potential impact of missing data is dependent on the underlying mechanism. In MCAR, neither the observed nor the unobserved data are related to the probability of dropout. This situation is unlikely in most clinical trial scenarios. There are two ways to think about the less restrictive MAR mechanism: (1) the missingness does not depend on missing data given observed data and (2) the distribution of unobserved future outcomes is the same as the distribution of observed future outcomes, conditional on earlier outcomes. If these conditions do not hold, then data are MNAR.

13

Simple and Ad Hoc Approaches for Dealing with Missing Data

13.1 Introduction

This chapter provides an overview of simple and ad hoc methods of dealing with missing data in longitudinal clinical trials. These methods are generally not recommended for use but are of historic interest and provide a useful starting point from which to differentiate the more principled methods described in subsequent chapters. It is assumed throughout this chapter that the estimand of interest is the treatment effect that would have been estimated in an infinitely large trial with no missing values; that is, estimand 3 as introduced in Table 2.1, the de jure (efficacy) estimand. Focus is on the difference between treatments in mean change from baseline to endpoint.

In this context, the complete data set is a random sample of subjects from the hypothetical infinitely large trial of all subjects. Therefore, evaluation of treatment effects from complete data (even using simple estimators such as the two sample t-test comparing unadjusted sample means) provides unbiased estimates of that estimand. In fact, this consideration motivates use of estimates from complete data as valid benchmarks for performance of methods applied to incomplete data. Bias in methods is with respect to the above estimand, understanding that a method with bias for this estimand may provide unbiased results for a different estimand. Methods are illustrated using the small example data set with dropout (see Section 4.3). Results from the various methods applied to the incomplete data are benchmarked against results from the corresponding complete data set.

As detailed in Section 4.3, missing data were created by applying to the complete data an MAR missingness process with the probability of dropout depending on the observed outcomes. Only monotone missingness patterns were generated; that is, if a subject had a missing value at a time $= t$ all assessments at time $> t$ were also missing.

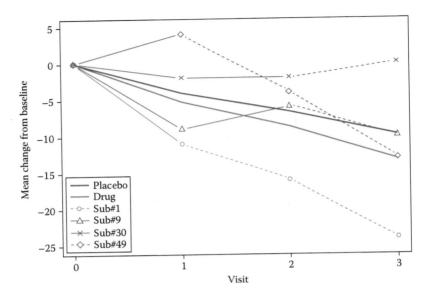

FIGURE 13.1
Response and missing data profiles for four selected patients. Solid lines are the observed outcomes and dotted lines show "unobserved" outcomes from complete data that were deleted to create the incomplete data.

Figure 13.1 illustrates incomplete and complete outcome profiles of four subjects (#1, #9, #30, and #49) that were selected to represent different response and missingness patterns. These subjects are used as case studies to illustrate features of each analytic approach.

13.2 Complete Case Analysis

In complete case analysis (also known as observed case or completers analysis) subjects with one or more missing values for the outcome being analyzed are discarded from the data set. Only subjects with complete data for the outcome being analyzed are included.

Completers analyses have serious drawbacks. The subset of subjects that complete the trial is seldom a random subset. For example, subjects with poor outcomes are often more likely to discontinue. In other words, the missing data seldom arise from an MCAR mechanism. In essence, including only completers creates selection bias. This bias typically causes overestimation of within group effects, particularly at the last scheduled visit.

When the selection process is the same for each treatment arm such that the bias to within-group point estimates is the same, this results in an unbiased estimate of the difference between treatments. However, such an assumption is difficult to justify a priori, especially when comparing active medications to placebo. If for example efficacy differs by treatment and efficacy influences adherence, the amount of selection bias will differ by treatment group, leading to a bias in the treatment contrast when analyzing completers. Moreover, even if the bias in change to last visit cancelled out between treatment groups, other aspects of the analysis are likely biased. For example, the completers are likely a more homogenous group than the initially randomized cohort of subjects, leading to underestimation of variance, which, in turn, leads to standard errors that are too small, confidence intervals that are too narrow, and test statistics that are biased toward inferences that the groups differ.

Setting aside the issue of bias, analyzing only completers results in a problematic loss of information because subjects who discontinued the trial are ignored. The partial information from incomplete sequences can still be valuable in estimating treatment effects. For example, if a subject discontinued just before the last scheduled visit t, his/her observed outcomes up to visit $t-1$ provide relevant information that could be utilized ("borrowed") for estimating the treatment effect at visit t.

As an illustration, consider the following simple, hypothetical scenario. Assume that the distribution of the change in efficacy scores from baseline to the last scheduled visit is normally distributed with means $\mu_A = -13$ and $\mu_B = -10$ for Drug A and Drug B (a larger negative change indicates greater improvement). Further assume a common standard deviation $\sigma = 5$. Therefore, the true treatment contrast (B–A) for the complete data = 3.

Now assume that subjects discontinue and therefore miss the final assessment with probability 1 if their change score is above the threshold value $k = -10$. The observed data at the last visit will follow a truncated normal distribution within each treatment arm with the mean given by the expression: $\mu - \sigma\phi\left(\dfrac{k-\mu}{\sigma}\right)\Big/\Phi\left(\dfrac{k-\mu}{\sigma}\right)$, where $\phi(.)$ and $\Phi(.)$ are standard normal PDF and CDF, respectively. These new means are about −15.3 for Drug A and −14.0 for Drug B, resulting in a treatment difference of 1.3 versus the difference of 3.0 for the complete data. The truncation causes a shift in the within-group means toward better outcomes. The impact of truncation is not the same in both groups; it is greater in the group with worse efficacy. In real clinical trial scenarios, discontinuations likely result from complex stochastic process(es). However, this simple example illustrates how dropouts due to lack of efficacy would differentially exaggerate observed efficacy within each treatment arm, thus inducing bias (likely dilution) in the contrast between treatments.

Figure 13.2 plots visit-wise least squares means from the small example data set with dropout based on the subset of subjects who completed Time 3 (solid lines) compared to the benchmark from complete (full) data (dotted line). The "complete case" estimates are those at the last visit (Time 3). Estimates were obtained using ANCOVA for visit-wise changes from baseline with treatment and baseline value as covariates in the model.

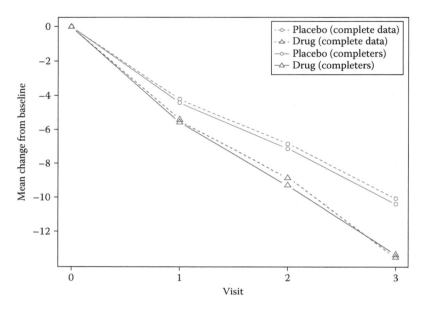

FIGURE 13.2
Comparison of "complete case" analysis with analysis based on complete (full) data.

In this example, visit-wise means for the active treatment arm (Treatment 2) are not affected much by dropouts, whereas in the placebo arm the means for completers consistently deviate from those based on complete data, indicating selection bias and dilution of the treatment contrast at the last visit.

13.3 Last Observation Carried Forward and Baseline Carried Forward

Last observation carried forward (LOCF) and baseline observation carried forward (BOCF) are methods for nonstochastic imputation. For subjects with monotone patterns of missing values, the outcomes are imputed using their earlier observed values. As the names imply, LOCF imputes all missing values for each subject using the last observed value for that subject and BOCF imputes all missing values for each subject using the baseline value for that subject.

Typically, when LOCF and BOCF are used the repeated measures nature of the data is ignored and a single outcome for each subject is analyzed. As initially noted in Chapter 12, use of LOCF and BOCF was in part justified because these methods were thought to provide conservative estimates of treatment effects and/or to be a composite measure of effectiveness that combined aspects of efficacy, safety, and tolerability. However, particularly LOCF can be considered as pursuing different estimands rather than as imputation methods for estimating treatment effects in the sense of a de jure (efficacy) estimand. Focus here is on estimates of efficacy.

If subjects on Drug A discontinue from a trial because of the side effects prior to achieving full benefit from the drug, their last observed values for efficacy outcomes would tend to be worse compared to those that would have been observed had the subjects remained in the trial until the last assessment. Carrying baseline values forward would often be a more conservative imputation because subjects who discontinued at any time, even one visit prior to end of the study, would be considered to have had no change.

Figure 13.3 plots the "visit-wise" LOCF and BOCF estimates by treatment arm as well as the benchmark estimate from the complete data set (shown as dotted line). All estimates are based on an ANCOVA model with treatment and baseline score as covariates. The estimates at visit (Time) 3 are what would be computed as the final LOCF or BOCF estimate of treatment effect. In the example, LOCF and BOCF yield smaller mean changes over time compared with the complete data reference.

Although it seems reasonable to consider LOCF and BOCF as providing conservative estimates of within-group mean changes, the impact on treatment contrasts is less clear. This lack of clarity on the direction of bias from LOCF and BOCF is compounded by the fact that these methods consistently

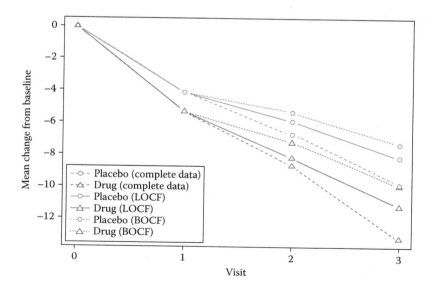

FIGURE 13.3
Mean changes from LOCF and BOCF in data with dropout compared with the analysis of the corresponding complete (full) data.

underestimate the variance. In fact, the power and Type I error rate control provided by LOCF and BOCF when assessing treatment contrasts is difficult to predict (Molenberghs et al. 2004). Many studies have shown that LOCF and BOCF can inflate treatment contrasts and markedly increase the rate of false-positive conclusions (Molenberghs et al. 2004; Lane et al. 2007; Barnes et al. 2008; Mallinckrodt et al. 2008; Sidiqui et al. 2009). Not surprisingly, the expert panel on missing data, convened at the request of FDA, stated that LOCF and BOCF are generally not appropriate means of dealing with missing data (NRC 2010).

Although it is not possible to be certain of the direction of bias, situations in which LOCF and BOCF are likely to overestimate treatment benefit include:

- When dropout in the control group is more frequent.
- When the difference between treatments is greatest at intermediate assessments. This bias would occur even if missingness were completely at random.
- In studies where the treatment goal is to maintain rather than improve outcomes.
- If LOCF and BOCF indeed provided a smaller estimate of the difference between treatments, this would not be conservative for safety outcomes. For example, if a drug causes weight gain, LOCF and BOCF will underestimate the magnitude of this unwanted side-effect.
- In noninferiority (NI) studies the null hypothesis is that the new treatment is worse than the standard treatment by a certain pre-specified amount (the noninferiority or Δ margin). Underestimating the difference between treatments in an NI study would be a bias in favor of the experimental arm.
- More generally, underestimating the inferiority of the inferior treatment would not be conservative.

13.4 Hot-Deck Imputation

Another single imputation approach is the so-called *hot-deck* method. Hot deck is of less historical interest, because it was not used as frequently in clinical trials as LOCF and BOCF. However, *hot-deck* imputation is useful to introduce, because it starts the movement toward more principled imputations. In *hot-deck* imputation, values are imputed by borrowing from an appropriate complete case (or *donor* case) that is in some sense similar to the missing case (Molenberghs and Kenward 2007).

Finding the appropriate donor for each subject with missing data involves finding the donor who is most similar. In longitudinal clinical trial data similarity can be based on observed outcomes and baseline covariates. Donors can also be matched based on estimates for the probability of dropout. The donor can be the subject with nonmissing outcomes whose estimated probability of being observed is closest to that of the subject with missing value(s). The model used to assess the probabilities can be fit using a logistic regression of the form $\Pr(R = 1 | X, Y_{obs})$.

In general, missingness must arise from an MCAR mechanism for *hot-deck* imputation to yield unbiased estimates of treatment effects. Besides, simple hot-deck methods typically underestimate standard errors of estimated treatment effects. Therefore, *hot-deck* imputation will not usually be valid, but the idea that imputation can be based on borrowed information is central to more principled approaches discussed in subsequent chapters.

13.5 Single Imputation from a Predictive Distribution

The approach illustrated in this section is not of historical interest, because it was not commonly used in clinical trials. However, this approach illustrates some key aspects of the more principled methods of analyzing incomplete data that are discussed in subsequent chapters. The approach takes a data set with missing values and makes it complete by imputing missing observations using a predictive model that is based on data from the longitudinal profiles of all subjects. The imputed-complete data set is then analyzed using a model that would have been appropriate had there been no missing data.

Recall that single imputation approaches do not account for the uncertainty in the imputation, resulting in underestimation of standard errors. Fundamental concepts in accounting for the uncertainty of imputation will be illustrated by introducing randomness in the predicted values; that is, imputed values are drawn from a distribution. Such an approach would be valid under MCAR and MAR if the imputation model properly accounted for the correlations between the repeated measurements within subjects.

A relatively straightforward way to implement this procedure is to first estimate the visit-wise marginal means for each treatment arm and the unstructured covariance matrix by fitting to the data an appropriate direct likelihood model, such as those described in Section II. Then, imputed values can be generated from the conditional normal distribution. A better approach would be to use subject-specific marginal means adjusted for baseline severity and other covariates, but for illustration the simpler imputation model is used here.

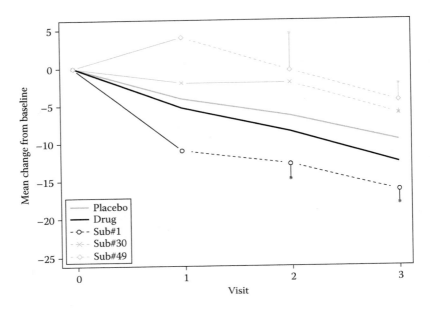

FIGURE 13.4
Illustration of single imputation from a predictive distribution for selected subjects. Subjects #1, #30, and #49 with observed data (solid lines), conditional means (dotted lines), and imputed values (asterisks). Treatment mean profiles (thick lines) are estimated via direct likelihood.

To obtain imputed values for a subject with missing data at Visits (Times) 2 and 3, such as placebo Subject #49 (see Figure 13.4), generate outcomes from the conditional distribution, $f(y_2, y_3|y_1)$, which is a bivariate normal distribution $N(\mu^*, \Sigma^*)$, with the mean vector μ^* and covariance matrix Σ^* given by

$$\mu^* = (\mu_2, \mu_3) + \frac{1}{\sigma_1^2}\Sigma_{23,1}(y_1 - \mu_1) = (-0.321, -4.454)$$

$$\Sigma^* = \Sigma_{23} - \frac{1}{\sigma_1^2}\Sigma_{23,1}(\Sigma_{23,1})^T = \begin{pmatrix} 9.964 & 7.635 \\ 7.635 & 18.578 \end{pmatrix}$$

where μ_1, μ_2, μ_3 are marginal means at Times 1, 2, and 3 for the placebo arm, Σ_{23} is the 2×2 error covariance matrix for Times 2 and 3, and $\Sigma_{23,1} = (\sigma_{21}, \sigma_{31})$ is a 2×1 vector with covariances between Times 2 and 1, and 3 and 1, respectively.

To obtain imputed values for a subject with missing data at Visit (Time) 3, such as Subject #30 (see Figure 13.4), generate imputed values from the conditional distribution $f(y_3|y_1, y_2)$ which is univariate normal with the mean μ^* and variance σ^{*2} given by

$$\mu^* = \mu_3 + \Sigma_{3,12}\Sigma_{12}^{-1}(y_1 - \mu_1, y_2 - \mu_2)^T = -6.182$$

$$\sigma^{*2} = \sigma_3^2 - \Sigma_{3,12}\Sigma_{12}^{-1}(\Sigma_{3,12})^T = 12.728$$

Predictive distributions for each missing value are obtained by replacing all these elements in the expressions for μ^* and Σ^* by the corresponding estimates from an appropriate likelihood-based analysis, resulting in the numerical values shown in the above equations.

Figure 13.4 plots the observed values and conditional means for the visits when the outcomes were unobserved for Subjects 1, 30, and 49.

The following observations and comments can be made

- The imputation model based on the conditional normal distributions estimated from the observed data likelihood effectively assumes that the distribution of future outcomes given earlier outcomes for subjects with observed future outcomes is the same as for those with missing future outcomes. This is equivalent to an MAR mechanism. Therefore, the point estimates from analysis of completed data with imputed missing values is consistent under MAR.

- The equality of the conditional distributions of missing and observed values given earlier values arises from use of marginal means and covariances estimated from the maximum likelihood analysis of observed data. Had estimates of the marginal means and covariances been obtained from a complete case analysis rather than a maximum likelihood analysis of all observed data, the imputation model would essentially reproduce the complete case analysis inducing similar biases in the final point estimates as the complete case analysis.

- Assuming positive within-subject correlations, which is typically the case, subjects whose observed outcomes were better than their treatment mean would also have conditional means better than the group mean for the future time points. That is, better (worse) than average outcomes at past visits predict better (worse) outcomes at future visits. For example, Subject 1 from the drug-treated group had greater change than the group mean at the time of discontinuation. The conditional means for Subject 1 were greater than the corresponding treatment group means. Similarly, placebo Subjects 30 and 49 were worse than (smaller changes) the corresponding group mean at the time of discontinuation and the projections for outcomes at future visits were worse (smaller changes) than the group means.

- Consistent with the weaker correlations between observations more distant in time, predicted individual conditional means get closer to the group mean (greater shrinkage) as the observation and the prediction time get farther apart. Refer to Section 5.4 for detailed explanation of how variance components influence shrinkage.

- Also consistent with the weaker correlations between observations more distant in time, the conditional distribution has greater variance as the time between the observation and the prediction time get more distant from each other. This makes intuitive sense in that when the source of information (the observed data) is more weakly correlated with what is to be predicted there is greater uncertainty in the prediction. In the example above, the conditional error variances for imputing outcomes at Time 3 using the data from Time 1 and Time 2 was 12.7 and the variance for imputing the Time 3 using only Time 1 was 18.6.

To further explain, consider a simple regression model with a single post-baseline outcome, y_1 regressed on baseline score y_0. Further assume equal variances $\sigma^2 = (\sigma_1)^2 = (\sigma_0)^2$. The conditional mean $E(Y_1|Y_0 = y_0)$ is $\mu_{1|0} = \mu_1 + \rho(y_0 - \mu_0)$. Therefore, the marginal mean μ_1 is adjusted by an additive term $\rho(y_0 - \mu_0)$. Assuming that within-subject error correlation (ρ) between the first and the second time points is positive, the adjustment would be positive or negative depending on whether the observed value y_0 was above or below the mean μ_0. The amount of adjustment is shrunk closer to zero by the factor of $|\rho| \le 1$. For example, no adjustment would be made if $\rho = 0$ (no within-subject correlation). The conditional variance $\sigma^2(1 - \rho^2)$ is smaller than the unconditional variance σ^2 by a factor $(1 - \rho^2) \le 1$. However, this factor will get closer to 1 with weaker within-subject correlation, such as when the future and observed time points are farther apart.

Once the missing values have been imputed, a completed data set is obtained and could be analyzed via standard complete data techniques. As previously noted, the point estimates from such an imputation strategy will be correct if the imputation model is based on consistent estimates of means and error covariance from the repeated measures likelihood.

Adding random noise to the predicted values when carrying out imputation (rather than taking the conditional mean for the predicted value "as is") adjusts the variance to account for the uncertainty due to imputation. However, standard errors would still be calculated with imputed values treated as observed values. This effectively assumes a larger sample size than that which was actually observed, resulting in artificially reduced standard errors that reflect greater precision than was actually the case. Although resampling methods (e.g., jackknife or bootstrap) could be used to obtain valid estimates of standard errors, the key concept for the present purpose is that single imputation, combined *with standard estimators of standard errors*, results in invalid inference.

An obvious question is why estimate treatment effects by imputing missing outcomes from a likelihood-based model when treatment effects can be estimated using the same assumptions directly from the likelihood model without imputation? In fact, the method illustrated in this subsection is of little practical value, but it is important for illustrating two key points.

First, imputing from the conditional normal distribution serves as a building block for more principled methods such as multiple imputation. And, as illustrated in Chapter 15, there are situations when breaking the estimation process into two steps: (1) generating a complete data set by imputing missing values and (2) estimating treatment effects from completed data may have advantages over directly estimating treatment effect from a single model applied to incomplete data.

13.6 Summary

The simple and ad hoc methods of dealing with missing data discussed in this chapter are generally not recommended for use. Nevertheless, the methods are of historic interest and provide a useful starting point from which to differentiate the more principled methods described in subsequent chapters. In particular, single imputation from a predictive distribution provides an important stepping stone for understanding multiple imputation and direct-likelihood analyses.

14

Direct Maximum Likelihood

14.1 Introduction

If missing data arise from an MCAR or MAR mechanism, a likelihood-based analysis can yield unbiased estimates and valid inferences from the available data such that the missing data can be ignored. With GEE and least squares estimation, for the missingness to be ignorable, it must arise from an MCAR mechanism. Therefore, the plausibility of ignorable missing data is greater with likelihood-based analyses than with GEE or least squares (Verbeke and Molenberghs 2000).

The technical explanation for why MCAR and MAR missingness can be ignored in likelihood-based analyses (such as those illustrated in Section II) is based on factorization of the likelihood function. This factorization explanation and other technical details are covered in the next section and examples in subsequent sections further illustrate how likelihood-based methods account for missing data.

14.2 Technical Details

Factorization of the likelihood function in this context means that the hypothetical "full" data are split into two parts: the actually observed part and the missing part, which are often described as the measurement process and the missingness process, respectively (Verbeke and Molenberghs 2000).

As a building block to factoring the full data likelihood, consider the observed data for subject i, denoted as an $1 \times n_i$ vector $Y_{i,obs}$ and the observed $1 \times n$ vector of missingness indicators R_i that indicate whether the subject has the outcome observed on jth occasion ($r_{ij} = 1$) or missing ($r_{ij} = 0$). The observed data likelihood can be written as the joint density of the random variables $Y_{i,obs}$ and R_i, $f(y_{i,obs}, r_i | x_i, \theta, \Psi)$, where X is the design matrix for fixed effects (e.g., baseline covariates, treatment, and time), θ is a vector of parameters for the outcome process, and Ψ is a vector of parameters for the missingness process.

The aim in clinical trials is typically to estimate θ, with ψ being of ancillary interest. As such, it would be desirable to partition the joint (log-) likelihood of $(Y_{i,obs}, R_i)$ so as to isolate the portion of the likelihood that is relevant for estimating θ. If such partitioning can be achieved, then the parts of the likelihood associated with missingness parameters are not relevant for maximizing the likelihood with respect to θ—and these missingness parameters could therefore be ignored.

The joint likelihood can be formally written as the product of marginal and conditional distributions

$$f(y_{i,obs}, r_i | x_i, \theta, \Psi) = f(y_{i,obs} | x_i, \theta, \Psi) f(r_i | y_{i,obs}, x_i, \theta, \Psi)$$

or on the log-likelihood scale as the sum

$$\log[f(y_{i,obs}, r_i | x_i, \theta, \Psi)] = \log[f(y_{i,obs} | x_i, \theta, \Psi)] + \log[f(r_i | y_{i,obs}, x_i, \theta, \Psi)].$$

In this decomposition, θ and Ψ are present in both pieces of the likelihood in the right-hand side, and thus Ψ is not ignorable. Fortunately, if missingness results from an MCAR or MAR mechanism and the parameters θ and Ψ are functionally separable (the so-called separability condition), a partitioning to isolate the parameters of interest is attainable.

To see how this is possible, consider the full data likelihood that includes both the observed and the missing data. Let a random variable $Y_{i,mis}$ denote the $1 \times (n - n_i)$ component vector of missing data for the ith subject. Although $Y_{i,mis}$ represents data that are not observed, it is a valid random variable representing the potential outcomes for subjects who discontinued from the trial that would have been observed had they remained.

The observed data likelihood can be written as the integral over the $Y_{i,mis}$. Under the integral sign, the joint density can be written as follows:

$$f\left(y_{i,obs}, r_i | x_i, \theta, \Psi\right) = \int f\left(y_{i,obs}, y_{i,mis}, r_i | x_i, \theta, \Psi\right) dy_{i,mis}$$

$$= \int f\left(y_{i,obs}, y_{i,mis} | x_i, \theta\right) f\left(r_i | y_{i,obs}, y_{i,mis}, x_i, \Psi\right) dy_{i,mis}$$

With the introduction of Y_{mis}, the joint likelihood for the full data can be factored into pieces that separate the parameters θ and Ψ because of the assumption that the complete outcome $(Y_{i,obs}, Y_{i,mis})$ does not depend on the missingness parameter Ψ, and the missingness process (R) does not depend on θ *after conditioning on the complete* data. By assuming MAR, the joint distribution of the *observed* data can be factored similarly.

Under MAR, $f(r_i|y_{i,obs}, y_{i,mis}, x_i, \Psi) = f(r_i|y_{i,obs}, x_i, \Psi)$. Therefore, this likelihood factor can be taken outside the integral and the desired factorization of the observed data likelihood is obtained as follows:

$$f(y_{i,obs}, r|x_i, \theta, \Psi) = f(y_{i,obs}|x_i, \theta)\, f(r_i|y_{i,obs}, x_i, \Psi)$$

Now parameter θ is associated only with the likelihood term containing $y_{i,obs}$. Therefore, we could estimate θ (and any functions of treatment effect of our interest) by using only contributions to the observed data likelihood of $y_{i,obs}$, $i = 1, ..., N$, because the parts associated with parameters of missingness (Ψ) would not be relevant for maximizing the likelihood with respect to θ.

This elegant proof (Little and Rubin 1987) is general and applies to *any* type of outcome as long as its likelihood can be written. The proof may be appealing to mathematically inclined readers. However, it is not intuitively obvious exactly how the missing data in the context of a longitudinal clinical trial (dropouts) are accounted for in this analytic framework. A more operational and instructive explanation of how direct likelihood methods, and in particular, methods based on an unstructured modeling of time and covariance, yield unbiased estimates under MAR can be given by a factorization of the likelihood for the observed part of the full repeated measures outcome $Y_i = (Y_{i1}, Y_{i2}, ..., Y_{in})$.

Consider the small example data set with three post-baseline outcomes, represented for the *i*th subject by the trivariate normal variate $Y_i = (Y_{i1}, Y_{i2}, Y_{i3})$ and further assume that all the missingness is due to dropouts (i.e., the missing data have a monotone pattern). Focus first, for simplicity, on the analysis of a single treatment arm because adding covariates does not change matters in principle. Thus, all time-fixed covariates are denoted collectively as X.

The trivariate normal distribution associated with random variate Y_i can be factored as a product of the conditional distributions that represent a sequence of regressions, where each component of the distribution is regressed on the previous outcomes and baseline scores. Subject indices (i) are suppressed for simplicity.

$$f(y|x, \theta) = f(y_1|x, \theta_1)\, f(y_2|x, y_1, \theta_2)\, f(y_3|x, y_1, y_2, \theta_3)$$

Here, parameter θ combines the vector of means and covariance matrix of multivariate normal distribution of Y conditional on X, and parameters θ_1, θ_2, and θ_3 contain regression coefficients and error variances associated with the three univariate conditional normal distributions (regressions): $[Y_1|X]$, $[Y_2|X, Y_1]$, and $[Y_3|X, Y_1, Y_2]$. With multivariate normal distributions, there is a one-to-one relation between parameters in θ and in $(\theta_1, \theta_2, \theta_3)$, therefore, θ can be obtained by simple matrix manipulations with $\theta_1, \theta_2,$ and θ_3, and vice versa.

It is instructive to think of obtaining maximum likelihood (ML) estimates of θ via sequentially fitting the above regression models, even though that is not how the likelihood maximization procedure is actually implemented in software packages. If the parameters θ_1, θ_2, and θ_3 estimated by the three regression models are unbiased under MAR, then θ would also be unbiased. The key question here is the following: why are the regression models based on observed data unbiased and not adversely affected by the presence of missing data?

Recall that the MAR assumption for monotone missingness patterns can be stated in two equivalent forms: (1) the missingness mechanism does not depend on missing data given observed data and (2) the distribution of unobserved future outcomes is the same as the distribution of observed future outcomes, conditional on earlier outcomes. The second condition means that the future outcomes for subjects who discontinued should be similar to the future outcomes of subjects who continued *if they had the same values of past outcomes, covariates, etc.* As a result of point 2 above, complete data are not needed to estimate any of the three regression models. For example, the model based on fitting $f(y_{3,obs} | x, y_{1,obs}, y_{2,obs}, \theta_3)$ to observed data should estimate the same parameter vector θ_3 as if somehow the model was fit to the actual missing data: $f(y_{3,mis} | x, y_{1,obs}, y_{2,obs}, \theta_3)$. Therefore, failing to observe $y_{3,mis}$ does not bias estimation results for θ_3.

14.3 Example

The small example data set that was introduced in Chapter 4 is used to illustrate how direct likelihood analyses account for missing data. Results are compared to those based on the corresponding complete data set. Selected individual subjects are used for further illustration. Data were analyzed as specified in Code Fragment 8.1, which featured an unstructured modeling of means and covariance. Recall that in this formulation of the mixed-effects model fitting versus not fitting a random intercept has no effect on fixed-effect estimates. The model with the random intercept and unstructured modeling is actually overspecified in that the residual covariance matrix fully captures all the information in the random effects. However, fitting the random intercept is useful here in order to obtain predictions for individual subjects. Therefore, the random intercept was included mindfully that fixed effects would be identical if the random intercept was not included. Results from the data with dropout and the corresponding complete data are summarized in Table 14.1.

Results at Time 1 were similar in complete and incomplete data. Differences in results between complete and incomplete data were greater at Time 3 than at Time 2. This pattern was not surprising, given that no data were missing at Time 1 and more data were missing at Time 3 than at Time 2.

As the amount of missing data increased, standard errors increased. Visitwise lsmeans for change from baseline were smaller for both treatment groups in the incomplete data than in the complete data. This disparity was

TABLE 14.1

Results from Likelihood-Based Analyses of Complete and Incomplete Data, with a Model Including Baseline as a Covariate

Treatment	Time	Complete Data		Incomplete Data	
		LSMEANS	SE	LSMEANS	SE
1	1	−4.13	0.91	−4.10	0.91
1	2	−6.70	0.93	−6.42	0.97
1	3	−9.86	1.05	−9.73	1.17
2	1	−5.32	0.91	−5.29	0.91
2	2	−8.70	0.93	−8.52	0.96
2	3	−13.26	1.05	−12.62	1.14
Endpoint Treatment Difference		3.39	1.49 ($p = 0.0274$)	2.90	1.64 ($p = 0.084$)

greater in Treatment 2, thereby yielding a smaller treatment contrast from incomplete data than from complete data.

It is important to interpret the results above as just one realization from a stochastic process. If the comparisons were replicated many times under the same conditions—with missing data arising from an MAR mechanism—the average of the lsmeans and treatment contrasts across the repeated samples would be the same for complete and incomplete data. Standard errors would be consistently greater in incomplete data, however.

To further clarify how missing data are handled in likelihood-based analyses, consider the observed and predicted values for selected subjects summarized in Table 14.2. First, consider the incomplete data for drug-treated (Treatment 2) Subject 1 who was dropped from the study after the first post-baseline visit. Although Times 2 and 3 were not observed, the parameters for the estimated treatment means factor-in the general dependency of Y_2 and Y_3 on Y_1, which can be used to generate predicted outcomes. This is because under MAR the future values of Y_2 and Y_3 for Subject 1 and other subjects who discontinued after Time 1 follow the relationships associated with the conditional distributions of $[Y_2|Y_1]$ and $[Y_3|Y_1,Y_2]$.

For Subject 1, it is predicted that the unobserved outcomes at Times 2 and 3 would have shown continued improvement, and the improvement for Subject 1 would have been greater than the group average. Factors influencing this prediction include the following: (1) the group to which Subject 1 belonged showed continued improvement over time and (2) the positive correlation between the repeated measurements suggested that subjects (such as Subject 1) with outcomes better (worse) than their group mean were likely to remain better (worse) than the group mean in the future.

Recall that the example data were created by first having complete data and then deleting observations according to an MAR mechanism. Therefore, the predicted outcomes from the incomplete data can be compared to

TABLE 14.2

Observed and Predicted Values for Selected Subjects
from Analyses of Complete and Incomplete Data

Time	Observed Change	Group Mean	Pred Change	SE Pred	Residual
Subject 1 Complete Data					
1	−11	−5.32	−12.36	2.16	1.36
2	−16	−8.70	−16.12	2.18	0.12
3	−24	−13.26	−19.20	2.27	−4.79
Subject 1 Incomplete Data					
1	−11	−5.29	−10.03	2.70	−0.96
2	.	−8.52	−13.49	3.34	.
3	.	−12.62	−15.39	4.58	.
Subject 30 Complete Data					
1	−2	−4.13	0.20	2.17	−2.20
2	−2	−6.70	−2.32	2.17	0.32
3	0	−9.86	−5.67	2.23	5.67
Subject 30 Incomplete Data					
1	−2	−4.10	−1.34	2.51	−0.65
2	−2	−6.42	−3.62	2.52	1.62
3	.	−9.73	−6.34	3.85	.

the actually observed complete data and to predicted values obtained from
the complete data. Predicted values for Subject 1 in the complete data deviate more from the group mean than in the incomplete data. For example, at
Time 3, the predicted value for Subject 1 is approximately 6 points above the
mean in complete data and only 3 points above the mean with incomplete
data. With incomplete data, there is less evidence for the superior improvement of Subject 1; therefore, the above average improvement seen at Time 1
yields a predicted value at Time 3 that is regressed (shrunk) more strongly
back to the group mean. The standard errors of the predicted values increase
substantially when the corresponding observation was missing. Refer to
Section 5.4 for a detailed examination of how variance components in the
mixed-effects model influence shrinkage of estimators.

Similar relationships exist for Subject 30, which came from the placebo
(Treatment 1) group. However, this subject had smaller improvements than
the group mean. In the incomplete data, the predicted values for Subject 30
were less than the group average, reflecting the anticipation of continued
below average performance. As with Subject 1, incomplete data resulted in
greater shrinkage of predicted values back to the group mean than in complete data. This increased shrinkage with incomplete data is because the evidence for the deviation in performance was weaker with fewer observations.

However, Subject 30 had two observations and the shrinkage in the incomplete data was less than if only one value had been observed. Correspondingly, the standard errors of the predicted values are smaller for Subject 30 than for Subject 1.

14.4 Code Fragments

Given the ignorability properties of direct likelihood, no special adjustments to accommodate missing data are required. All the likelihood-based analyses described in Section II of this book can be implemented exactly to incomplete data.

14.5 Summary

If missing data arise from an MCAR or MAR mechanism, a likelihood-based analysis yields unbiased estimates and valid inferences from the available data such that the missing data process can be ignored. Factorization of the full data likelihood into parts that isolate the missingness parameters from the parameters underlying the outcome process provides the technical explanation for why MCAR and MAR missingness can be ignored in likelihood-based analyses.

A more intuitive explanation for ignorability arises from the definition of MAR. Recall the following two ways to consider MAR: (1) the missingness mechanism does not depend on missing data given observed data and (2) the distribution of unobserved future outcomes is the same as the distribution of observed future outcomes, conditional on earlier outcomes. The second condition means that the future outcomes for subjects who discontinued should be similar to the future outcomes of subjects who continued *if they had the same values of past (observed) outcomes, covariates, etc.* As a result of point 2 above, models can be formulated from only the observed data that yield unbiased estimates of parameters describing the full data.

15

Multiple Imputation

15.1 Introduction

Multiple imputation (MI) is a popular and accessible method of model-based imputation. Standard references for MI include Rubin (1987) and Little and Rubin (2002). Multiple imputation is flexible and therefore has a number of specific implementations. However, the three basic steps to MI are:

1. Impute the missing data (typically) using Bayesian predictive distributions of missing data, conditional on observed data, resulting in multiple (m) completed data sets.

2. Analyze the m completed data sets using an analysis that would have been appropriate for complete data. This results in a set of m estimates (e.g., treatment contrasts).

3. Combine (pool) the m estimates into a single inferential statement by using combination rules (or "Rubin's rules") that account for uncertainty due to imputation of the missing values, therefore providing valid inference.

These steps can be applied to continuous outcomes that follow a normal distribution, categorical outcomes, or time to event (e.g., exponentially distributed) outcomes where missingness is created by censoring.

If MI is implemented using the same imputation and analysis model, and the model is the same as the analysis model used in a maximum likelihood-based (ML) analysis, MI and ML will yield asymptotically similar point estimates. That is, as the size of the data set and the number of imputations in MI increase, results from MI and ML converge to a common estimand for the 2-point estimates. Although ML is somewhat more efficient (smaller standard errors) Wang and Robins (1998), MI is more flexible, the distinct steps for imputation and analysis in MI yields flexibility that, as explained in subsequent sections, can be exploited in a number of situations. A down side to MI is that if interest exists in a number of parameters, the three-step process must be applied for each parameter. Alternatively, multiple parameters can

be handled simultaneously using a multiparameter version of the combination rules in step 3, with the additional burden of estimating the variance
covariance matrix associated with estimated parameters.

15.2 Technical Details

Point estimates in MI are computed as a simple average of the estimates
from the m completed data sets. The precision of these estimates is evaluated using simple formulas that incorporate both between-imputation and
within-imputation variability in the calculation of standard errors. In the following, we provide technical details assuming, for simplicity, the test statistics (and associated estimates) are univariate; however, the formulas readily
generalize for multivariate statistics.

Let $\hat{\theta}_i$, $i = 1,...,m$ be univariate estimates (e.g., treatment contrasts at the last
scheduled visit) obtained by applying an appropriate analysis model to the
m completed data set and U_i, $i = 1,...,m$ are their estimated (squared) standard errors. The MI point estimate is

$$\hat{\theta}_{MI} = \frac{\sum_{i=1}^{m} \hat{\theta}_i}{m}$$

The total variance is computed by combining the between-imputation
variability, $B = (m-1)^{-1} \sum_{i=1}^{m} (\hat{\theta}_i - \hat{\theta}_{MI})^2$, and the within-imputation variability,
$W = m^{-1} \sum_{i=1}^{m} U_i$

$$V = W + \left(1 + \frac{1}{m}\right) B$$

Inference on θ is based on the test statistic $T = \frac{\hat{\theta}_{MI}}{\sqrt{V}}$. As with ML, the $\hat{\theta}_{MI}$ estimator is unbiased if missing data arise from an MCAR or MAR mechanism.

The null distribution of T is not normal. Therefore, standard Wald-based
inference assuming T has the standard normal null distribution is not valid.
This is because for finite $m < \infty$ the total variance V is an inconsistent estimate of the true variance of the point estimator, $var(\hat{\theta}_{MI})$. That is, when the
sample size N increases to infinity, NV does not converge to a constant but
remains a random variable following a nondegenerate (chi-squared) distribution. This is in contrast to, for example, the variance of a sample mean:

$$N\left[\widehat{var}(\bar{x})\right] = \frac{N}{N}\hat{\sigma}^2 \xrightarrow{p} \sigma^2 = const.$$

To account for this extra variability, Rubin (1987) proposed using a student's t distribution instead of a normal distribution, with the number of degrees of freedom computed as

$$v = (m-1)\left(1 + \frac{1}{1+m^{-1}} \frac{W}{B}\right)^2$$

The price paid for the generality of the MI estimator is a degree of conservatism (sometimes negligible). This overestimation of variability has three sources (Wang and Robins 1998 and Robins and Wang 2000):

- The asymptotic variance of the MI point estimator (for finite m) exceeds that of the ML estimator
- The standard error of the MI point estimator obtained by Rubin's rules may exceed its true value, the square root of the asymptotic variance (i.e., overestimation of the standard error)
- Inconsistency of Rubin's variance estimator requiring use of the wider confidence intervals based on the t distribution rather than the normal distribution.

The MI procedure outlined above is essentially an extension of the single imputation model using a conditional normal distribution that was introduced in Section 13.5. There are two important differences, however. First, each missing value is imputed *multiple* times, which allows for explicit accounting for uncertainty due to the imputation/missing data. This is accomplished by incorporating the between-imputation variability.

The second difference is more subtle. In MI, imputations are simulated from the Bayesian predictive distribution of missing data given observed data $f(y_{mis}|y_{obs})$ rather than from the density $f(y_{mis} \mid y_{obs}, \hat{\theta})$ with parameters θ estimated at specific values (e.g., by maximum likelihood), as shown in Section 13.5. The predictive distribution is obtained by integrating (averaging) out parameters from the likelihood using the posterior distribution of parameters.

$$f(y_{mis} \mid y_{obs}) = \int f(y_{mis} \mid y_{obs}, \theta) f(\theta \mid y_{obs}) d\theta$$

Therefore, imputed values are sampled from distributions that incorporate uncertainty in estimating model parameters and uncertainty due to sampling data from the estimated model.

As a simple example, when estimating the mean and variance of a univariate normal distribution $N(\theta, \sigma^2)$, MI accounts for uncertainty in the estimated θ and σ^2 as well as uncertainty of sampling missing values from $Y_{mis} \sim N(\hat{\theta}, \hat{\sigma}^2)$.

It is instructive to think of imputing (sampling) from a predictive distribution as a two-stage procedure that is repeated m times. Repeat the following two steps m times for $i = 1,...,m$:

1. Draw a single random sample from the posterior distribution of parameters given observed data $\tilde{\theta}_i \sim f(\theta \mid y_{obs})$.
2. Draw random samples from the observed-data likelihood model $Y_{mis} \sim f(y \mid \tilde{\theta}_i)$ to produce a single completed data set.

The single imputation scheme considered in Section 13.5 essentially implements only the second step for $m = 1$ with $\tilde{\theta}_1$ set to the ML estimate $\tilde{\theta}_1 = \hat{\theta}_{ML}$.

It is useful to consider the consequences of creating m completed data sets using only the second step (i.e., without re-sampling from the posterior of θ). In this approach, point estimates would still be valid, essentially reproducing the ML estimates. However, the total variance V computed using Rubin's rules would be too small because the between-imputation variability would not include the uncertainty due to parameter estimation. As a result, the confidence intervals based on V would be too narrow, failing to maintain the nominal Type I error rates. Such imputation models have been termed *improper* (Rubin 1987).

With complex models, analytic formula for the posterior distribution $f(\theta \mid y_{obs})$ often do not exist and Markov Chain Monte Carlo (MCMC) methods can be used (Tanner and Wong 1987; Schafer 1997).

The MCMC algorithms are widely used in Bayesian inference to sample from joint posterior distributions of parameters when analytical expressions are not available. Sampling from the predictive distribution of missing data can be incorporated within this general approach through data augmentation algorithms. In the Bayesian framework there is no fundamental difference between missing data and parameters; both are unobserved quantities and are dealt with similarly. Although application of MCMC appears different from the two-stage sampling outlined above, they implement sampling from the same target distribution: $f(y_{mis} \mid y_{obs})$.

For example, the Gibbs method alternates between sampling from full conditionals $\tilde{y}_{mis}^{(k+1)} \sim f\left(y_{mis} \mid \tilde{\theta}^{(k)}, y_{obs}\right)$ and $\tilde{\theta}^{(k+1)} \sim f\left(\theta \mid \tilde{y}_{mis}^{(k+1)}, y_{obs}\right)$ through a large number of iterations $k = 0,...,K$, starting with some initial values for parameters $\tilde{\theta}^{(0)}$. As a result, after some initial (burn-in) draws, the samples of $\tilde{y}_{mis}^{(k+1)}$ and $\tilde{\theta}^{(k+1)}$ will be drawn approximately from the unconditional target distributions of $f(y_{mis} \mid y_{obs})$ and $f(\theta \mid y_{obs})$, respectively.

In the context of repeated measures analysis with a multivariate normal model, when the pattern of missingness is arbitrary, generic MCMC sampling must be used for imputation. When the pattern is monotone, sampling can be based on factorization of the joint normal distribution into a sequence of conditionals and using analytical formulas for the posterior distribution of parameters associated with each factor.

For the small example data set with dropout, the factorization of the likelihood is

$$f(y|x, \theta) = f(y_1|x, \theta_1) f(y_2|x, y_1, \theta_2) f(y_3|x, y_1, y_2, \theta_3)$$

Then, imputation can be organized sequentially

- Draw $\tilde{\theta}_1 \sim f(\theta_1 | x, y_1)$ and impute missing values for $Y_1, Y_{mis} \sim f(y_1 | x, \tilde{\theta}_1)$ (in the example data set no y_1 are missing and this step is not needed)
- Draw $\tilde{\theta}_2 \sim f(\theta_2 | x, y_1, y_2)$ and impute missing Y_2 based on observed and imputed Y_1 with $Y_{mis} \sim f(y_2 | x, \tilde{y}_1, \tilde{\theta}_2)$, where $\tilde{y}_1$ indicates that the value can be observed or imputed
- Draw $\tilde{\theta}_3 \sim f(\theta_3 | x, y_1, y_2, y_3)$ and impute missing Y_3 based on observed and imputed Y_1 and Y_2, $Y_{mis} \sim f\left(y_3 | x, \tilde{y}_1, \tilde{y}_2, \tilde{\theta}_3\right)$

Therefore, imputation of missing values is done via estimated Bayesian regression models where parameters are drawn from posterior distributions. In this case of normal linear regression, missing values for y_2 (Time 2) are imputed by sampling values from the regression model $Y_{mis} = \tilde{\beta}_0 + \tilde{\beta}_1 X + \tilde{\beta}_2 \tilde{Y}_1 + e\tilde{\sigma}$, where X is the baseline score, $\tilde{Y}_1$ is observed or imputed value of the change from baseline at Time 1 and $\tilde{\beta}_0, \tilde{\beta}_1, \tilde{\beta}_2, \tilde{\sigma}^2$ are drawn from their respective posterior distributions. Random error e is sampled from the standard normal distribution, $e \sim N(0,1)$. Here we omit details on specification of prior distributions for the parameters of the imputation model and corresponding posterior distributions, which for this case of normally distributed data are fairly straightforward and can be found, for example, in Schafer (1997) or SAS technical documentation for PROC MI.

As an illustration, Figure 15.1 depicts the observed data and the means from 100 imputations using the above sequential Bayesian regression for Subjects 1, 30, and 49 from the small example data set with dropout. The SAS and R code for this analysis is listed in Section 15.8 (Code Fragment 15.1). Results for treatment groups are discussed later. The focus here is on the individual subjects. Thin solid lines depict the observed data and dotted lines depict means of the imputed values for the focus subjects. Thick solid lines depict the treatment group means. The error bars indicate standard deviation of imputed values.

The trajectory for means of the imputed values resembles the conditional means based on a direct likelihood analysis as depicted Figure 13.4 and Table 14.2. Subjects with observed changes that were less than the average of their group have mean imputed values that are less than the corresponding group mean; subjects with observed changes that were greater than the group average have mean imputed values that are greater than the corresponding group mean. Also, similar to the direct-likelihood analysis, the

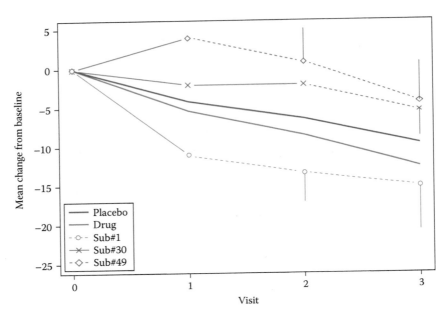

FIGURE 15.1
Illustration of multiply imputed values for Subjects #1, #30, and #49 from the small example
data set with dropout. The error bars represent the between imputation variability (standard
deviation based on the 100 imputed values at each time point).

standard deviation bars indicate greater variability in imputed values at
Time 3 for Subjects 1 and 49, who had only one observed value (at Time 1)
compared with Subject 30 who had two observed values.

The concordance between direct-likelihood and MI results is not coinci-
dental; these similarities are expected in all circumstances when the methods are implemented using similar models. Multiple imputation can also be
compared with direct Bayesian inference. Rubin (1987) showed that MI is
compatible with Bayesian analysis in the sense that the MI point estimate
and variance are approximating the posterior expectation and posterior
variance of a Bayesian analysis.

In that regard, MI is somewhat circular. First, the Bayesian posterior distribution of parameters is sampled. Next, the distribution of missing values is simu-
lated, and in the end the posterior sample of parameters is discarded. Hence,
the posterior distribution of parameters serves merely as an intermediate step
in imputation. Alternatively, sampling from posterior distribution could continue and be used for purely Bayesian inference about parameters based on
the output from posterior distribution of θ's (and any of their functions).

As noted earlier in this section, when implemented with similar models, MI
and ML yield asymptotically similar point estimates, but MI has greater variance and is therefore less efficient, meaning that ML would be somewhat more
powerful. However, MI has other advantages, such as when some covariate

values are missing. In likelihood-based analyses, if a covariate is missing for a subject, all post-baseline data for that subject are discarded. In MI the missing covariates can be imputed, thereby preserving inclusion of the post-baseline data. An example of imputing missing covariates is provided in Section 15.5.

Other advantages of MI stem from having separate steps for imputation and analysis. This flexibility does not exist in ML because ML has only the analysis step, thereby implying that only the analysis variables can be used to account for the missing data.

In MI, the imputation model can include additional covariates not present in the analysis model. These covariates may be predictive of outcomes and/or the probability of dropout. Meng (1994) and Collins et al. (2001) provide examples of and rationale for these so-called inclusive modeling strategies. An example of inclusive modeling is provided in Section 15.6 and additional details of inclusive modeling were discussed in Section 12.3.4.

The consequences of an analysis model that is richer (has more variables) than the imputation model is very different. Consider an imputation model that does not include treatment. The imputation model in essence assumes no *direct* treatment effect and is capable of capturing *indirect* treatment effect that may be mediated via intermediate outcomes (if included in the model). As a result, imputed outcomes across treatment arms are likely to be more similar than should be the case. Analyses based on such imputed data sets therefore would be biased whenever a direct treatment effect existed (additionally to the effect mediated via intermediate outcomes).

Although the model in the example above is misspecified—in the context of MAR—it can also be thought of as a specific form of MNAR. In the above example, the imputed values systematically deviate from unbiased MAR estimates in a manner that decreases the magnitude of the estimated treatment contrast. This points to what is becoming an important usage of MI—as a convenient tool for conducting sensitivity analyses. The imputation models can be set up to generate specific departures from MAR, thereby fostering a sensitivity analysis for an MAR-based primary analysis. These implementations of MI are considered in Chapter 18 and further illustrated in Chapter 21.

15.3 Example—Implementing MI

15.3.1 Introduction

This section provides details on implementing several multiple imputation strategies using readily available statistical software applied to data from the small example data set with dropout. Focus is on relevant SAS procedures because they are commonly used in practice; however, some examples using R are also provided.

In SAS, multiple imputation can be implemented via the following steps:

1. Use PROC MI to generate m completed data sets.
2. Analyze each data set, resulting in m point estimates and standard errors.
3. Pass the point estimates and standard errors from Step 2 to PROC MIANALYZE that implements Rubin's rules for combining results.

The output from PROC MIANALYZE includes the upper and lower limits of the confidence interval and associated p-value for the two-sided null hypothesis that the parameter is at the specified value (e.g., $\theta = 0$). The parameter of interest for MI inference can be multivariate, although scalar parameters of treatment effects at specific time points will be considered in the examples here.

The procedure outlined above is easy to implement and is a common approach in conducting multiple imputation analysis in SAS. However, variations on the approach are possible and sometimes needed. For example, the first step can be divided into two steps: (1) sampling from posterior distributions of parameters estimated by an appropriate likelihood-based model using a SAS procedure (different from PROC MI); (2) given each posterior draw, impute missing values from the posed imputation model with custom programming code. An example could be imputing missing counts (such as in the analysis of recurrent events) from a Bayesian Poisson regression, which can be fitted separately using SAS PROC GENMOD with the BAYES statement. In some situations (in particular, when modeling growth curves in repeated measures data) multiple draws from posterior predictive distributions can be conveniently obtained via SAS PROC MCMC (available from SAS Version 9.3). Performing MI using the above procedures is not covered as we focus here on imputation from general multivariate distributions via PROC MI.

In some cases (particularly, for nonparametric and semiparametric models) sampling from posterior distributions can be replaced with nonparametric bootstrap. For example, data can be sampled with replacement, resulting in m bootstrap samples from the original data. Posterior draws $\tilde{\theta}_1, \tilde{\theta}_2, \ldots, \tilde{\theta}_m$ are mimicked with parameter estimates from bootstrap samples $\hat{\theta}_1^*, \ldots, \hat{\theta}_m^*$. The imputed values are then generated from conditional distributions, $Y_{mis} \sim f\left(y \mid \hat{\theta}_i^*\right), i = 1, \ldots, m$.

As an example, consider imputing time to event for a subject censored at time t_{cens}. Imputations can be based on Kaplan-Meier estimates of a survival distribution computed for m bootstrap samples: $\tilde{T} \sim \hat{S}_i^*\left(t \mid t > t_{cens}\right), i = 1, \ldots, m$.

Bootstrap is also often used in conjunction with hot-deck procedures. As stated in Chapter 13, single hot-deck imputation is generally not valid because it fails to fully account for uncertainty due to missing data. However, using approximate Bayesian bootstrap (such as in "Monotone Propensity Score Method" implemented in SAS PROC MI) allows constructing more valid hot-deck procedures. First observed values are sampled with replacement (stratified by the propensity of missingness) to generate sets of "donors". Then missing values are replaced by resampling from "donors" within propensity score groups that have similar probability of missingness. In this case, the bootstrap is used to mimic sampling from predictive posterior distribution of missing data.

Using bootstrap to mimic posterior sampling of parameters—or the predictive distribution of missing data—was termed "approximate Bayesian bootstrap" in Little and Rubin (1987, section 14.5). This should not be confused with standard uses of bootstrap as a method for obtaining standard errors and confidence intervals (e.g., via percentile or ABC methods). For example, 95% confidence interval for the treatment contrast θ can be constructed in the familiar manner of using the 2.5% and 97.5% percentiles of the bootstrap distribution of the MI point estimator $\hat{\theta}_{MI}$ as the confidence interval bounds.

Bootstrap confidence intervals are more computationally intensive than the usual confidence intervals based on Rubin's rules, but can be useful when the latter have questionable validity. When using the bootstrap for confidence intervals, multiple imputation should be carried out on each bootstrap sample and the MI point estimate computed from the m completed data sets. Efron (1994) presented different methods of using bootstrap with missing data and in conjunction with multiple imputation. However, the following details focus only on the traditional three-step process for MI that does not include bootstrapping.

Example SAS code to implement MI for the small example data set with dropout is provided in Code Fragment 15.1 (Section 15.8). The most commonly used R package for MI is *mice*. Example R code to implement MI is provided in Code Fragment 15.2.

15.3.2 Imputation

To use PROC MI, the data should be prepared in the so-called "multivariate" (or "wide" or "horizontal") format with data from each time point in a separate column. Longitudinal data are typically stored as a "stacked" (or "long") data set, which is the format anticipated by SAS PROC MIXED. Converting data from the stacked format to the wide format can be accomplished by using SAS PROC TRANSPOSE. The transposed data set is passed to PROC MI and missing data are imputed using a multivariate normal model with treatment fitted as a covariate or imputations done separately by treatment.

The example data have a monotone missingness pattern. Therefore, a Bayesian regression for multivariate normally distributed data can be used, thus avoiding the MCMC methods that are needed for imputing data with arbitrary missingness patterns. Checking whether the pattern is monotone can be conveniently done by running PROC MI with parameter NIMPUTE = 0. Table 15.1 shows the missing data patterns by treatment group that are produced as default output from PROC MI. The output makes it easy to see that the response patterns in the example data are indeed monotone. If a subject has a missing value at a given visit, all subsequent observations are also missing.

TABLE 15.1

Missing Data Patterns for the Small Example Data Set with Dropout

Treatment	Group	Basval	Yobs1	Yobs2	Yobs3	Freq	Percent
	1	X	X	X	X	18	72.0
1	2	X	X	X	.	2	8.0
1	3	X	X	.	.	5	20.0
2	1	X	X	X	X	19	76.0
2	2	X	X	X	.	3	12.0
2	3	X	X	.	.	3	12.0

[a] "X" indicates presence of the outcome score at baseline (Basval) and three post-baseline visits (Yobs1, Yobs2, Yobs3). "." indicates the value is missing. "Groups" identifies the distinct patterns present in the data set.

The order of variables listed in the VAR statement of PROC MI should correspond to the order of imputations. For the example data, the order of variables corresponds to the assessment times. Alternatively, the sequential orientation can be made explicit using multiple statements. The code for this explicit specification is also provided in Code Fragment 15.1. The explicit specification is not needed for this example, but provides flexibility that can be utilized in other situations that will be illustrated in subsequent examples.

In this example, data are imputed by treatment arm. This is equivalent to having a single imputation model that includes treatment, treatment-by-visit and all treatment-by-covariate interactions. However, having separate imputation models by treatment arm is simple and yields the same result as the more parameter-rich single, saturated imputation model (with the minor difference that separate covariance structures would be fitted when using by-treatment processing, whereas a single pooled error covariance matrix will be used in case of a single imputation model).

The number of imputations (specified by the parameter NIMPUTE) chosen for this example is 1000. In the early MI literature it was recommended that as few as $m = 5$ imputations was sufficient to achieve good precision of MI estimates. This recommendation was based on the argument of relative efficiency of MI estimates compared to that based on maximum likelihood estimates. However, this recommendation was later challenged. The decrease in power due to small m may substantially exceed that expected from the theoretical argument based on relative efficiency (Graham et al. 2007). With modern computing power, generating hundreds and even thousands of imputations can be done in reasonable time. The case for using a small number of imputations is obsolete. For a summary of recent literature on choosing the number of imputations see van Buuren (2012, pp. 49–50).

As a practical tool for selecting a reasonable number of imputations, the MI point estimates can be plotted against the number of imputations, as done in Figure 15.2 for the small example data set with dropout. This plot allows visual

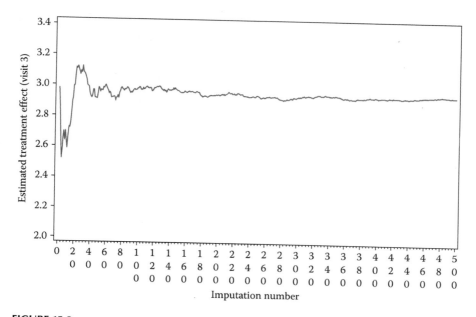

FIGURE 15.2

MI estimator $\hat{\theta}_m$ for the treatment contrast at visit 3 computed over the first m completed data sets versus the number of imputations (m).

assessment of the stability of MI estimator $\hat{\theta}_m$ for smaller m and its "convergence" to $\hat{\theta}_\infty$. In Figure 15.2 after $m_0 = 200$, the point estimator is stable, which ensures the *reproducibility* of MI analyses for this data set with $m \geq m_0$. The sufficient number of imputations will of course vary from one data set to another. In all examples for this Chapter, $m = 1000$, although this may be larger than needed.

In PROC MI, the output data set has the same "multivariate" structure as the input data set. However, the now completed multiple data sets are *stacked* and the variable named _Imputation_ (assuming values 1,..., <*nimpute*>) is automatically generated to indicate to which data set each observation belongs. Figure 15.3 shows a fragment of the imputed (completed) data set. Imputed values can be clearly discerned in this example as they have a larger number of decimal points. Sometimes auxiliary variables (with values 0 and 1) that indicate whether values were actually observed or imputed may be needed. This should be done by writing custom SAS code prior to calling PROC MI.

15.3.3 Analysis

After completing the imputation step, an appropriate analysis model can be applied to each completed set. For longitudinal data, as in the example data set, it is natural to consider applying the same direct likelihood analysis of repeated measures via PROC MIXED to each completed data set as

	Imputation	trt	subject	basval	Yobs1	Yobs2	Yobs3
1	1	1	2	20	−6	−5.371893093	−10.27327664
2	1	1	5	12	−6	−3	−9
3	1	1	6	14	−6	−10	−10
4	1	1	8	21	−2	−9	−9
5	1	1	9	19	−9	−6	−12.78127318
6	1	1	13	20	−9	−12	−13
7	1	1	14	19	−6	−12	−16
8	1	1	16	19	−3	−11	−17
9	1	1	18	23	−7	−10	−15
10	1	1	19	26	−5	−5	−11
11	1	1	24	20	1	−1	−6
12	1	1	25	22	0	−4	−9
13	1	1	27	21	−1	−2	−3
14	1	1	28	21	−2	−2	−2
15	1	1	30	19	−2	−2	−6.425250822
16	1	1	32	24	−10	−14	−20
17	1	1	34	21	−2	−1	−6
18	1	1	36	20	−4	−7.120718604	−14.13814589
19	1	1	38	22	−3	−5	−6
20	1	1	40	18	−5	−6.057750783	−2.045101917
21	1	1	42	15	0	−2	−8
22	1	1	43	19	−3	−6.167970307	−10.26103763
23	1	1	45	20	−9	−11	−9
24	1	1	48	17	−10	−14	−14
25	1	1	49	23	4	4.4830432444	2.5435936604
26	2	1	2	20	−6	−11.29465031	−11.65938348
27	2	1	5	12	−6	−3	−9
28	2	1	6	14	−6	−10	−10
29	2	1	8	21	−2	−9	−9
30	2	1	9	19	−9	−6	−16.37321523
31	2	1	13	20	−9	−12	−13
32	2	1	14	19	−6	−12	−16

FIGURE 15.3
Fragment of complete data set produced by PROC MI.

for the analysis of incomplete data. While this analysis approach is useful for assessing the longitudinal response profiles, it is also now possible to implement a simple visit-wise ANOVA or ANCOVA if interest is only on the cross-sectional contrasts. This is possible because imputation fully accounts for the missing data (if assumptions hold true) and there is no benefit from further accounting for the missing data via a repeated measures analysis.

When applying the analysis model to imputed data it is useful to take advantage of SAS "BY-processing" capability using the "by _Imputation_"

	Imputation	Label	Estimate	StdErr	DF	tValue	Probt	time
267	67	trt effect at vis 3	−1.7813	1.4729	47	−1.21	0.2325	3
268	68	trt effect at vis 3	−3.4297	1.4091	47	−2.43	0.0188	3
269	69	trt effect at vis 3	−3.1104	1.5551	47	−2.00	0.0513	3
270	70	trt effect at vis 3	−2.3183	1.5762	47	−1.47	0.1480	3
271	71	trt effect at vis 3	−2.5356	1.4717	47	−1.72	0.0915	3
272	72	trt effect at vis 3	−4.4898	1.6927	47	−2.65	0.0109	3
273	73	trt effect at vis 3	−2.9977	1.4591	47	−2.05	0.0455	3
274	74	trt effect at vis 3	−3.4374	1.5221	47	−2.26	0.0286	3
275	75	trt effect at vis 3	−1.8695	1.7225	47	−1.09	0.2833	3
276	76	trt effect at vis 3	−3.6741	1.5684	47	−2.34	0.0234	3
277	77	trt effect at vis 3	−3.5779	1.4950	47	−2.39	0.0207	3
278	78	trt effect at vis 3	−3.8548	1.5870	47	−2.43	0.0190	3
279	79	trt effect at vis 3	−3.5465	1.4240	47	−2.49	0.0163	3
280	80	trt effect at vis 3	−4.0039	1.7441	47	−2.30	0.0262	3
281	81	trt effect at vis 3	−4.0162	1.4955	47	−2.69	0.0100	3
282	82	trt effect at vis 3	−4.0411	1.3845	47	−2.92	0.0054	3
283	83	trt effect at vis 3	−3.5701	1.4470	47	−2.47	0.0173	3
284	84	trt effect at vis 3	−2.3854	1.3850	47	−1.72	0.0916	3

FIGURE 15.4

Fragment of results from the analyses of multiply imputed data sets to be used as input for PROC MIANALYZE.

statement in the analysis procedure. If a repeated measures analysis of the imputed data is desired, an additional data manipulation step is needed to transpose the PROC MI output data set back to the "stacked" format required with repeated measures data in PROC MIXED. In this example, the simple ANCOVA model is implemented to analyze the Time 3 variable (Yobs3 in the imputed data set). The point estimates and standard errors from the analyses of some of the imputed data sets are shown in Figure 15.4.

15.3.4 Inference

The last step in MI is to combine estimates and standard errors to obtain a single inferential statement. Code Fragment 15.3 shows the SAS code for PROC MIANALYZE to accomplish this step. The "by time" statement is used here because the input data set contains treatment contrasts for Time 2 and Time 3. Note that Time 1 did not have missing values; therefore, all estimates for the treatment contrast at Time 1 obtained from the multiply imputed data set are identical and, of course, it does not make sense to run PROC MIANALYZE for Time 1. The results are shown in Table 15.2.

The lsmeans, treatment contrasts, and standard errors from the MI analysis of the incomplete data are, as expected, similar to the corresponding results from direct likelihood (see Table 14.1). Compared with the complete data, the

TABLE 15.2

Treatment Contrasts and Least-Squares Means Estimated by Multiple
Imputation from the Small Example Data Set with Dropout

Treatment	Time	Complete Data		Incomplete Data (MI), $m = 1000$	
		LSMEANS	SE	LSMEANS	SE
1	2	−6.70	0.93	−6.36	1.01
1	3	−9.86	1.05	−9.61	1.19
2	2	−8.70	0.93	−8.50	0.99
2	3	−13.26	1.05	−12.56	1.23
Endpoint Treatment Difference		3.39	1.49 ($p = 0.0274$)	2.95	1.73 ($p = 0.0971$)

MI results show a smaller treatment contrast, larger standard errors, and a
larger *P*-value for the endpoint treatment contrast. It is important to interpret
these results as just one realization from a stochastic process. If the comparisons were replicated many times under the same conditions—with missing data arising from an MAR mechanism—the average of the lsmeans and
treatment contrasts across the repeated trials would be (approximately) the
same for complete and incomplete data. Standard errors would be consistently greater in incomplete data, however.

15.3.5 Accounting for Nonmonotone Missingness

Thus far, only monotone missingness has been addressed. When the pattern
of missing data is nonmonotone, PROC MI with the addition of the MCMC
statement can be used. To illustrate these procedures, intermittent missingness
was introduced into the example data by deleting some outcomes at Time 2 for
subjects that had no other missing data. The Time 2 data were deleted for three
subjects in the treated group (2) and for two subjects in the placebo group (1).

The top panel (a) of Code Fragment 15.4 (Section 15.8) provides an example
of PROC MI code for imputation from a multivariate normal distribution
using MCMC. Missing values are imputed from a single chain of the MCMC
algorithm. Recall that MCMC samples converge to the target posterior distribution as the number of samples becomes large. Therefore, to ensure
that the draws occur sufficiently close to the target distribution, a number
of initial samples are skipped. This skipping is specified in the number of
burn-in iterations (NBITER = 200). Also because of serial correlation in sampled values within the same chain, a thinning period should be specified
as the number of iterations between imputations in a chain. In the example, (NITER = 100) and PROC MI skips 100 samples after each imputation.
The values NBITER = 200 and NITER = 100 are defaults that would be used
if these options are omitted but are explicitly specified here for illustration.

The various MCMC diagnostics (e.g., autocorrelation plots) should be
inspected. Imputations should be rerun with increased values of NBITER and

NITER if issues exist with MCMC convergence (see PROC MI help for more details). The example code explicitly specified that the initial values for the MCMC chain are posterior modes of parameters obtained by the EM (expectation-maximization) algorithm, with the maximum number of iterations set at MAXITER = 200. This number should be increased if the EM algorithm fails to converge within the specified limit. Nonconvergence is more likely in data sets with larger fractions of missing data or if there are sparse patterns of missing values. The SAS log file includes a warning if convergence was not achieved.

The MCMC approach may be rather cumbersome. It (typically) requires more computing time compared with regression methods. The additional layer of approximation inherent in MCMC requires monitoring for convergence to the desired target distributions. In contrast, the regression methods for monotone data sample *directly* from the target distributions and so there is no worry about convergence.

Often, only a few intermittently missing values cause the patterns to deviate from monotone as a result of a few patients with missed outcomes while remaining in the study. In these situations it is efficient to first impute the intermittent missing values using PROC MI to complete the pattern to monotone; then, methods for monotone missingness can be applied, such as the Bayesian regression from the previous example.

The SAS code for implementing this two-stage imputation strategy is presented in the bottom panel (b) of Code Fragment 15.4 (Section 15.8). Two runs of PROC MI are required. The first run produces partially completed data sets, each having a monotone pattern of missing values. The second run takes the output data set from the first run as input, processed by _Imputation_, and completes each data set with a single imputation from Bayesian regression for monotone data.

15.4 Situations Where MI Is Particularly Useful

15.4.1 Introduction

This section outlines situations when MI-based analyses provide certain advantages compared to direct likelihood (ML) or present a reasonable analytic strategy in absence of appropriate direct likelihood methods. Detailed examples are provided in subsequent sections.

15.4.2 Scenarios Where Direct Likelihood Methods Are Difficult to Implement or Not Available

One general area where MI can be particularly useful is situations where direct likelihood methods are hard to implement or not available. Several scenarios when this may be the case for analysis of clinical data are outlined below.

Missing baseline covariates make direct likelihood methods (e.g., via SAS PROC MIXED) sub-optimal because all subjects with a missing covariate are discarded from the analysis. In contrast, MI can be used to impute baseline covariates jointly with outcome variables (see Section 15.5 for examples).

Repeated categorical outcomes are hard to analyze using direct likelihood methods because—in contrast to multivariate normal distributions for repeated continuous outcomes—multivariate distributions for binary or count data do not have simple and natural formulations. Details on analyses of incomplete categorical data are provided in Chapter 19. Imputing missing categorical data is relatively easy, especially for data with monotone missingness when sequential imputation strategies can be applied.

For outcomes of mixed types (continuous and categorical), MI can be implemented either by sequential imputation (for monotone patterns of missing data) or in the case of arbitrary missingness by repeatedly sampling from full conditional distributions (van Buuren 2007). The method of "fully conditional specification" (FCS) is implemented in the R package *mice* (Multivariate Imputation by Chained Equations; van Buuren and Groothuis-Oudshoorn 2011) and recently in SAS PROC MI (via FCS statement available from SAS Version 9.3 and later).

Unlike joint modeling, FCS specifies the multivariate distributions through a sequence of conditional densities of each variable given the other variables. With FCS it is even possible to specify models for which no joint distribution exits — a situation referred to as incompatibility. Although incompatibility is not desirable, in practice it is a relatively minor problem, especially if the missing data rate is modest (van Buuren 2012, p. 112).

15.4.3 Exploiting Separate Steps for Imputation and Analysis

Other situations where MI is particularly useful are those in which the separation of the imputation and analysis stages can improve efficiency (compared to direct likelihood methods).

Recall that the original motivation for MI in Rubin (1978) was for analysis of complex surveys where the *imputer* had access to more information than the *analyst*. The idea was that once the missing data has been imputed using the richer set of data, completed data sets with a limited number of variables would be made publicly available for analysts. Several clinical trial situations are considered where the imputation model can be based on more information than is included in the analysis model.

Sometimes clinical endpoints specified in the primary analysis are *derived* outcomes based on underlying outcomes. In such situations, an efficient MI strategy could include four steps:

1. Impute missing data for the underlying outcome measures.

2. Compute derived outcomes from the completed data sets.

3. Analyze completed data.

4. Combine (pool) results for inference.

An example of a derived variable is the analysis of "clinical response," defined as x% improvement in some continuous scale (or a combination of several scales). Imputing the underlying continuous measures may improve efficiency compared to analysis (or imputation and analysis) of the binary outcome.

As noted in Section 15.3.4, MI can utilize auxiliary variables in the imputation model that help predict the outcome and/or the dropout process. These auxiliary variables may not be available or are undesirable for use in analysis model (Meng 1994; Collins et al. 2001). For example, the analysis model should not include intermediate outcomes or *mediators* of treatment effect, which would result in diluting the estimated treatment effect in a likelihood-based analysis. Classic examples of such variables would be time-varying post-baseline variables that are influenced by treatment, such as secondary efficacy outcomes.

The following situations are examples of inclusive imputation strategies that can be useful.

- Pretreatment covariates (demographic and illness characteristics), and perhaps their interactions with treatment, are included in the imputation model. The selection of covariates can be based on their ability in predicting the outcome or in predicting dropout. This can be evaluated in separate modeling steps and a subset of covariates can be selected from a broader set of candidate covariates using appropriate model selection techniques such as stepwise selection, LASSO, or other machine learning methods.

- Post-baseline time-varying covariates. Inclusive imputation models can be used to *jointly* impute two related outcomes, such as two efficacy scales, Y1 and Y2. This may be two clinical rating scales that reflect different aspects of the disease and "borrowing" from Y2 may improve imputation of Y1. An example is given in Section 15.6, where joint imputations of the clinician-rated HAMD severity scale and a patient-reported outcome scale (Patient Global Impression of Improvement) are conducted. The basic idea is that incorporating both the clinician's and patient's perspective on response may help explain subsequent HAMD outcomes and/or better inform the missingness process.

- When the outcome of interest is collected at sparse visit intervals or only at the last scheduled evaluation whereas other outcomes are observed more frequently. Examples include efficacy and safety scales collected at scheduled time points and spontaneously recorded outcomes (occurrences of hospitalizations, adverse events).

An approach that at first may seem counterintuitive but can be useful is to use safety assessments to help impute efficacy outcomes. Suppose that dropouts are predicted by both previous outcomes and future (unobserved outcomes) so the missingness is MNAR. Then MI using only earlier outcomes is inadequate and may result in biased estimates. However, suppose that conditional on both recent safety assessments (occurrence of specific adverse events) and earlier efficacy outcomes the dropouts *do not* depend on future outcomes. This may be the case when AEs are early signs/predictors of emerging changes (sudden worsening, say) in the outcome that cannot be predicted from the efficacy outcome alone. In this scenario, adding safety assessments in the imputation model may help satisfy the MAR assumption.

15.4.4 Sensitivity Analysis

The flexibility of separate analysis and imputation steps can be used to create relevant departures from MAR, thereby facilitating a sensitivity analysis for an MAR primary analysis. Alternatively, the same imputation approaches can be conceptualized as modeling plausible outcomes after treatment discontinuation or switching treatment when assessing an effectiveness estimand. Such MNAR analyses can be implemented via MI by controlling the imputation procedures or done by manipulating imputed outcomes prior to data analysis. Extensive examples are provided in Chapters 18 and 19.

It is important to appreciate the point raised earlier in this chapter that when implemented in similar manners, MI and ML have similar assumptions and yield similar results. Therefore, MI implemented similarly to ML is not a sensitivity analysis. The point here is that something "different" is done during the imputation step that facilitates the sensitivity assessment.

15.5 Example—Using MI to Impute Covariates

15.5.1 Introduction

In the small example data set with missing values, there were no missing baseline values. In well-conducted clinical trials, missing data in baseline covariates are usually minimal. However, occasionally some subjects may have missing baseline values. In addition, analysis models may include stratification covariates or other covariates that could be missing. In such scenarios the chance that at least one covariate is missing for a given subject can be appreciable (say 5–10%). In these situations, typical likelihood-based analyses are not optimal because subjects with missing covariates are excluded from the analysis, resulting in loss of efficiency and potentially biased estimates.

15.5.2 Implementation

Multiple imputation provides several strategies for imputing missing covariates. An obvious route is to use a two-stage strategy similar to that demonstrated in Section 15.3 for data with nonmonotone missingness. First, MCMC-based imputation is used to impute missing covariates. Then the missing post-baseline values can be imputed to create the complete data sets. The SAS code for imputing covariates and missing post-baseline covariates in a scenario with baseline severity and three covariates (X1, X2, and X3) is presented in Code Fragment 15.5 (Section 15.8). The approach is similar to that in Code Fragment 15.4, thereby illustrating that only minor modification is required to impute missing covariates.

Another potential strategy may be to impute only missing baseline covariates using MCMC (PROC MI) and then applying a direct likelihood repeated measures analysis to multiple data sets with imputed baseline covariates and using Rubin's combination rules as we would normally do when imputing all missing values. Results from this MI approach can be compared with the analysis where all subjects with missing covariates were excluded in order to isolate the impact of missing baseline covariates on the estimated treatment effect and associated standard errors. Imputing missing covariates should improve efficiency and lead to smaller standard errors when compared to deleting records with missing covariates. Also, if baseline covariates are not missing completely at random, estimates of the treatment effect may be biased if subjects with missing covariates are excluded.

To illustrate the efficiency of multiply imputing covariates alone, artificial missingness in baseline severity was created in the small example data set with dropout by deleting the baseline scores of five subjects who had unfavorable outcomes in HAMD changes at the last scheduled visit. Lsmeans and treatment contrasts from a direct likelihood analysis (SAS PROC MIXED) of the 45 subjects with nonmissing baseline scores in the small example data set with dropout are compared to results from MI of the missing covariates in Table 15.3. The left-side columns are results from the direct likelihood analysis that excluded subjects with missing covariates. The right-side columns are results based on the same repeated measures model fitted to data sets with baseline scores imputed using all available outcome variables (via PROC MI, MCMC statement with IMPUTE=MONOTONE option). As mentioned, normally both baseline and post-baseline values would be imputed. However, the approach used here is valid under MAR and allows explicit assessment of the impact of having to exclude subjects with missing covariates in the likelihood-based analysis.

The results with MI of the missing covariates, as expected, had smaller standard errors. Excluding the five patients with missing baseline scores also resulted in approximately a one-half point increase in the endpoint treatment contrast. Of course, this is just one contrived example from a small example data set. It is not possible to know how including versus not including subjects with missing covariates will impact point estimates in actual clinical trial scenarios. However, regardless of scenario, including subjects with missing covariates increases the plausibility of MAR and reduces the standard

TABLE 15.3

Treatment Contrasts and Least-Squares Means with and without Imputation of Missing Covariates in the Small Example Data Set with Dropout

Treatment	Time	Covariates Missing[a]		Covariates Imputed[b]	
		LSMEANS	SE	LSMEANS	SE
1	1	−4.08	0.90	−4.21	0.94
1	2	−6.55	1.05	−6.56	1.00
1	3	−9.79	1.21	−9.78	1.12
2	1	−6.05	0.92	−5.25	0.94
2	2	−9.05	1.05	−8.45	0.98
2	3	−13.36	1.21	−12.79	1.09
Endpoint Treatment Difference		3.56	1.71 (p = 0.0443)	3.01	1.56 (p = 0.0606)

[a] Direct likelihood analysis with five subjects having missing covariates who are therefore excluded from the analysis.
[b] Direct likelihood analysis after multiple imputation of missing baseline covariates.

errors compared with excluding those subjects and allows following the ITT principle in terms of including all randomized subjects in the analysis.

This hypothetical example also helps to illustrate why imputation models for covariates should include post-baseline outcomes. Including post-baseline outcomes for imputing covariates may at first seem counterintuitive in that the model is predicting the past from the future. However, the approach can be justified theoretically and was also shown to be appropriate in simulation studies (Crowe et al. 2009).

The imputation model does not have to be a causal model. In fact, if the missingness mechanism is such that subjects with poorer outcomes are more likely to have missing baseline scores, failing to include future outcomes when imputing baseline covariates may result in biased estimates of the fixed effects associated with these covariates.

Whether this bias would translate into biased estimates of treatment contrasts is not a clear-cut issue. Treatment may seem independent of baseline covariates due to randomization, in which case bias in estimates of covariates would not bias treatment contrasts. However, an incorrect imputation model (provided it includes post-baseline measures) may induce correlation between the treatment variable and covariates. Treatment contrasts could be biased indirectly through the biased estimates of the fixed effects associated with covariates. See Section 5.3.1 for examples and illustration of how changes that directly affect one parameter also indirectly affect another parameter—that is, correlation between estimates of fixed effect parameters.

In general, the imputation model should be compatible with the analysis model. That is, if an effect is included in the analysis model it should also be used in the imputation model.

15.6 Examples—Using Inclusive Models in MI

15.6.1 Introduction

Section 12.3.4 introduced and contrasted inclusive and restrictive modeling frameworks. This section provides an example of an inclusive imputation strategy for the small example data set with dropouts. In this example, as elsewhere in this book, the primary outcome of interest is change in the HAMD scale. The difference here is that the Patient Global Impression of Improvement (PGIIMP) scale is used in addition to HAMD scores to "improve" the imputation of the missing HAMD scores.

Recall from the descriptions in Chapter 4 that the HAMD is a clinician-rated symptom severity score that focuses explicitly on specific symptoms and combines responses on the 17 individual items into a total score. The PGIIMP scale is a patient-rated measure of global improvement taken at each post-baseline visit. The PGIIMP assesses patient's overall feeling since they started taking medication and ranges from 1 ("very much better") to 7 ("very much worse"). The process used to delete data to create the small example data set with dropout was such that if a HAMD value was deleted, the corresponding PGIIMP value was also deleted.

The clinical and statistical justification for this inclusive strategy stems from the PGIIMP reflecting *patients'* overall perspective, which may capture aspects not fully captured by the *clinician*-rated HAMD scale.

15.6.2 Implementation

The first step in jointly imputing HAMD and PGIIMP using SAS PROC MI is to transpose data for both outcomes from the "stacked" to the "horizontal" format. That is, the output data set has three columns for changes in HAMD (CHG1, CHG2, CHG3) and three columns for PGIIMP1, PGIIMP2, PGIIMP3 that correspond to post-baseline Times 1, 2 and 3. Columns are also included for baseline severity on the HAMD and treatment group. There are no baseline assessments for PGIIMP because it is inherently a measure of change.

The next step is to check for monotonicity of missingness patterns on *both* outcomes. For this purpose, the following order of the outcome variables is assumed: CHG1 PGIIMP1 CHG2 PGIIMP2 CHG3 PGIIMP3. Table 15.4 displays the missing data patterns produced by SAS PROC MI that indicate the joint patterns are indeed monotone. One patient with a HAMD score at Time 3 had a missing Time 3 PGI–Improvement (Group 2, Treatment 2 in Table 15.4). The pattern is still monotone because PGIIMP3 goes after CHG3 in the ordering of variables. Imputation of values for PGIIMP3 is not needed because focus is on HAMD and PGIIMP3 does not inform imputation for CHG3. Hence, the PGIIMP3 column could be omitted with no impact on HAMD results.

TABLE 15.4

Missingness Patterns for Joint Imputation of Changes in HAMD and PGI-Improvement

Group				Missing Data Patterns				Frequency	Percent
	Basval	CHG1	PGIIMP1	CHG2	PGIIMP2	CHG3	PGIIMP3		
Treatment = 1 (Placebo)									
1	X	X	X	X	X	X	X	18	72.00
2	X	X	X	X	X	.	.	2	8.00
3	X	X	X	.	.	.	.	5	20.00
Treatment = 2 (Treatment)									
1	X	X	X	X	X	X	X	18	72.00
2	X	X	X	X	X	X	.	1	4.00
3	X	X	X	X	X	.	.	3	12.00
4	X	X	X	.	.	.	.	3	12.00

Note: "X" indicates presence of the outcome score at baseline (Basval). "." indicates the value is missing. "Groups" identifies the distinct patterns present in the data set.

Two imputation approaches can be considered. All outcomes can be treated as continuous and sequential Bayesian regression for multivariate normal data used to impute both HAMD changes and PGI–Improvement. In this approach, it is possible to impute missing values for PGIIMP that are outside the scales range of 1 to 7. Therefore, the validity of applying a normal distribution to categorical PGIIMP data may be questioned. Schafer (1997) showed that imputation is fairly robust to some deviations from multivariate normality. Also, Lipkovich et al. (2014) provide simulation evidence in favor of using a multivariate normal distribution for imputing categorical data.

The second approach avoids assuming multivariate normality for PGI–Improvement. The process is to sequentially implement: (1) linear regression to impute changes in HAMD conditional on earlier HAMD changes and on PGI–Improvement and (2) ordinal logistic regression to impute missing PGIIMP values conditional on earlier (observed or imputed) HAMD changes and PGIIMP scores.

Implementing this second approach in SAS PROC MI requires specifying PGIIMP1 and PGIIMP2 as class variables in both linear and logistic regression models. Recall that a PGIIMP score of 4 corresponds to "no change," and scores > 4 indicate worsening. In these data, PGIIMP scores > 4 are uncommon. Therefore, all scores > 4 were combined with scores of 4 (i.e., recoded as "level 4") and the rescaled PGI scores for Time 1 and Time 2 were named PGIIMPGR1 and PGIIMPGR2, respectively.

The SAS code to implement the imputation strategy using multivariate normal is provided in the top panel (a) of Code Fragment 15.6 (Section 15.8) and the code to implement the normal-ordinal model is in the bottom panel (b). In PROC MI, it is possible to sample from truncated marginal distributions when imputing PGIIMP2 scores, thereby ensuring the scores are within the scale range 1 to 7. However, this approach was shown to be inferior to nontruncated imputation (Lipkovich et al. 2014). Therefore, truncation is not used here.

Imputation of categorical outcomes by an ordinal logistic model is similar in spirit to imputation by linear regression (explained in Section 15.2). Code Fragment 15.6 implements Bayesian ordinal logistic regression fitted separately for each treatment arm to predict PGIIMP scores at Time 2 given PGIIMPGR1 (class variable), CHG1 (continuous variable) and baseline HAMD score (continuous variable). Then, for a single draw from the posterior distribution of model parameters, the probability for each of the four categories, P1, P2, P3, P4 (adding up to 1), is estimated and imputed values are generated as a multinomial random variable.

For example, the probability of category "2" is computed as the difference Prob(PGIIMP2="2")=Prob(PGIIMP2≤"2")−Prob(PGIIMP2≤"1") whereas Prob(PGIIMP2≤"2") and Prob(PGIIMP2≤"1") are directly estimated from the assumed logistic model

$$logit\left[\text{Prob}(Y_i \leq l_k)\right] = a_k + \sum x_{ij}\beta_j$$

TABLE 15.5

Treatment Contrasts and Least-Squares Means Estimated by Multiple Imputation: Changes in HAMD Using Joint Model for HAMD and PGIIMP

Treatment	Time	Incomplete Data (MI) (Joint Multivariate Normal Model)		Incomplete Data (MI) (Joint Modeling using Normal Model for HAMD and Ordinal Logistic for PGIIMP)	
		LSMEANS	SE	LSMEANS	SE
1	2	−6.37	1.02	−6.35	1.01
1	3	−9.72	1.22	−9.76	1.38
2	2	−8.45	0.99	−8.59	1.00
2	3	−12.41	1.20	−12.63	1.30
Endpoint Treatment Difference		2.69	1.71 (p = 0.1248)	2.87	1.90 (p = 0.1393)

where Y_i denotes the PGI Improvement score for the *i*th patient, l_k, $k = 1,...,3$ correspond to the categories "1", "2", "3" of the outcome variable, and x_{ij} represents the observed or imputed score for the *j*th covariate. The time dimension and specific covariate structure (including for this case BASVAL and CHG1) is suppressed to simplify notation.

Results from the two models are summarized in Table 15.5. The treatment contrasts from the normal and logistic-normal imputation models were 2.69 and 2.87, respectively. Recall the treatment contrast from "standard" MI in Table 15.2 was 2.95. It is important to interpret these results as an illustration. The intent is to show the potential usefulness of, and the process for, inclusive multiple imputation models. Results from this small example data set do not inform expectation of results for actual clinical trial scenarios.

The Code Fragment 15.7 illustrates using the R package MICE for multiply imputing continuous outcomes jointly with categorical PGIIMP scores.

15.7 MI for Categorical Outcomes

As explained in Chapter 10, likelihood-based analyses can be difficult to implement for categorical outcomes. Therefore, multiple imputation provides an important framework for MAR-based analyses of categorical data.

See Chapter 19 for a general discussion of accounting for categorical missing data. This discussion includes multiple imputation examples for analysis of a binary outcome derived from an underlying continuous scale and for an ordinal categorical variable.

15.8 Code Fragments

CODE FRAGMENT 15.1 SAS Code for Multiple Imputation Analysis. Creating Completed Data Sets with PROC MI Using Monotone Imputation

```
/* transpose original data resulting in WIDE data with
   outcome columns Yobs1 Yobs2 Yobs3 corresponding to
   post-baseline visits 1,2,3 */
PROC SORT DATA=ALL2; BY TRT SUBJECT BASVAL; RUN;
PROC TRANSPOSE DATA=ALL2 OUT= ALL2_TRANSP2 (DROP=_NAME_)
   PREFIX=YOBS;
   BY TRT SUBJECT BASVAL;
   VAR CHGDROP;
   ID TIME;
RUN;

/* check whether pattern is monotone */
PROC MI DATA = ALL2_TRANSP2 NIMPUTE =0;
   BY TRT;
   VAR BASVAL YOBS1 YOBS2 YOBS3;
RUN;

/* perform multiple imputation for monotone data */
PROC MI DATA = ALL2_TRANSP2 OUT = ALL2_MIOUT NIMPUTE=1000
   SEED=123;
   BY TRT;
   MONOTONE METHOD=REG;
   VAR BASVAL YOBS1 YOBS2 YOBS3;
RUN;

/* multiple imputation of monotone data with explicit model
   statement*/
PROC MI DATA = ALL2_TRANSP2 OUT = ALL2_MIOUT_2
   NIMPUTE=1000 SEED=123;
   BY TRT;
   VAR BASVAL YOBS1 YOBS2 YOBS3;
   MONOTONE REG (YOBS1 =BASVAL);
   MONOTONE REG (YOBS2 =YOBS1 BASVAL);
   MONOTONE REG (YOBS3 =YOBS2 YOBS1 BASVAL);
RUN;
```

CODE FRAGMENT 15.2   Example R Code for Multiple Imputation Analysis of Continuous Outcome with Arbitrary Missingness: Change from Baseline on HAMD

```
library(mice)
# assumes transposed data set in multivariate format
head(hamdchng)

    trt   basval  CHG1    CHG2     CHG3
1    1     20     −6      NA       NA
2    1     12     −6      −3       −9
3    1     14     −6      −10      −10
4    1     21     −2      −9       −9
5    1     19     −9      −6       NA
6    1     20     −9      −12      −13

# performs MI, using imputation sequence: CHG2, CHG3
imp<-mice(hamdchng, seed=123,visitSequence=c(4,5))

# creates data with imputed sets stacked (if need to look
  at data)
# columns are trt, basval CHG1, CHG2,CHG3
stacked<-complete(imp,"long",)

# fits a linear model for changes in HAMD at vis3 to each
completed set
fit<-with(imp, lm(CHG3~trt+basval))

# pooles inference using Rubin's rules
est<-pool(fit)
summary(est)
```

CODE FRAGMENT 15.3   SAS Code for Multiple Imputation Analysis.* Combined Inference Using PROC MIANALYZE

```
/* combined inference for estimated treatment contrasts */
 ODS OUTPUT PARAMETERESTIMATES=ES_MI;
  PROC MIANALYZE DATA=ES_MI_M ;
    BY TIME;
    MODELEFFECTS ESTIMATE;
    STDERR STDERR;
  RUN;
/* combined inference for lsmeans */
 ODS OUTPUT PARAMETERESTIMATES=LS_MI;
  PROC MIANALYZE DATA=LS_MI_M ;
    BY TIME TRT;
```

---

* Code Fragment 15.3 assumes that data analysis was ran on imputed data and the estimates and associated standard errors of time- specific treatment contrast are saved in SAS data set ES_MI_M.

```
   MODELEFFECTS ESTIMATE;
   STDERR STDERR;
RUN;
```

CODE FRAGMENT 15.4 SAS Code for Multiple Imputation Analysis. Imputing Data from Nonmonotone Pattern Using MCMC

```
a) /* using MCMC to impute data from non-monotone patterns */

PROC MI DATA = ALL2_TRANSP3 OUT = ALL2_MIOUT NIMPUTE=1000
   SEED=123;
   BY TRT;
   MCMC CHAIN=SINGLE NBITER=200 NITER=100 INITIAL=EM (ITPRINT
   MAXITER=200);
   VAR BASVAL YOBS1 YOBS2 YOBS3;
RUN;

b) /* using MCMC to first complete data to monotone and
     then perform a single imputation to each monotone set by
     Bayesian regression to produce complete data sets */

PROC MI DATA = ALL2_TRANSP3 OUT = ALL4_MIOUT NIMPUTE=1000
SEED=123;
   BY TRT;
   MCMC IMPUTE = MONOTONE;
   VAR BASVAL YOBS1 YOBS2 YOBS3;
RUN;


PROC SORT DATA=ALL4_MIOUT; BY _IMPUTATION_ TRT; RUN;
PROC MI DATA = ALL4_MIOUT OUT = ALL5_MIOUT NIMPUTE =1 SEED
   =123;
   BY _IMPUTATION_ TRT;
   MONOTONE METHOD=REG;
   VAR BASVAL YOBS1 YOBS2 YOBS3;
RUN;
```

CODE FRAGMENT 15.5 SAS Code for Multiple Imputation Analysis. Imputing Data for Baseline Covariates Using MCMC

```
/* using MCMC to first impute baseline covariates X1, X2,
X3, basval and other missing values deviating from monotone
pattern and then perform a single imputation to each
monotone sets by Bayesian regression to produce complete
data sets */

PROC MI DATA = ALL2_TRANSP3 OUT = ALL4_MIOUT NIMPUTE=1000
   SEED=123;
   BY TRT;
   MCMC IMPUTE = MONOTONE;
   VAR X1 X2 X3 BASVAL YOBS1 YOBS2 YOBS3;
```

```
RUN;
PROC SORT DATA=ALL4_MIOUT; BY _IMPUTATION_ TRT; RUN;
PROC MI DATA = ALL4_MIOUT OUT = ALL5_MIOUT NIMPUTE=1
  SEED=123;
BY _IMPUTATION_ TRT;
MONOTONE METHOD=REG;
VAR X1 X2 X3 BASVAL YOBS1 YOBS2 YOBS3;
RUN;
```

CODE FRAGMENT 15.6   SAS Code for an Inclusive Multiple Imputation Strategy: Joint Imputation of Changes in HAMD and PGIIMP

```
a) Imputing from joint multivariate normal distribution

PROC MI DATA = ALL3_TRANSP OUT = ALL3_MIOUT NIMPUTE=1000
  SEED=123;
BY TRT;
MONOTONE METHOD=REG;
VAR BASVAL CHG1 PGIIMP1 CHG2 PGIIMP2 CHG3 ;
RUN;

b) multiple imputation using normal regression for changes
   in HAMD and ordinal logistic regression for PGIIMP*/
PROC MI DATA = ALL3_TRANSP OUT = ALL3_MIOUT NIMPUTE=1000
  SEED=123;
BY TRT;
CLASS PGIIMPGR1 PGIIMPGR2;
VAR BASVAL CHG1 PGIIMPGR1 CHG2 PGIIMPGR2 CHG3;
MONOTONE REG (CHG1=BASVAL);
MONOTONE LOGISTIC (PGIIMPGR1 =CHG1 BASVAL);
MONOTONE REG (CHG2= PGIIMPGR1 CHG1 BASVAL);
MONOTONE LOGISTIC (PGIIMPGR2= CHG2 PGIIMPGR1 CHG1 BASVAL/
   DETAILS);
MONOTONE REG (CHG3= PGIIMPGR2 CHG2 PGIIMPGR1 CHG1 BASVAL);
RUN;
```

CODE FRAGMENT 15.7   Example of R Code for an Inclusive Multiple Imputation Strategy: Joint Imputation of Changes in HAMD and PGIIMP

```
#### joint imputation of continuous and
  categorical(ordered) outcomes

hamdpgi<-widedata[,c("trt","basval","CHG1","PGIIMPGR1","CHG
  2","PGIIMPGR2","CHG3")]

# make PGIIMP ordered factors
hamdpgi$PGIIMPGR1<-ordered(hamdpgi$PGIIMPGR1)
```

```
hamdpgi$PGIIMPGR2<-ordered(hamdpgi$PGIIMPGR2)

imp<-mice(hamdpgi, seed=123,visitSequence=c(5,6,7))
# fits linear model for change in HAMD at Time 3 to each
   imputed data set
fit<-with(imp, lm(CHG3~trt+basval))

# pooled inference using Rubin's rules

est<-pool(fit)
summary(est)
```

15.9 Summary

Multiple imputation (MI) is a popular and accessible method of model-based imputation. The three basic steps to MI include imputation, analysis, and inference. These steps can be applied to outcomes with a variety of distributions, including normally distributed, categorical, and time to event (e.g., with piece-wise exponential hazard) outcomes.

If MI is implemented using the same imputation and analysis model, and the model is the same as the analysis model used in a maximum likelihood-based (ML) analysis, MI and ML will yield asymptotically similar point estimates, but ML will be somewhat more efficient. However, with distinct steps for imputation and analysis, MI has more flexibility than other methods. This flexibility can be exploited in a number of situations.

Scenarios where MI is particularly useful include those when covariates are missing, when data are not normally distributed such that likelihood-based analyses are difficult to implement, and when inclusive modeling strategies are used to help account for missing data. Multiple imputation is also very useful for sensitivity analyses. See Chapter 18 for further details on using MI for sensitivity analyses.

16

Inverse Probability Weighted
Generalized Estimated Equations

16.1 Introduction

Although inverse probability weighting (IPW) can be applied in a variety of settings, focus here is on using IPW in conjunction with generalized estimating equations (GEEs) to construct weighted GEE (wGEE). Technical details on estimating parameters via GEE were presented in Section 5.5.3. A standard reference for wGEE is Robins et al. (1995).

GEEs are nonlikelihood-based equations and parameter estimates (e.g., of treatment effect) are biased under MAR (Robins et al. 1995). The stronger assumption of MCAR is required because the root of the estimating equation expectation is not equal (in general) to the true parameters underlying the outcome process, unless the missingness is MCAR. The requirement of MCAR stems from the parameters of the working correlation matrix in GEE being estimated based on what is essentially a complete case analysis. Only subjects that were observed at both visits t_1 and t_2 contribute to the estimate of within-subject correlation between visits t_1 and t_2. When within subject correlations are not used in computing point estimates (the case of "independent working correlation structures"), bias under MAR is even more apparent since GEE point estimates of treatment effect at each time point are merely treatment contrasts evaluated for complete cases at a given evaluation visit.

The bias in GEE from MAR missingness can be removed by incorporating weights into the GEE (wGEE). The weights are based on the inverse probability of observing the dropout patterns that were present in the data. The idea of weighting can be traced back to the well-known Horvitz and Thompson (1952) inverse probability (IP) estimator.

16.2 Technical Details—Inverse Probability Weighting

16.2.1 General Considerations

The motivation behind IPW is to correct for bias caused by nonrandom selection (dropout). Assume interest is in computing the expected value of discrete random variable, Y, in a finite population of N elements, and Y can assume only two possible values: y_1 and y_2. The population mean is computed as a weighted average

$$\mu = E(Y) = \frac{N_1 y_1 + N_2 y_2}{N}$$

Now assume that a selection mechanism is applied to the population that removes some elements y_1 with probability of selection $\pi_1 = 1/2$, while not affecting the selection of y_2 ($\pi_2 = 1$). Therefore, only $\frac{N_1}{2}$ occurrences of y_1 are expected to be observed, while N_2 occurrences of y_2 are observed. Assume that the relative frequencies of y_1 and y_2 in the population equal these expected values (i.e., ignoring the randomness in the dropout process). Then, when estimating the population mean based on the mean from incomplete data ("observed case" or "complete case" estimator, $\hat{\mu}_{cc}$) the expectation of this estimator is

$$E(\hat{\mu}_{cc}) = \frac{\frac{1}{2} N_1 y_1 + N_2 y_2}{\frac{1}{2} N_1 + N_2}.$$

Of course, this estimator is biased because in general $E(\hat{\mu}_{cc}) \neq E(Y)$. In this example, the selection probabilities are known and adjustments for the selection bias can be made by associating y_1 and y_2 with weights computed as the inverse of their respective selection probabilities, $w_1 = \frac{1}{\pi_1} = 2, w_2 = \frac{1}{\pi_2} = 1$. Thus

$$E(\hat{\mu}_{IPW}) = \frac{\frac{1}{2} N_1 y_1 w_1 + N_2 y_2 w_2}{\frac{1}{2} N_1 w_1 + N_2 w_2} = \frac{\frac{1}{2} N_1 y_1 2 + N_2 y_2 1}{\frac{1}{2} N_1 2 + N_2 1} = \frac{N_1 y_1 + N_2 y_2}{N} = E(Y)$$

With $\pi_1 = 1/2$ the inverse is $2/1$, which amounts to essentially counting each observed value of y_1 twice because the probability of observing each instance of y_1 from the population is $1/2$. If $\pi_1 = 2/3$, then each occurrence of y_1 would be given a weight of $3/2 = 1.5$. In actual clinical trial data the probabilities are unknown and must be estimated from sample data.

If the selection probability for elements y_1 were $\pi_1 = 0$ then all y_1 are missing and IPW cannot be used. Hence, an important requirement of IPW is that all possible values of the outcome variable have nonzero probability of being in the observed population. If some values have very low probabilities it is unlikely that these values would be observed in a sample. In such cases IPW may lead to bias (if some values are not observed in the sample) and/or high variance (if some values are observed but have low estimated probabilities resulting in very large weights).

To illustrate a general use of IPW, let y_i, $i = 1,..., N$ denote realizations of an outcome variable Y in a complete data set, $y_{i,obs}$, $i = 1,..., N_1$ and r_i is the observed values of missingness indicator variable R so that for subject i.

$$y_i = \begin{cases} y_{i,obs}, if \ \ r_i = 1 \\ y_{i,mis}, if \ \ r_i = 0 \end{cases}$$

Assume that the true selection probabilities (or probabilities of nonmissingness) are known, $\pi_i = \Pr(R_i = 1)$. Note that in general π_i may be a function of y_i; therefore, π_i's are conditional probabilities $\pi_i = \Pr(R_i = 1 | Y = y_i)$. The IPW estimator can be defined as

$$\hat{\mu}_{IPW} = \frac{1}{N} \sum_{i=1}^{N_1} y_{i,obs} \frac{1}{\pi_i}$$

Equivalently, the expression can be written in terms of the complete data outcome as

$$\hat{\mu}_{IPW} = \frac{1}{N} \sum_{i=1}^{N} y_i r_i \frac{1}{\pi_i}$$

Although some values of y_i are not observed, the product $y_i r_i$ is fully observed. To show that $\hat{\mu}_{IPW}$ is an unbiased estimator of $\mu = E(Y)$ its expectation with respect to the joint distribution of Y and R is needed. The law of conditional iterated expectations can be exploited to allow decomposition of the joint expectation as $E_{Y,R}() = E_Y\{E_{R|Y}()\}$. Then

$$E(\hat{\mu}_{IPW}) = \frac{1}{N} \sum_{i=1}^{N} E(Y_i R_i) \frac{1}{\pi_i} = \frac{1}{N} \sum_{i=1}^{N} \frac{1}{\pi_i} E\left(Y_i E_{R|Y} R_i\right)$$

$$= \frac{1}{N} \sum_{i=1}^{N} \frac{1}{\pi_i} \Pr\left(R = 1 | Y = y_i\right) E(Y_i)$$

$$= \frac{1}{N} \sum_{i=1}^{N} \frac{\pi_i}{\pi_i} E(Y_i) = \frac{1}{N} \sum_{i=1}^{N} E(Y_i) = E(Y) = \mu$$

Therefore, as seen from the third line, assigning weights that are the inverse of the probability of selecting the observations recovers the mean expected in the complete data. In practice, the weighted sum of observed values is divided by the sum of weights rather than by N.

$$\hat{\mu}_{\text{IPW}} = \frac{1}{\sum_{i=1}^{N_1} \frac{1}{\pi_i}} \sum_{i=1}^{N_1} y_{i,\text{obs}} \frac{1}{\pi_i}$$

In expectation, these are equivalent:

$$E\left(\sum_{i=1}^{N_1} \frac{1}{\pi_i}\right) = E\left(\sum_{i=1}^{N} \frac{R_i}{\pi_i}\right) = E\left(\sum_{i=1}^{N} \frac{\pi_i}{\pi_i}\right) = N.$$

Therefore, the relative subject-specific weights (summing up to 1) can be defined as

$$\hat{\mu}_{\text{IPW}} = \sum_{i=1}^{N_1} y_{i,\text{obs}} w_i$$

$$w_i = \frac{\frac{1}{\pi_i}}{\sum_{i=1}^{N_1} \frac{1}{\pi_i}}$$

Once IPW estimates of the expected outcome for each treatment group $\left(\hat{\mu}_{\text{IPW}}^{(t)}, t = 0, 1\right)$ are obtained, treatment effects can be estimated as, $\hat{\theta}_{\text{IPW}} = \hat{\mu}_{\text{IPW}}^{(1)} - \hat{\mu}_{\text{IPW}}^{(0)}$.

As an initial illustration, consider estimating treatment effect via inverse probably weighting of the completers (subjects with no missing data) in the small example data set with dropout. For this illustration, subjects are considered to have only one observation, the Time 3 assessment. The IPW weights are not known, but can be estimated using logistic regression. For this example probability of dropout was estimated using a model applied to data pooled across visits with the dropout indicator as the response variable. Predictor variables included change from baseline at the previous visit, baseline score, and treatment. The inverse weights estimated from this model were applied to the subset of subjects that completed the trial (sometimes called inverse probability weighted complete case or IPWCC estimator) in order to estimate the mean that would have been observed if all patients had completed.

For this example, the probabilities of completing the trial are computed as a product of conditional probabilities of completing each of the visits. That is,

$$\pi_i = \Pr(R_{1i} = 1) \Pr(R_{2i} = 1 | R_{1i} = 1) \Pr(R_{3i} = 1 | R_{1i} = 1, R_{2i} = 1)$$

Because all subjects completed the first post-baseline visit it is assumed the $\Pr(R_{1i} = 1) = 1$. Estimates of conditional probabilities are obtained as functions of observed outcomes and other baseline covariates (e.g., using logistic regression) as will be shown in detail in the next sections.

Weighting removes selection bias by giving larger weight to outcomes that are underrepresented in the observed data compared to what would have been observed if there were no dropouts. Conversely, smaller weights are given to observed values that are "overrepresented." Typically, as is the case with the small example dataset with dropout, subjects with poorer efficacy are less likely to be observed. Therefore, subjects with poor outcomes are underrepresented in the observed data and their weight should be larger compared to those who had larger improvements.

As expected, weights estimated from the small example data set are larger for subjects with worse outcomes (changes from baseline closer to zero) and smaller for subjects with better outcome (larger negative changes from baseline). The left panel of Figure 16.1 illustrates this relationship. The right panel is a plot of visit-wise mean changes from baseline for subjects who completed the trial divided into two strata; the first stratum is subjects whose estimated weights were less than the median and the second stratum is subjects with weights larger than the median. The figure clearly shows subjects with larger weights had worse marginal means than those with smaller weights.

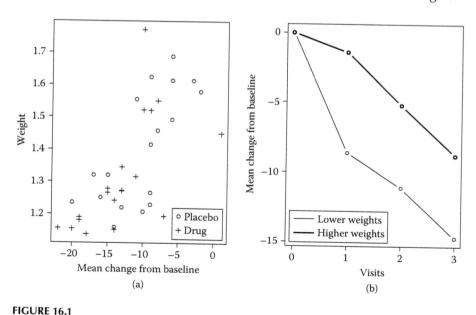

FIGURE 16.1

Relationship between weights and changes from baseline for completers. (a) Scatter plot of subject weights versus changes from baseline to visit 3 and (b) right panel is mean change profiles for completers with weights larger than median (thick line) and lower than the median (thin line).

16.2.2 Specific Implementations

The previous section illustrated IPW for an ANCOVA model with a single outcome per subject. Inverse probability weighting is now considered in the context of repeated measures analysis via weighted GEE. Inverse probability weights are commonly calculated in one of the two ways. Either one weight is given per subject and applied to all visits, thus reflecting the probability of the observed dropout pattern; or, each subject gets a unique weight at each visit, thus reflecting the visit-wise probabilities of dropout.

Robins and Rotnitzky (1995) proposed inverse probability weights that change by visit (observation-level weighting). The weights can be incorporated in the working covariance model as the elements of a diagonal $n_i \times n_i$ weight matrix W_i

$$V_i = \phi A_i^{\frac{1}{2}} W_i^{-\frac{1}{2}} R(\alpha) W_i^{-\frac{1}{2}} A_i^{\frac{1}{2}}$$

The weights are computed for each subject at each time point in a manner similar to how the weights for the last visit were computed in the weighted analysis of completers in the previous section. For example, Subject 9 had two completed visits; hence the matrix W is a 2×2 diagonal matrix with weights based on estimated probabilities as follows (subject index omitted whenever it does not cause confusion)

$$w_1 = \frac{1}{\hat{\pi}_1}, w_2 = \frac{1}{\hat{\pi}_2}$$

$$\hat{\pi}_1 = \Pr\left(R_1 = 1 \middle| x\right)$$

$$\hat{\pi}_2 = \widehat{\Pr}(R_1 = 1 \middle| x) \, \widehat{\Pr}\left(R_2 = 1 \middle| R_1 = 1, x, y_1\right)$$

Here again $\hat{\pi}_1 = 1$, and correspondingly, $\hat{\pi}_2 = \widehat{\Pr}(R_2 = 1 | R_1 = 1, x, y_1)$, because no dropouts had occurred prior to the first post-baseline visit. [Note we use $\Pr(R_2 = 1 | R_1 = 1, x, y_1)$ as a shorthand for $\Pr(R_2 = 1 | R_1 = 1, X = x, Y_1 = y_1)$]. The weights can change from visit to visit reflecting the changing probability of a subject remaining in the study given the previous data.

Fitzmaurice et al. (1995) proposed subject-level weighting wherein a single weight is computed for each subject that is used at every visit (repeated for all diagonal elements of the W_i matrix). The weight is an inverse of the estimated probability $\hat{\pi}^{(d)}$ of observing the dropout pattern d that was actually observed for that subject. Here the pattern $d = 1,..., T + 1$ indicates the *next* time point after patient was observed for the last time. That is, for a subject who was last seen at time t, $d = t + 1$. For completers, $d = T + 1$, where T indicates the last scheduled visit.

The working covariance model is then expressed as

$$V_i = \hat{\pi}_i^{(d)} \phi A_i^{\frac{1}{2}} R(\alpha) A_i^{\frac{1}{2}}$$

As a result, the weighted estimating equations are obtained from the original estimating equations simply by multiplying each subject's contributions to the estimating equations by the inverse probability of his/her observed dropout pattern $w_i = 1/\hat{\pi}_i^{(d)}$.

To illustrate, for a subject that completed all the scheduled visits, the weight is computed exactly as weights for completers at the last visit were computed in the previous section. That is,

$$\hat{\pi}^{(d)} = \widehat{\Pr}(R_1 = 1 | x)\, \widehat{\Pr}(R_2 = 1 | R_1 = 1, x, y_1)\, \widehat{\Pr}(R_3 = 1 | R_1 = 1, R_2 = 1, x, y_1, y_2)$$

For subjects who did not complete the trial, the probability of the observed pattern is computed as the probability of that subject remaining in the trial until the last observed visit and discontinuing right after. As an example, for Subject 9, the probability of the observed dropout pattern is computed as

$$\hat{\pi}^{(d)} = \widehat{\Pr}(R_1 = 1 | x)\, \widehat{\Pr}(R_2 = 1 | R_1 = 1, x, y_1) \left[1 - \widehat{\Pr}(R_3 = 1 | R_1 = 1, R_2 = 1, x, y_1, y_2) \right]$$

16.3 Example

With the building blocks of IPW in place, a wGEE analysis of the small example dataset with dropout can be considered. The goal is to estimate treatment effects using a weighted GEE model, with weights reflecting the selection probability; that is the probability of completing all three visits. This example uses the approach of Fitzmaurice et al. (1995) introduced in 16.2.2. Subject weights are computed based on inverse probability of observed dropout pattern $\hat{\pi}_i^{(d)}$.

After estimating the probabilities $\hat{\pi}_i$, the weights are computed as $w_i = \dfrac{1}{\hat{\pi}_i^{(d)}}$.

The weights are then included in the dataset as additional variable and the weighted analysis is conducted, for example, via SAS PROC GENMOD (SAS 2013). The weights are data-dependent, but the analysis assumes the weights are known, similar to the assumption that variance components are known in a standard mixed-effects model analysis. The robust sandwich estimates of standard errors provided by the GEE are still valid, although conservative (Robins et al. 1995). Resampling methods can be used to obtain non conservative estimates.

It is important to recognize that wGEE provides valid estimates under MAR, assuming that the model for dropout is correctly specified. As previously noted, estimating weights can be challenging when some of the true probabilities of observed patterns are close to 0. This can result in large weights and unstable estimates of treatment effects. Truncation and stratification can be used to stabilize weights. Also more stable versions of weights have been proposed (Hernàn et al. 2000).

SAS code for obtaining subject-level and observational-level inverse probability weights are listed in Section 16.4 (Code Fragment 16.1). SAS code to implement wGEE analyses via PROC GENMOD using the calculated IPW weights is listed in Section 16.4 (Code Fragment 16.2), followed by a code fragment for experimental procedure PROC GEE that is available in SAS/STAT 13.2 (SAS 2013) wherein the weights are obtained as part of the PROC.

Results for the wGEE analyses using subject-level weights are compared to results from an unweighted GEE and results from complete data in Table 16.1. It is important to interpret these results as just one realization from a stochastic process. If the comparisons were replicated many times under the same conditions—including missing data arising from an MAR mechanism—the average of the lsmeans and treatment contrasts across the repeated samples would be asymptotically equal for complete data, incomplete data analyzed via direct likelihood, MI, or wGEE with an appropriate dropout model. Standard errors would be consistently greater in incomplete data.

The wGEE analysis yielded a point estimate for the treatment contrast at Time = 3 in-between the result obtained from the analysis of complete cases

TABLE 16.1

Results from GEE and wGEE Analyses of the Small Example Data Set

		Complete Data		GEE Incomplete Data		wGEE Incomplete Data	
Treatment	Time	LSMEANS	SE	LSMEANS	SE	LSMEANS	SE
1	1	−4.13	0.91	−4.10	0.76	−4.38	0.83
1	2	−6.70	0.93	−6.70	1.04	−5.64	0.87
1	3	−9.86	1.05	−10.17	1.11	−9.58	1.08
2	1	−5.32	0.91	−5.29	0.97	−4.88	0.88
2	2	−8.70	0.93	−8.29	0.96	−6.09	1.10
2	3	−13.26	1.05	−13.10	1.27	−12.71	1.28
Endpoint Treatment Difference		3.39	1.49 ($p = 0.0274$)	2.92	1.73 ($p = 0.0905$)	3.13	1.71 ($p = 0.0670$)

and from complete data. As expected, the standard error for the Time 3 treatment contrast from wGEE with incomplete data was larger than the standard error from complete data and slightly larger than the standard error from the direct likelihood analysis of incomplete data (see Table 14.1). The relaxed distributional assumptions of GEE results in a slightly less efficient analyses than likelihood-based methods.

16.4 Code Fragments

CODE FRAGMENT 16.1 SAS Code for Obtaining Inverse Probability Weights

```
/* Create change at previous visit variable and dropout
   indicator variable */
PROC SORT DATA=ALL2; BY SUBJECT TIME; RUN;
DATA FOR_WGEE;
 SET ALL2;
 RETAIN DROP CHANGE_LAG1;
 BY SUBJECT TIME;
 IF FIRST.SUBJECT THEN DO;
   DROP=0;
      CHANGE_LAG1=.;
 END;
 IF DROP=1 THEN DELETE;
 IF CHGDROP=. THEN DROP=1;
 OUTPUT;
 CHANGE_LAG1=CHGDROP;
RUN;

/* Logistic regression analysis to obtain probabilities of
dropping, Pr(DROP=1)*/
PROC LOGISTIC DATA=FOR_WGEE DESC;
 CLASS TRT;
 MODEL DROP=TRT BASVAL CHANGE_LAG1;
 OUTPUT OUT =PRED P=PRED;
RUN;

/* Calculate and merge weights into data set */
DATA WEIGHTS_SUB (DROP=WEIGHT_OBS PB_OBS)
   WEIGHTS_OBS (DROP=WEIGHT_SUB PB_SUB);
SET PRED;
BY SUBJECT TIME;
RETAIN PB_SUB PB_OBS;
IF FIRST.SUBJECT THEN DO;
```

```
   PB_OBS =1; /* PROB. OF OBSERVING SUBJECT AT GIVEN TIME
     - FOR OBSERVATIONAL WEIGHTS */
   PB_SUB =1; /* PROB. OF OBSERVED DROPOUT PATTERN - FOR
     SUBJECT WEIGHTS */
 END; ELSE DO;
   IF DROP THEN PB_SUB =PB_SUB * PRED; ELSE PB_SUB =PB_SUB
     *(1-PRED);
   PB_OBS =PB_OBS * (1-PRED);
 END;

 WEIGHT_OBS=1/PB_OBS ;
   OUTPUT WEIGHTS_OBS;
   IF LAST.SUBJECT THEN DO;
     WEIGHT_SUB =1/PB_SUB;
     OUTPUT WEIGHTS_SUB;
   END;
 RUN;

 PROC SORT DATA=FOR_WGEE; BY SUBJECT; RUN;
 PROC SORT DATA=WEIGHTS_SUB; BY SUBJECT; RUN;

 DATA FOR_WGEE;*
   MERGE FOR_WGEE
     WEIGHTS_SUB (KEEP=SUBJECT WEIGHT_SUB);
   BY SUBJECT;
 RUN;
```

CODE FRAGMENT 16.2   SAS Code for Weighted GEE Analysis Using the PROC GENMOD

```
 ODS OUTPUT ESTIMATES=ES_CHDR_WGEE_IND
     LSMEANS=LS_CHDR_WGEE_IND;
 PROC GENMOD DATA=FOR_WGEE (WHERE=(CHGDROP NE .));
   CLASS TRT TIME SUBJECT;
   MODEL CHGDROP= BASVAL TRT TIME TRT*TIME /LINK=ID
     DIST=NORMAL;
   WEIGHT WEIGHT_XXX¹;
   REPEATED SUBJECT=SUBJECT /TYPE=IND;
   ESTIMATE "TRT EFFECT AT VIS 3" TRT -1 1 TRT*TIME 0 0 -1 0 0 1;
   LSMEANS TRT*TIME;
 RUN;
```

1. Use WEIGHT_SUB for subject-level weights and WEIGHT_OBS for observation-level weights

---

* Here we show creating analysis data set for wGEE using subject weights. Analysis data with observation-level weights is created similarly by merging with WEIGHTS_OBS data set.

CODE FRAGMENT 16.3 SAS Code for Weighted GEE
Analysis Using the Experimental PROC GEE

```
PROC GEE DATA=ALL2 DESC PLOTS=HISTOGRAM;
  CLASS SUBJECT TRT TIME;
  MISSMODEL PREVY TRT BASVAL / TYPE=SUBLEVEL;
  MODEL CHGDROP = BASVAL TRT TIME TRT*TIME BASVAL*TIME /
    DIST=NORMAL LINK=ID;
  REPEATED SUBJECT=SUBJECT / WITHIN=TIME CORR=IND;
RUN;
```

16.5 Summary

Although GEE is valid only under MCAR, inverse probability weighting (IPW) can correct for MAR, provided an appropriate model for the missingness process (dropout) is used whereby missingness depends on observed outcomes but not further on unobserved outcomes. The weights are based on the inverse probability of dropout and in effect create a pseudo-population of data that would have been observed with no missing data in an infinitely large trial.

Weighting can be at the subject level, with one weight per subject reflecting the inverse probability of observing the dropout pattern; or, weighting can be at the observation level, with one weight per subject per visit that reflects the changing probability of dropout as outcomes evolve over time.

As with standard GEE, in wGEE no assumptions about the correlation structure are required and therefore wGEE yields semi-parametric estimators. The wGEE estimates are generally not as efficient as maximum likelihood (parametric) estimators obtained using the correct model, but they remain consistent whereas maximum likelihood estimators from a misspecified parametric model are inconsistent.

17

Doubly Robust Methods

17.1 Introduction

Common references for the emerging area of doubly robust (DR) methods include Carpenter et al. (2006) and Tsiatis (2006). The genesis of DR methods can be seen by building from the properties of weighted generalized estimating equations (wGEEs), which are briefly reviewed below.

Although GEE is valid only under missing completely at random (MCAR), inverse probability weighting (IPW) can correct for missing at random (MAR), provided an appropriate model for the missingness process (dropout) is used whereby missingness depends on observed outcomes but not further on unobserved outcomes (Molenberghs and Kenward 2007). The wGEEs yield semi-parametric estimators because they do not model the entire distribution of the outcome values. These semi-parametric estimates are generally not as efficient as maximum likelihood estimators obtained using the correct model, but they remain consistent when maximum likelihood estimators from a misspecified parametric model are inconsistent (Molenberghs and Kenward 2007).

Therefore, a motivation for DR methods is to improve the efficiency of wGEEs by augmenting the estimating equations with the predicted distribution of the unobserved data, given the observed data (Molenberghs and Kenward 2007). Although augmentation is motivated by efficiency, it also introduces the property of double robustness.

To understand double robustness, consider that efficient IPW estimators require three models: (1) a substantive (analysis) model that relates the outcome to explanatory variables and/or covariates; (2) a model for the probability of observing the data (usually a logistic model of some form); and (3) a model for the joint distribution of the partially and fully observed data, which is compatible with the substantive model (1) (Molenberghs and Kenward 2007).

If model (1) is wrong, for example, because a key confounder is omitted, then estimates of all parameters will typically be inconsistent. The intriguing property of augmented wGEE is that if either model (2) or model (3) is wrong, but not both, the estimators in model (1) are still consistent (Molenberghs and Kenward 2007). However, DR methods are fairly new with few rigorous simulation studies or real data applications in the literature. Refer Robins et al. (1995), Carpenter et al. (2006), Tsiatis (2006) and Daniel and Kenward (2012) for additional details.

17.2 Technical Details

In Section 16.2, inverse probability estimation was explained starting with the simple case of estimating the sample mean of an outcome variable Y when some of its values y_i, $i = 1,...,N$, are missing (indicated with $r_i = 0$). Subsequently, IPW was extended to repeated measures. A similar approach is used here, with the ideas of DR estimation building on the results of Chapter 16.

To fix ideas, assume that missingness is MAR and the probability that Y is missing does not depend on unobserved vales of Y, given covariates $\mathbf{X}$ (that includes various pretreatment covariates). Recall that an unbiased estimate of treatment means can be obtained using the inverse probability estimator:

$$\hat{\mu}_{\text{IPW}} = \frac{1}{N} \sum_{i=1}^{N} y_i r_i \frac{1}{\pi_i}$$

where π_i are probabilities of having observed outcome (known or estimated from available data). Note that under MAR (for this example) $\pi_i = \pi(x_i) = \Pr(R = 1 | X = x_i)$ is a known or estimated function of covariates; therefore, we can write $\pi = \pi(x)$. The consistency of the IPW estimator follows from the assumption that the model for probability of missingness was correctly specified. If that is not the case, probabilities $\hat{\pi}_i$ estimated from an incorrect model will converge (as N becomes large) to some "misspecified" function $\tilde{\pi}(x)$. As a result, the estimate of population mean would in general be biased. The *augmented inverse probability weighted estimator* of sample mean $\hat{\mu}_{\text{AIPW}}$ aims to protect against bias due to misspecification of the weight by combining IPW with an outcome (or imputation) model $m(x)$

$$\hat{\mu}_{\text{AIPW}} = \frac{1}{N} \sum_{i=1}^{N} \tilde{y}_i = \frac{1}{N} \sum_{i=1}^{N} \left\{ \frac{r_i}{\hat{\pi}_i} y_i - \left(\frac{r_i}{\hat{\pi}_i} - 1 \right) \hat{m}_i \right\}.$$

We emphasize that this requires estimation of models for (1) probability of being observed and (2) outcome value (whether missing or observed) by placing hats over $\hat{\pi}_i$ and $\hat{m}_i$. Therefore, the estimator is an average of N "augmented values", $\tilde{y}_i, i = 1,...,N$. Note that, unlike the IPW estimator, the augmented IPW (AIPW) estimator receives nonzero contribution from patients with missing values ($r_i = 0$), specifically such patients contribute with their imputed or predicted value, $\widehat{m}_i$, estimated from the outcome model $m(x)$.

The AIPW estimator is often written in the following alternative forms that can be easily obtained from the original one by re-arranging terms:

$$\hat{\mu}_{\text{AIPW}} = \frac{1}{N} \sum_{i=1}^{N} \left\{ \frac{r_i}{\hat{\pi}_i} y_i - \left(\frac{r_i}{\hat{\pi}_i} - 1 \right) \widehat{m}_i \right\} = \frac{1}{N} \sum_{i=1}^{N} \left\{ \frac{r_i}{\hat{\pi}_i} \left(y_i - \widehat{m}_i \right) + \widehat{m}_i \right\}$$

$$= \frac{1}{N} \sum_{i=1}^{N} \left\{ y_i + \left(\frac{r_i}{\hat{\pi}_i} - 1 \right) \left(y_i - \widehat{m}_i \right) \right\}.$$

The last representation is particularly useful for demonstrating the *double robustness* property of the AIPW estimator: the estimator is consistent as long as at least one of the two models is correctly specified. To illustrate, assume that the sample size is large so that the estimators $\hat{\pi}_i$ and $\widehat{m}_i$ converge (in probability) to their large sample counterparts, whether they are correctly or incorrectly specified functions of observed data.

Also assume that the model for probability of missingness is correctly specified, $\pi(x)$ and the outcome model is a (possibly) misspecified function $\ddot{m}(x)$. Applying the law of conditional iterated expectations to a joint distribution of random variables R, X, Y as $E_{R,X,Y} = E_{X,Y}\{E_{R|X,Y}()\}$, the expectation of individual augmented values can be written as follows (after factoring out $Y - \ddot{m}(X)$, which is a constant conditional on X and Y):

$$E(\tilde{Y}) = E(Y) + E\left\{ E\left(\frac{R}{\pi(X)} - 1 \,\middle|\, X, Y \right) (Y - \ddot{m}(X)) \right\}$$

$$= \mu + E\left\{ \left(\frac{E(R \mid X, Y)}{\pi(X)} - 1 \right) (Y - \ddot{m}(X)) \right\}$$

$$= \mu + E\left\{ \left(\frac{\pi(X)}{\pi(X)} - 1 \right) (Y - \ddot{m}(X)) \right\}$$

$$= \mu + 0$$

The second term vanishes regardless of what $E_{XY}(Y - \ddot{m}(X))$ may be because under MAR $E(R \mid X = x, Y = y) = \Pr(R = 1 \mid X = x) = \pi(x)$, resulting in consistent estimation of the population mean μ.

Similarly, assuming that the model for probability of missingness is possibly misspecified $\ddot{\pi}(x)$ and for outcome model the true function $m(x)$ is estimated, after applying the law of conditional iterated expectations

$E_{R,X,Y} = E_{R,X}\{E_{Y|R,X}()\}$, the expectation of individual augmented values can be written as follows

$$E(\tilde{Y}) = E(Y) + E\left\{\left(\frac{R}{\hat{\pi}(X)} - 1\right)E(Y - m(X))|R,X)\right\}$$

$$= \mu + E\left\{\left(\frac{R}{\hat{\pi}(X)} - 1\right)\left(E(Y|X,R) - m(X)\right)\right\}$$

$$= \mu + E\left\{\left(\frac{R}{\hat{\pi}(X)} - 1\right)\left(m(X) - m(X)\right)\right\}$$

$$= \mu + 0$$

Again, the second term vanishes in expectation because under MAR the distribution of outcomes conditional on observed data is the same for subjects with observed ($R = 1$) and unobserved ($R = 0$) outcome values; hence, $E(Y|X = x, R = r) = E(Y|X = x) = m(x)$.

To summarize, the idea of DR estimation is to combine the strengths of two models: for probability of missingness and for imputing missing values. Both models can be estimated under the assumption of MAR utilizing observed patient-level data which, however, may be undesirable or awkward to include in the direct maximum likelihood-based modeling of the parameter of interest (e.g., treatment contrast at specific time point). The DR estimation via AIPW results in two types of gain: (1) protection against one of the two models being misspecified (doubly robustness) and (2) increased efficiency. While intuitively the increase in efficiency may appear a natural outcome of using additional information (predicted values for subjects with missing outcomes), it relies on sophisticated theory of semi-parametric estimation (Robins and Rotnitzky 1995; Tsiatis 2006), which is outside the scope of this book.

Despite its intuitive appeal the DR estimators also received a great deal of criticism, its opponents arguing that in situations when both models may be "slightly" misspecified (a typical situation with real data) the doubly robustness property may not translate in any gain, especially given inherent instability of IPW. For example, as argued in Kang and Schafer (2009), "two wrong models are not better than one" (see also a different view in Cao et al. 2009 and Tsiatis et al. 2011 who proposed improved DB estimators).

As in the case of IPW, AIPW estimator previously introduced in the context of estimating population means gives rise to AIPW-based (generalized) estimating equations. Their general form is quite simple, it starts with IPW estimated equations (Chapter 16) and adds some function of the data with zero expectation

$$\sum_{i=1}^{N}\left\{\frac{r_i}{\pi_i}U(y_i, x_i, |\theta) - \left(\frac{r_i}{\pi_i} - 1\right)\phi(y_i, x_i)\right\} = 0$$

Like the AIPW estimator of population mean, the AIPW estimating equations have two terms: one is based on contributions from observed data only (inversely weighted by π_i) and the second is based on contributions from both observed and unobserved cases. The zero mean function $\phi(y,x)$ is then constructed to have minimal variance following semi-parametric theory of Robins and Rotnitzky (1995), resulting in conditional expectation of the score function $U(y_i, x_i | \theta)$ on the observed data Y_{obs}, X, that can be loosely termed "imputation model". However, particular implementations, especially extensions for longitudinal data, are not straightforward and selection of the best augmented function may be not obvious (see Karpenter and Kenward 2006 for applying DR estimators in the context of missing covariate and Tsiatis et al. 2011 for modeling longitudinal outcomes).

17.3 Specific Implementations

Specific implementation of AIPW requires the selection of (1) a substantive model of interest; (2) a missing data model for computing IPW; and (3) an outcome (imputation) model. In the context of data analysis from clinical trials, the substantive model would be the one for evaluating the treatment effect (e.g., treatment contrast at the last scheduled visit). The missingness process can be modeled using logistic regression. The outcome model typically would be estimated using repeated measures analysis. Both (2) and (3) can be modeled using "inclusive" strategies, incorporating a large number of potentially relevant covariates, whereas model (1) is typically focused on the primary estimand (parameter) of interest.

Consider a simple application of AIPW estimating equations in the context of the small example data set that has three post-baseline visits, which is a natural extension of the example of the IPW estimator of treatment effect in completers (IPW complete-case, or IPWCC) from Section 16.2.1 (see Seaman and Copas 2009, for other implementation).

Here, the substantive model (1) will be an ANCOVA for outcome at Time 3 with terms for intercept, baseline covariate (Y_0) and treatment indicator (Z),

$$E(Y_3 | Z, Y_0) = \beta_0 + \beta_1 Z + \beta_2 Y_0.$$

Let x_i be a row vector comprising the constant 1 and two covariates: $x_i = \{1, Y_{i0}, Z_i\}$. A possible augmented estimating equations can be

$$\sum_{i=1}^{N} \left\{ \frac{r_i}{\hat{\pi}_{i3}} x_i^T \left(y_{i3} - x_i^T \beta \right) - \left(\frac{r_i}{\hat{\pi}_{i3}} - 1 \right) \hat{E}\left(X_i^T \left(Y_{i3} - X_i^T \beta \right) \mid x_i, y_{i1}, y_{i2} \right) \right\} = 0$$

Here (similarly to computing IPW weights for completers for the example shown in Section 16.2), the probability of being observed at the last visit $\hat{\pi}_{i3}$ is estimated as a function of baseline and available post-baseline data

$$\pi_3(x_i, y_{i,obs}) = \Pr(R_{i3} = 1 \mid R_{i2} = 1, x_i, y_{i1}, y_{i2}) \Pr(R_{i2} = 1 \mid x_i, y_{i1})$$

The probabilities in the chain product can be estimated from two separate logistic regressions for dropouts at Times 2 and 3 (recall that there are no dropouts in the first post-baseline visit, $\Pr(R_{i1} = 1) = 1$).

Solving the above augmented estimating equations can be challenging. Let $\hat{m}_{i3} = \hat{E}(Y_{i3} \mid x_i, y_{i1}, y_{i2})$. It is easy to see that the equations can be written by rearranging terms as

$$\sum_{i=1}^{N} \left\{ \frac{r_{i3}}{\hat{\pi}_{i3}} x_i^T \left(y_{i3} - \hat{m}_{i3} \right) + x_i^T \left(\hat{m}_{i3} - x_i^T \beta \right) \right\} = 0$$

If the outcome model $m_3(x, y_1, y_2)$ is correctly specified, the first term vanishes in expectation and the roots of the equations (in expectation) must be the true values of the parameter vector β. With some particular choices of estimated mean function $\hat{m}_3$, the elements of the first term (shown below as a 3×1 vector S) can be made *exactly* equal to zero which, as seen shortly, would greatly simplify the estimation of parameter β

$$S = \sum_{i=1}^{N} \left\{ \frac{r_{i3}}{\hat{\pi}_{i3}} x_i^T \left(y_{i3} - \hat{m}_{i3} \right) \right\} = 0$$

Obviously, $S = 0$ can be enforced by choosing $\hat{m}_{i3}$ to be the solution of the above-mentioned IPW estimating equations. However, note that $\hat{m}_{i3}$ is sought as a function of a broader set of covariates *including all observed post-baseline outcomes*, not just those included in the covariate set X. To this end, m_{i3} is estimated as $\hat{m}_{i3}^{IPW} = \hat{m}_3(x_i, y_{i1}, y_{i2})$ by using the weighted estimating equations as a linear function in X, Y_1, and Y_2

$$\sum_{i=1}^{N} \left\{ \frac{r_{i3}}{\hat{\pi}_{i3}} (x_i, y_{i1}, y_{i2})^T \left(y_{i3} - m_3(x_i, y_{i1}, y_{i2}) \right) \right\} = 0$$

Now that the elements of S are made exactly zero, the original augmented equations for estimating $\beta's$ simplify to (unweighted) estimating equations

$$\sum_{i=1}^{N} x_i^T \left(\hat{m}_{i3}^{IPW} - x_i^T \beta \right) = 0$$

where $\hat{m}_{i3}^{IPW}$ are predicted outcomes at post-baseline visit 3 for each subject, either with observed or missing outcomes.

However, one caveat is that the predictive model m_3 includes as covariates (possibly missing) intermediate outcomes at Time 2, Y_2. Now, we can apply (recursively) the same idea and use similar weighted estimating equations for estimating $\widehat{m}_{i2}^{\text{IPW}}$

$$\sum_{i=1}^{N}\left\{\frac{r_{i2}}{\widehat{\pi}_{i2}}\left(x_i,y_{i1}\right)^T\left(y_{i2}-m_2\left(x_i,y_{i1}\right)\right)\right\}=0$$

Here, $\widehat{\pi}_{i2}$ is the estimated probability of the i-th subject not missing at Time 2. Since no outcomes Y_1 are missing at Time 1, our "recursion" stops here and we will be able to compute $\widehat{m}_{i3}^{\text{IPW}}=\widehat{m}_3\left(x_i,y_{i1},y_{i2}\right), i=1,...,N$, where the missing values for Y_2 will be replaced with predicted $\widehat{m}_{i2}^{\text{IPW}}=\widehat{m}_2\left(x_i,y_{i1}\right)$.

This gives rise to the following general algorithm, suggested by Vansteelandt et al. (2010) for analysis of data with missing covariates and very similar to that implemented for repeated measures recently in O'Kelly and Ratitch (2014, section 8.4, pp. 377–378).

1. Compute subject-specific probabilities of being observed at the specific time point $\widehat{\pi}_{it}\left(x_1,x_2\right)$ using a full set of covariates partitioned into two subsets: X_1 (intended for modeling treatment effect) and X_2 (including baseline and post-baseline variables observed prior to the time point t when treatment assessment is made).

2. Predict outcome $\widehat{m}_{it}^{\text{IPW}}\left(x_1,x_2\right)$ at time point t for all subjects, whether observed or missing the outcome, using the full set of covariates and inverse probability weights from Step 1 (e.g., via appropriate generalized linear model). If some post-baseline covariates in the set X_2 are missing, iterate Steps 1 and 2 to impute them taking advantage of monotone patterns of missing data.

3. Use predicted values $\widehat{m}_{it}^{\text{IPW}}$ from Step 2 as new responses to fit a generalized linear model (GLM) on covariates from the set X_1 and obtain estimates of the coefficients.

4. Compute standard errors for coefficients of the model in Step 3 via bootstrapping the entire modeling strategy (Steps 1–3).

Details of this analytic strategy are illustrated in the next section using application to the example data set.

17.4 Example

In this section, DR estimation outlined in Section 17.3 is applied to the small example data set to evaluate the treatment effect at the last scheduled visit.

This analysis involves the following steps (the SAS code is included in Section 17.5).

1. Estimating probabilities of discontinuation (and remaining on treatment) at Times 2 and 3 using logistic regression models. Specifically, the model for probability $\hat{\pi}_{i2} = \widehat{\Pr}(R_{i2} = 1 \mid x_i, y_{i1})$ of remaining on treatment by Time 2 included terms for baseline severity score, changes in outcome from baseline at Time 1, treatment indicator and all interactions of treatment with other covariates. Only subjects who completed the first post-baseline visit contributed to this estimate (which in our case were all randomized subjects). Probability of remaining on treatment at Time 3 was estimated as a product of conditional probabilities $\hat{\pi}_{i3} = \hat{\pi}_{i2} \times \widehat{\Pr}(R_{i3} = 1 \mid R_{i2} = 1, x_i, y_{i1}, y_{i2})$, where the second conditional probability was estimated from a separate logistic regression with terms for the baseline score, changes from baseline at Times 1 and 2, treatment indicator and all treatment-by-covariate interactions. Only subjects completing the first two post-baseline visits contributed to this model.

2. Imputing missing values for the changes in outcome variable at Time 2 with its predicted values from the linear regression model $m_2(x_i, y_{i1})$ estimated using inverse probability weights, $w_i = 1/\hat{\pi}_{i2}$, with the same terms that were used for modeling $\hat{\pi}_{i2}$ (although this is not essential).

3. Fitting a linear regression model for completers (patients with non-missing outcomes at visit 3) $m_3(x_i, y_{i1}, y_{i2}^*)$ with weights, $w_i = 1/\hat{\pi}_{i3}$, and with the same terms that were used for modeling $\hat{\pi}_{i3}$. Missing outcomes for changes from baseline to Time 2 were replaced with predicted values from the previous step (which is emphasized in the notation with an asterisk, y_{i2}^*).

4. Finally, we use predicted values $\hat{m}_{i3}$, $i = 1, ..., N$, obtained at previous step as "new data" to fit an ANCOVA model with baseline score and treatment indicator as covariates.

5. The point estimate for the treatment contrast from the model in #4 is the final estimate of treatment effect at Time 3 (shown in Table 17.1), $\hat{\theta}_{AIPW}$. Clearly, the standard errors and p-values reported by ANCOVA (on the basis of full sample of N subjects) are severely biased downward, as they do not account for the estimation done in previous steps, in particular, the uncertainty due to imputation of missing values.

6. We obtain valid standard errors and confidence intervals by bootstrap (shown in Table 17.1). Each bootstrap sample of size N is formed by sampling with replacement subject records (rows) of the observed $N \times p$ data matrix. Any subject irrespective of his/her missingness pattern has the same probability $1/N$ to be selected

TABLE 17.1

Estimating Treatment Contrast and Least-Squares Means Using a Doubly Robust AIPW Method for Completers (Bootstrap-Based Confidence Intervals and Standard Errors)

Treatment	Time	Complete Data			Incomplete Data (AIPWCC)		
		LSMEANS	SE	95% CI	LSMEANS	SE	95% CI
1	3	−9.86	1.05	(−11.98, −7.75)	−9.70	1.11	(−11.62, −7.17)
2	3	−13.26	1.05	(−15.37, −11.14)	−12.58	1.26	(−15.19, −10.23)
Endpoint Treatment Difference		3.39	1.49	(0.39, 6.39)	2.88	1.71	(0.18, 6.82)

in each draw and may appear multiple times in each bootstrap data set. We form 2000 bootstrap data sets, and each gives rise to the same analysis Steps 1–5 as were applied to the observed data (including re-fitting models for computing weights) resulting in point estimates $\hat{\theta}_{\text{AIPW}}^{(b)}, b = 1,...,2000$, which is the bootstrap distribution of our AIPW estimate. A valid estimate of standard error can be obtained as the standard deviation of the bootstrap distribution. We further construct a 95% confidence interval by using the percentile method; that is, by taking as confidence limits the 2.5% and 97.5% percentile points of the bootstrap distribution. Other more sophisticated methods for bootstrap intervals can be used (e.g., BCa, bias-corrected and accelerated bootstrap intervals, available in SAS %BOOTCI macro and R package *boot*). Because the example data set is rather small, in some bootstrap samples modeling probability of discontinuation using logistic regression may be challenging because of quasi-complete or even complete separation making maximum likelihood estimation of parameters not possible. In many situations, this can be fixed by using a variant of penalized regression known as Firth's (1993) penalized likelihood (available in SAS logistic regression procedure). A small number of particularly unfortunate bootstrap samples (e.g., with no missing values) can be skipped.

17.5 Code Fragments

Here, we implemented a simple version of AIPW estimator similar in spirit to Vansteelandt et al. (2010). To obtain bootstrap-based standard errors, we used %BOOT and %BOOTCI macros available at http://support.sas.com/kb/24/982.html. These macros require that the computation of estimates subjected to bootstrapping was implemented by the user in a separate macro called %ANALYZE. To facilitate "by-processing" when computing bootstrap distribution of estimates, %BYSTMT macro is called within each procedure and data step inside %ANALYZE macro. The code may be not most efficient and specific to the data set at hand but easy to follow and (as we hope) generalize to other examples the reader may encounter.

CODE FRAGMENT 17.1   SAS Code for Implementing Augmenting Inverse Probability Weighting

```
%macro analyze(data= , out= );
/* predicting prob of dropping at vis 2 */
   ODS LISTING CLOSE;
   PROC LOGISTIC DATA=&DATA DESC;
   %BYSTMT;
   MODEL R2 =TREAT BASVAL YOBS1 TREAT*YOBS1 TREAT*BASVAL/
     FIRTH MAXITER=100 ;
   OUTPUT OUT =PREDR2 P=PROB_V2;
 RUN;

/* predicting prob of dropping at vis 3 */
   PROC LOGISTIC DATA=PREDR2 DESC;
   %BYSTMT;
   MODEL R3 =TREAT BASVAL YOBS1 YOBS2 TREAT*YOBS1
     TREAT*YOBS2 TREAT*BASVAL/FIRTH MAXITER=100 ;
   OUTPUT OUT =PREDR3 P=PROB_V3;
 RUN;

/* computing weights at vis 2 and 3 */
   DATA WEIGHTS_OBS ;
    SET PREDR3;
    %BYSTMT;
    IF R2 =0 THEN DO;
      WEIGHT2=1/(1-PROB_V2);
    END;
    IF R3 =0 THEN DO;
      WEIGHT3=1/(1-PROB_V2)*1/(1-PROB_V3);
    END;
 RUN;

/* predict missing outcomes for vis 2 using IPW model*/
   PROC GENMOD DATA=WEIGHTS_OBS ;
    %BYSTMT;
    MODEL YOBS2= TREAT BASVAL YOBS1 TREAT*BASVAL
    TREAT*YOBS1;
    WEIGHT WEIGHT2;
    OUTPUT OUT=PREDY2 PRED=PRED_Y2;
 RUN;
```

```
/* replace missing values for vis 2 with predicted */
   DATA PREDY2;
    SET PREDY2 ;
   %BYSTMT;
    IF YOBS2= . THEN YOBS2=PRED_Y2;
  RUN;

/* predict outcomes for vis 3 using IPW model */
   PROC GENMOD DATA=PREDY2;
   %BYSTMT;
   MODEL YOBS3= TREAT BASVAL YOBS1 YOBS2 TREAT*BASVAL
     TREAT*YOBS1 TREAT*YOBS2;
   WEIGHT WEIGHT3;
   OUTPUT OUT=PREDY3 PRED=PRED_Y3;
  RUN;


ODS OUTPUT LSMEANS=LSDR1
       ESTIMATES=ESDR1;
PROC GENMOD DATA=PREDY3;
   %BYSTMT;
   CLASS TREAT;
   MODEL PRED_Y3= BASVAL TREAT;
   LSMEANS TREAT;
   ESTIMATE "DR ESTIMATE OF TRT" TREAT -1 1;
  RUN;


PROC TRANSPOSE DATA=LSDR1 OUT= LSMEANS_TRANSP (DROP=_NAME_)
   PREFIX=LSMEANS;
   %BYSTMT;
   VAR ESTIMATE;
   ID TREAT;
  RUN;


   DATA &OUT;
    MERGE ESDR1 (KEEP=MEANESTIMATE &BY RENAME=(MEANESTIMATE
      =TRTDIFF3))
      LSMEANS_TRANSP;
   %BYSTMT;
   RUN;
   ODS LISTING;
%MEND;

/* construct analysis data with single record per subject */
  PROC TRANSPOSE DATA=DATALONG OUT= DATAWIDE (DROP=_NAME_)
   PREFIX=YOBS;
   BY TRT SUBJECT BASVAL;
   VAR CHGDROP;
   ID TIME;
  RUN;
```

```
DATA FOR_ANALYSIS;
   SET DATAWIDE;
   R2=(YOBS2=.);
   R3=(YOBS3=.);
   TREAT=(TRT="2");
RUN;

/* applying analyze macro to observed data */
 %LET BY=;
   %ANALYZE(DATA=FOR_ANAL, OUT=OUT_EST);

   %BOOT(DATA=FOR_ANAL, ALPHA=.05, SAMPLES=2000,
      RANDOM=123, STAT = TRTDIFF3 LSMEANS0 LSMEANS1,
      CHART=0, BIASCORR=1);

   %BOOTCI(METHOD=PERCENTILE);
```

17.6 Summary

One motivation for DR methods is to improve the efficiency of wGEEs by augmenting the estimating equations with the predicted distribution of the unobserved data, given the observed data. This augmentation also introduces the property of double robustness.

Efficient IPW estimators require three models: (1) a substantive (analysis) model that relates the outcome to explanatory variables and/or covariates of interest; (2) a model for the probability of observing the data (usually a logistic model of some form); and (3) a model for the joint distribution of the partially and fully observed data, which is compatible with the substantive model (1).

With augmented wGEEs if either model (2) or model (3) is wrong, but not both, the estimators in model (1) are still consistent. If model (1) is wrong, then estimates of all parameters will typically be inconsistent.

DR methods are fairly new and our understanding of how to best apply these methods in clinical trial scenarios is emerging.

18

MNAR Methods

18.1 Introduction

Analyses in the MNAR framework try in some manner to model or otherwise take into account the missingness process and its impact on outcomes of interest. However, moving beyond MAR to MNAR poses fundamental problems. In MAR, it is assumed that the statistical behavior of the unobserved data is the same as it had been observed, such that the unobserved data can be predicted from the observed data. Of course, the characteristics and statistical behavior of the missing data are unknown (Mallinckrodt 2013). Therefore, it is impossible to know if MAR is valid and it is impossible to know if any specific MNAR model is correct.

Moving beyond MAR to MNAR can only be done by making assumptions. Conclusions from MNAR analyses are therefore conditional on the appropriateness of the assumed model (Verbeke and Molenberghs 2000). While dependence on assumptions is not unique to MNAR analyses, an important feature of MNAR analyses (as with MAR analyses) is that (some of) the assumptions are not testable (Molenberghs et al. 1997) because the data about which the assumptions are made are missing (Laird 1994). Hence, no individual MNAR analysis can be considered definitive and multiple MNAR models can yield the same fit but imply very different dropout processes (Verbeke and Molenberghs 2000; Molenberghs and Kenward 2007). Therefore, MNAR methods are evolving to be used as sensitivity analyses more so than as primary analyses (Mallinckrodt 2013; Molenberghs et al. 2015).

18.2 Technical Details

18.2.1 Notation and Nomenclature

General classes of MNAR methods arose from different factorizations of the likelihood functions for the joint distribution of the outcome variable and the indicator variable for whether or not a data point was observed, which are often described as the measurement process and the missingness process, respectively (Verbeke and Molenberghs 2000). In this context, outcome variable indicates the hypothetical "complete" data, which are split into two parts: the actually observed part and the missing part. The "full data" consist of the complete data and missingness indicators. The following terminology is used to describe and compare the methods.

Subject $i = 1,..., N$ is to be measured at times $j = 1,..., n$

Y_{ij} is the random variable measured on Subject i at time j, where j can take on the values $1,..., n$

R_{ij} is an indicator random variable taking on the value of 1 if Y_{ij} is observed, 0 otherwise.

Group Y_{ij} into a vector $Y_i = (Y_{i,obs}, Y_{i,mis})$

$Y_{i,obs}$ contains Y_{ij} for which $R_{ij} = 1$,

$Y_{i,mis}$ contains Y_{ij} for which $R_{ij} = 0$.

Group R_{ij} into a vector R_i that is commensurate with Y_{ij} such that all 1s are paired with the $Y_{i,obs}$ and the 0s are paired with the $Y_{i,mis}$

D_i is the time of dropout

Ψ = Parameters describing the missingness process

θ = Parameters describing the measurement process

18.2.2 Selection Models

A standard reference for selection models is Diggle and Kenward (1994). For a more recent reference, see Molemberghs et al. (2015, chapter 4).

In selection models, the joint distribution of the ith subject's outcomes (Y_i) and the missingness indicators (R_i) is factored as the marginal distribution of Y_i and the conditional distribution of R_i given Y_i.

$$f(y_i, r_i | \theta, \Psi) = f(y_i | \theta) f(r_i | y_{i,obs}, y_{i,mis}, \Psi)$$

A selection model can be thought of as a multivariate model, where one variable is the continuous efficacy outcome from the primary analysis and the second variable is the binary outcome for dropout modeled via logistic regression (Mallinckrodt 2013). In ignorable models, it is assumed that the missingness process is independent of the measurement process (conditional on the measurements). An MNAR selection model explicitly ties together the measurement and missingness processes as the outcome variable (Y) from the measurement model is a predictor variable in the dropout (missingness) model (Mallinckrodt 2013).

Parametric selection models can be fit to observed data, even though there is no empirical information about the association between the values of R

(0 or 1) and Y_i. By definition, Y_i is missing in all instances when $R_i = 0$. The parametric and structural assumptions imposed on the full data distribution allow the model to be fit. However, the appropriateness of the model and its assumptions cannot be verified from the data (Verbeke and Molenberghs 2000). Interestingly, Molenberghs et al. (2015) demonstrated that multiple selection models can be fit to the same data, yielding the same fit to the data, but implying different dropout processes, which in turn alter parameters describing the observed data. In other words, there is no definitive selection model that can be fit to a data set.

An example of a selection model used in a sensitivity analysis context is provided in Chapter 21.

18.2.3 Shared-Parameter Models

Standard references for shared-parameter models include Wu and Carroll (1988) and Wu and Bailey (1989). In a shared-parameter model, a set of latent variables, latent classes, and/or random effects is assumed to drive both the Y_i (measurement) and D_i (missingness, in this case time to dropout) processes. An important version of this model further asserts that, conditional on the latent variables, Y_i and D_i are independent. A shared-parameter model can be thought of as a multivariate model, where one variable is the continuous efficacy outcome from the primary analysis and the second is (typically) a proportional hazards time to event analysis for dropout (Mallinckrodt 2013).

Specifically, the full data likelihood can be factored similarly to a selection model as the product of the marginal outcome distribution $f(y_i \mid b_i)$ and the conditional distribution of D_i given Y_i and b_i (for simplicity, the dependence on fixed parameters associated with these distributions is suppressed).

$$f(y_i, d_i, b_i) = f(y_i \mid b_i) f(d_i \mid y_i, b_i) f(b_i)$$

$$= f(y_i \mid b_i) f(d_i \mid b_i) f(b_i)$$

Note that dependence of dropout on Y_i in the last equation can be dropped because of the assumption that the outcome and dropout processes are conditionally independent given the shared random effects, b.

Therefore, the dropout and measurement models are linked by having the same random effects in both the outcome and dropout models. As in selection models, there are again untestable assumptions, namely that conditional on the latent (i.e., unobserved) random effects, Y_i and D_i are independent. This assumption is untestable because Y_i is missing in each instance when D_i is prior to the end of the trial.

18.2.4 Pattern-Mixture Models

Standard references for pattern mixture models (PMMs) include Little (1993, 1994, 1995). PMMs as originally proposed were based on the reverse factorization of the full data likelihood as compared with the selection model factorization. In PMMs, the full data likelihood is the product of the measurement process conditional on the dropout pattern and the marginal density of the missingness process.

$$f(y_i, r_i|\theta, \Psi) = f(y_i|r_i, \theta)f(r_i|\Psi)$$

As originally proposed, PMMs fit a response model for each pattern such that the observed data are a mixture of patterns weighted by their respective probabilities. Results are pooled over the various patterns for final inference. These models can be viewed from an imputation perspective in which missing values Y_{mis} are imputed from their predictive distribution.

PMMs in this imputation context are by construction under-identified, that is, over-specified. For example, in the small example data set with dropout, say the goal is to estimate the difference between treatments at Time = 3. Although more dropout patterns are possible, only the three monotonic dropout patterns were actually present; that is, there were no intermittent missing data. Hence, the three patterns were last observations at Time 3 (completer), last observation at Time 2, and last observation at Time 1. Missing values for Time 3 can be imputed separately for each of the two noncompleter dropout patterns. However, information must be borrowed because there is no information about Time 3 within the noncompleter groups. This problem can be resolved through the use of identifying restrictions wherein inestimable parameters of the incomplete patterns are set equal to (functions of) the parameters describing the distribution of other patterns (Molenberghs and Kenward 2007).

Three specific and common identifying restrictions all use data from subjects that remained in the study at time t to identify the distribution for those subjects that discontinued (NRC 2010). These restrictions are:

- CCMV: Complete Case Missing Values, where information is borrowed from the completers group.
- NCMV: Neighboring Case Missing Values, where information is borrowed from the nearest dropout pattern.
- ACMV: Available Case Missing Values, where information is borrowed from all patterns in which the information is available.

ACMV is important because it corresponds to MAR, thereby providing a benchmark from which deviations can be judged (Mallinckrodt 2013).

Although not commonly seen thus far in the literature, it is also possible to define patterns by reason for dropout rather than time of dropout; or, as described in the next section, patterns can be defined by treatment group using the so-called controlled imputation approaches (Carpenter et al. 2013; O'Kelly and Ratitch 2014).

18.2.5 Controlled Imputation Approaches

Recently, another family of methods referred to as controlled imputation has been discussed in the literature and used in practice (Mallinckrodt 2013). Little and Yao (1996), Carpenter and Kenward (2007), Ratitch and O'Kelly (2011), Carpenter et al. (2013), Ayela et al. (2014) and Lipkovich et al. (2016) proposed imputation approaches that can be thought of as specific versions of PMMs. The common idea in each of these approaches is to construct a principled set of imputations that are controlled in a manner that creates a specific departure from MAR.

Controlled imputation approaches benefit from having assumptions—such as specific departures from MAR—that are transparent and therefore easy to understand and debate. This is an important feature given that accounting for departures from MAR must be purely assumption driven. Therefore, controlled imputation approaches are especially useful for sensitivity analyses and are therefore explained in some detail, with example analyses in the following Section 18.4.

Two general families of controlled imputation can be considered. In the delta-adjustment approach, it is assumed that subjects who discontinued had outcomes that were worse than otherwise similar subjects that remained in the study. The difference (adjustment) in outcomes between dropouts and those who remain can be a shift in mean or slope, an absolute value, or a proportion. The adjustment is referred to as delta (Δ). The delta-adjustment can be implemented in manners resulting in increasing, decreasing, or constant departures from MAR. Recent references for delta-adjustment methods include O'Kelly and Ratitch (2014) and Molenberghs et al. (2015, chapter 19).

The second general approach to controlled imputation is the so-called reference-based imputations. In this family of approaches, after dropout (or discontinuation of randomized study drug, or initiation of rescue medication), values are imputed by making qualitative reference to another arm in the trial (Molenberghs et al. 2015, chapter 19). In other words, deviations from MAR are created by assuming that after deviating from the initially randomized treatment (either via dropout, discontinuation of study drug, and/or initiation of rescue medication), imputed values take on the characteristics of a reference group.

The intent for sensitivity analyses is to generate a conservative estimate of an MAR-based estimand. This approach can be especially useful when the reference arm can be seen as a worst plausible case departure from MAR for the treatment group (Mallinckrodt et al. 2014). In some instances, reference-based imputation has been proposed as the primary approach to estimating effectiveness that reflects change in or discontinuation of treatment (Mallinckrodt et al. 2014).

Reference-based imputations can be implemented in a manner such that the transition to the reference arm is immediate or gradual, or the deviation from reference at the time of discontinuation can be maintained. A common approach is for missing values of drug-treated subjects to be imputed such that the post-deviation imputed values take on the statistical behavior of placebo-treated subjects. That is, the benefit of the drug is assumed to immediately disappear if study drug is discontinued (and/or rescue medication is initiated).

18.3 Considerations

Review papers that describe in detail, compare, and critique selection models, and shared parameter models and PMMs by identifying restrictions include Little (1995), Hogan and Laird (1997), Little and Rubin (2002), Diggle et al. (2002), Fitzmaurice et al. (2004), and Molenberghs and Kenward (2007). The NRC guidance on prevention and treatment of missing data summarizes the advantages and disadvantages of selection models and PMMS as follows (NRC 2010).

The basic idea behind selection models is intuitive: specify a relationship between the probability of discontinuation and the outcome of interest, including the unobserved outcomes. However, operationalizing that idea can be problematic. The predictive distribution of missing responses is typically intractable, making it difficult to understand exactly how the missing observations are being treated for a given selection model. This is especially the case given that the outcomes and probability of discontinuation are linked on the logit scale. Moreover, selection models are sensitive to parametric assumptions about the full data distribution. This concern can be alleviated to some degree via semi-parametric selection models. Many of these same comments can be applied to shared-parameter models.

Like selection models, PMMs start from an intuitive premise: conditional on the observed data, subjects with complete data have different outcome distributions than subjects with incomplete data. PMMs with identifying restrictions are transparent with respect to how missing observations are being imputed because the within-pattern models specify the predictive distributions directly.

However, PMMs can be computationally difficult. Ironically, this issue is especially problematic when, as would be hoped, the rates of missing data are low such that the parameters associated with sparse patterns cannot be estimated reliably. In addition, although the identifying restrictions are transparent, it is not necessarily easy for nonstatisticians to understand exactly what they imply about the missing values.

One of the NRC expert panel's recommendations (NRC 2010) was that methods for handling missing data be explained in protocols in a manner easily understood by clinicians. Others have questioned if, and if so, how this can be done. For example, Permutt (2015b) stated:

> No doubt there are clinicians who understand the assumptions of inverse probability weighting, pattern mixture models, and multiple imputation along with clinicians who do not. However, much of the language in the NRC report is inaccessible to many of the clinicians who serve as study investigators or who evaluate new drug applications. Furthermore, a general understanding of the methods does not suffice: what is required is to understand, so as to evaluate their plausibility, the specific assumptions being made by a specific model with specific covariates in a specific setting.

For example, consider trying to explain to clinicians how the various MNAR methods work. It is known that all methods rely on untestable assumptions. But explaining exactly what those assumptions are in a selection model, shared-parameter model, or even a PMM with traditional identifying restrictions (e.g., ACMV, CCMV, NCMV) is not straight-forward. Simply put, it is hard to understand exactly how these methods treat missing data, especially for nonstatisticians.

Therefore, for sensitivity analyses of confirmatory trials in a regulatory setting, selection models, shared-parameter models, and PMMs with traditional identifying restrictions may have limited utility.

Transparency and ease of understanding are far easier with delta-adjustment and reference-based imputations. For example, in a reference-based imputation, it is easier to understand the implications of assuming that drug-treated patients after early discontinuation of study medication have outcomes similar to placebo-treated patients; or, for delta-adjustment, that drug-treated patients after early discontinuation have outcomes worse than otherwise similar drug-treated patients who did not dropout by an amount equal to delta.

These advantages over earlier MNAR methods are leading to a wider use of controlled imputations, especially in regulatory settings (Permutt 2015b). Therefore, means to implement controlled imputations are covered in the next section.

18.4 Examples—Implementing Controlled Imputation Methods

18.4.1 Delta-Adjustment

Typically, only the experimental arm is delta-adjusted while the control arm is handled using an MAR-based approach. However, it is easy to delta-adjust each arm, using the same or different deltas. Whether or not to apply different dropout models by treatment arm is an important consideration for all MNAR approaches, not just delta-adjustment.

The magnitude of the deviation from MAR in an MNAR model is generally proportional to the amount of missing data. Therefore, unless dropout rates vary widely between treatments, fitting the same MNAR model to all treatment groups will typically have a relatively small effect on treatment contrasts. However, different MNAR models for each treatment arm provides greater opportunity for changes to estimated treatment contrasts compared with the corresponding MAR result. Delta-adjustment has thus far typically been implemented by applying delta to only the drug-treated arm(s) of the trial, leaving the control arm unadjusted.

Two general families of delta-adjustment can be applied: marginal and conditional. In the marginal approach, the delta-adjustment is applied after imputation of all missing values and the adjustment at one visit does not influence imputed values at other visits. Therefore, the marginal approach with a constant delta will result in a constant departure from MAR over time.

In the conditional approach, the delta-adjustment is applied in a sequential, visit-by-visit manner. In this approach, missing values are imputed as a function of both actually observed and previously imputed delta-adjusted values. In the conditional approach with delta applied to each visit, the deltas accumulate over time, resulting in a departure from MAR that increases over time. Alternatively, delta applied to only the first missing visit results in a departure from MAR that decreases over time (O'Kelly and Ratitch 2014).

A single delta-adjustment analysis allows testing if a specific departure from MAR overturns the MAR result. However, the delta-adjustment method can also be applied repeatedly as a progressive stress test to find how extreme the delta must be to overturn the MAR result. This is the so-called tipping point approach (O'Kelly and Ratitch 2014).

To illustrate the delta-adjustment approach, consider the small example data set with dropout. The SAS code fragment to implement the delta-adjustment controlled imputation approach is listed in Section 18.5 (Code Fragment 18.1). The SAS implementation of delta-adjustment uses the conditional approach where delta-adjustment at previous imputations influences the current imputation.

The top panel of Table 18.1 summarizes results from applying a delta-adjustment of 3 points to the drug-treated arm only using several approaches. First, adjustment was applied to only the endpoint visit (Time 3). That is, delta = 0 at Time 2. Even though the SAS implementation uses the conditional method, this implementation yields the same result as a marginal approach. That is, using delta = 0 at Time 2 is equivalent to a Time 2 delta that does not influence Time 3 imputed values. The bottom panel of Table 18.1 summarizes results from assuming progressively larger values of delta applied to only the endpoint visit, which again is equivalent to a marginal approach.

TABLE 18.1

Results from Various Delta-Adjustment Approaches to the Small Example Data Set with Dropout

Delta	Endpoint Contrast	Standard Error	P	Deviation from MAR
Delta = 3				
No adjustment[a]	2.98	1.71	0.082	0.00
Time 2 only	2.70	1.73	0.119	0.28
Time 3 only	2.25	1.76	0.201	0.73
Time 2 and Time 3	1.97	1.79	0.271	1.01
Delta Applied to Endpoint Visit Only				
No adjustment[a]	2.98	1.71	0.082	0.00
Delta = 1	2.74	1.73	0.103	0.24
Delta = 2	2.49	1.74	0.152	0.49
Delta = 3	2.25	1.76	0.201	0.73
Delta = 4	2.01	1.79	0.260	0.97
Delta = 5	1.77	1.82	0.323	1.21

[a] Delta = 0, the MAR result. Results do not exactly match previous multiple imputation results due to different seed values.

In both panels of Table 18.1, results from using delta = 0, that is no adjustment, is the MAR result to which delta-adjustment results are compared. In addition, interpretation of results is further facilitated by noting the (monotone) missing data patterns of the treatment arm to which the various deltas were applied. In the drug-treated arm (trt 2), three subjects had missing values at Time 2; those same three subjects plus three additional subjects had missing values at Time 3.

The top panel illustrates that applying the same delta to the endpoint visit has greater impact on the endpoint contrast than applying that delta to missing values at Time 2 only. This stems from two reasons. First, fewer patients have missing data at Time 2 than at Time 3. Hence, delta-adjustment is applied to fewer patients. In addition, applying delta to Time 2 imputed values impacts the endpoint contrast only indirectly via the correlation implied by the imputation model between Time 2 outcomes and Time 3 outcomes. This is another example of "shrinkage estimation" that was explained in Section 5.4.

Applying delta to Time 2 and Time 3 had a greater impact on the endpoint contrast than applying delta to Time 3 only. This is because the total effect of the delta-adjustment on the endpoint contrast—in the conditional approach—is essentially the sum of the effect from directly adjusting imputed values for Time 3 and the indirect effect on Time 3 imputed values by having adjusted the Time 2 imputed values that are used as part of the Time 3 imputations.

The bottom panel of Table 18.1 illustrates that increasing the delta applied to the endpoint visit has a consistent and therefore predictable effect for a given missing data pattern. In this example, for each 1-point increment of delta, the endpoint contrast was reduced by 0.24 points. This result is intuitive in that 24% of the values were missing for Treatment 2 at Time 3. In this simple illustration of applying what is essentially a marginal delta, the effect of delta-adjustment on the endpoint contrast can be analytically determined as follows: Let π = the percentage of missing values at the endpoint visit, and Δ = the delta-adjustment applied to the endpoint visit only. The change to the endpoint contrast = $\Delta \times \pi$.

From this simple, marginal approach to delta-adjustment it is easy to appreciate several important factors. First, it shows directly the impact of the fraction of missing values on the sensitivity of the MAR result to departures from MAR. If π is cut in half, Δ must double in order for the adjustment to have the same net effect on the endpoint contrast. It is also easy to see how progressively increasing delta can be used as a stress test to ascertain how severe departures from MAR must be in order to overturn inferences from the MAR result. However, the progressive stress test is not needed here because in this small example data set, results with dropout were not significant in the MAR result.

18.4.2 Reference-Based Imputation

Reference-based imputations can be tailored to specific scenarios. One variant of reference-based imputation, termed jump to reference (J2R), is implementation such that imputed values for subjects who discontinue the active arm immediately take on the attributes of the reference arm (placebo). That is, the treatment benefit in subjects who discontinue the active arm disappears immediately upon discontinuation. In a second approach, called copy reference (CR), the imputations result in a treatment effect that gradually diminishes after dropout in accordance with the correlation structure implied by the imputation model. In a third approach, called copy increment from reference (CIR), the treatment effect after discontinuation is maintained by matching changes after withdrawal to changes in the reference arm (Carpenter et al. 2013). With regard to assessing sensitivity, J2R results in the greatest departure from MAR.

Reference-based imputations as described above can also be interpreted as estimates of certain effectiveness estimands in that they explicitly model change in or discontinuation of treatment. In the effectiveness context, the J2R approach would be useful for symptomatic treatments with short duration of action where the benefits of the drug rapidly disappear after discontinuation. The CR approach would be useful for symptomatic treatments with long duration of action. The CIR approach would be appropriate for treatments thought to alter the underlying disease process (disease modification) (Mallinckrodt 2013).

It is perhaps easiest to understand these approaches by graphically depicting what they do in comparison to traditional multiple imputation based on MAR. These depictions are in Figures 18.1 through 18.4. Additional technical details can be found in Molenberghs et al. (2015, chapter 19).

Conceptually, consider traditional MI based on MAR as involving a regression on residuals (illustrated in Figure 18.1). Each subject's deviation from their respective group mean, while that subject was observed (shown as brown vertical segments extending from the line designating the treated mean), is used to impute the missing residuals. The actual imputed value (shown as "X" placed at the end of the red vertical segments) is the sum of the imputed residual and the group mean. In MAR, the imputed value is based on the mean of the group to which the subject was originally randomized. In J2R, the regression on residuals is again applied. However, imputed values are based on adding the imputed residuals to the reference arm mean—not the arm to which the subject had been randomized.

In CR (Figure 18.3), as in J2R (Figure 18.2), the regressed residuals are again added to the reference arm. However, in CR, the residual is determined by the deviation of observed values from the reference arm (shown as the upper blue line)—not the arm to which the subject was initially randomized, as is the case for MAR-based MI and J2R. This feature has the effect of giving credit to the drug arm for any benefit resulting from the drug while the subject adhered to treatment; that benefit declines over time in accordance with the correlations implied by the imputation model.

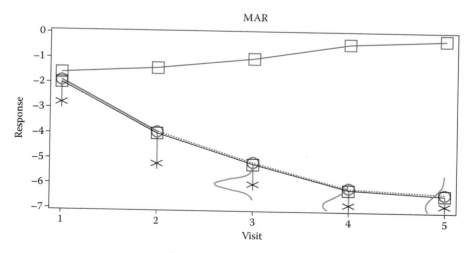

FIGURE 18.1
Illustration of multiple imputation based on MAR.

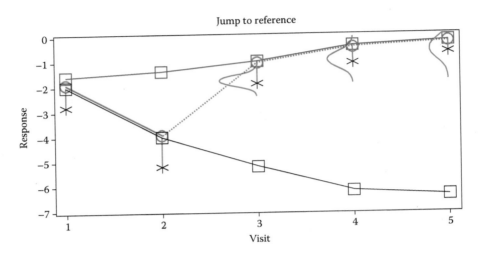

FIGURE 18.2
Illustration of jump to reference-based imputation.

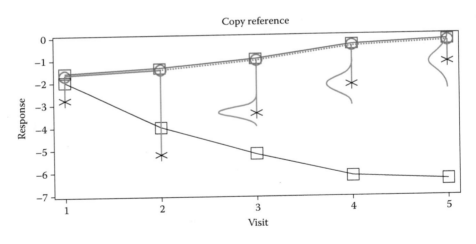

FIGURE 18.3
Illustration of copy reference-based imputation.

In CIR (Figure 18.4), residuals are determined as in MAR-based MI and J2R. However, missing values are imputed based on adding the regressed residuals to a hypothetical mean (shown as the dotted green line on the graph) that maintains the same deviation between the reference mean and the randomized group that was seen at the time of discontinuation.

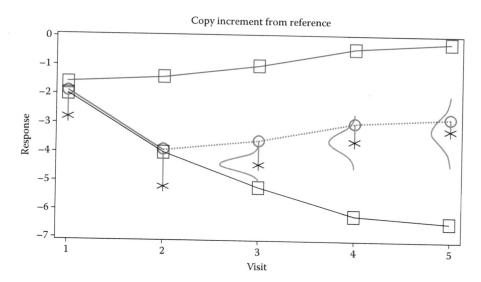

FIGURE 18.4

Illustration of copy increment from reference-based imputation.

Commercially available software to implement reference-based imputations is limited. It is possible to implement the CR approach in SAS. However, other variants must be implemented using specialty software. The Drug Information Association's (DIA) Scientific Working Group on missing data has SAS macros available at missingdata.org.uk, under the DIA working group tab, to implement a variety of reference-based imputation approaches, along with other specialty software tools. The code fragment to implement CR in SAS for the small example data set with dropout is listed in Section 18.5 (Code Fragment 18.2), and results are summarized in Table 18.2.

The deviation from MAR, based on difference in treatment contrast from the MAR analysis, when applying CR was 0.31 (2.98 versus 2.69). This deviation is smaller than would usually be the case in actual scenarios because only two post-baseline visits had missing values and these outcomes were strongly correlated.

TABLE 18.2

Results from Copy Reference Analyses of the Small Example Data Set with Dropout

Method	Endpoint Contrast	Standard Error	P	Deviation from MAR
MAR-based MI	2.98	1.71	0.082	0.00
Copy reference	2.69	1.64	0.103	0.31

18.5 Code Fragments

CODE FRAGMENT 18.1   SAS Code for Delta-Adjustment Controlled Multiple Imputation

```
/* 3 point adjustment at last visit only. No missing values
   At first post-baseline visit */
PROC MI DATA=y1 SEED=1214 OUT=outmi round=1 NIMPUTE=1000;
       by trt;
       class trt;
       monotone method=reg;
       var basval y1 y2 y3;
          mnar adjust(y2 /delta=0 adjustobs=(trt='2'));
          mnar adjust(y3 /delta=3 adjustobs=(trt='2'));
run;

ods output diffs = diffs;
proc Mixed data=finalY;
       class trt time subject;
       model y= basval trt time trt*time basval*time/ddfm=kr
          outp=check;
       repeated time / subject=subject type = un;
       by _Imputation_;
       lsmeans trt*time/diffs;
       id subject time ;
run;

data diffs2;
  set diffs;
  if time = _time and _time = 3;
run;

proc mianalyze data=diffs2;
  modeleffects estimate;
  stderr stderr;
run;
```

CODE FRAGMENT 18.2   SAS Code for the Copy Reference Method of Reference-Based Imputation

```
PROC MI DATA=y1 SEED=1214 OUT=outmi round=1 NIMPUTE=1000;
       class trt;
       monotone method=reg;
       var basval y1 y2 y3;
          mnar model (y2 / modelobs=(trt='1'));
          mnar model (y3 / modelobs=(trt='1'));
```

```
run;

ods output diffs = diffs;
proc Mixed data=finalY;
      class trt time subject;
      model y= basval trt time trt*time basval*time/ddfm=kr
         outp=check;
      repeated time / subject=subject type = un;
      by _Imputation_;
      lsmeans trt*time/diffs;
         id subject time ;
run;

data diffs2;
   set diffs;
   if time = _time and _time = 3;
run;

proc mianalyze data=diffs2;
   modeleffects estimate;
   stderr stderr;
run;
```

18.6 Summary

MNAR analyses model or otherwise take into account the missingness process and its impact on outcomes of interest. It is impossible to know if MAR is valid and it is impossible to know if any specific MNAR model is correct. Moving beyond MAR to MNAR can only be done by making (untestable) assumptions. Therefore, MNAR methods are evolving to be used as sensitivity analyses in support of an MAR-based primary analysis more so than as primary analyses.

In selection models, the joint distribution of the ith subject's outcomes (Y_i) and the missingness indicators (R_i) is factored as the marginal distribution of Y_i and the conditional distribution of R_i given Y_i. Selection models can be thought of as multivariate models, where one variable is the continuous efficacy outcome from the primary analysis and the second variable is the binary outcome for dropout modeled via logistic regression.

In a shared-parameter model, a set of latent variables, latent classes, and/or random effects is assumed to drive both the Y_i (measurement) and D_i (missingness) processes. Conditional on the latent variables, Y_i and D_i are assumed independent. A shared-parameter model can be thought of as a multivariate model, where one variable is the continuous efficacy outcome from the primary analysis and the second is (typically) a proportional hazards time to event analysis for dropout.

PMMs as originally proposed were based on the reverse factorization of the full data likelihood as for the selection model. Hence, the full data likelihood is the product of the measurement process conditional on the dropout pattern and the marginal density of the missingness process. As originally proposed, PMMs fit a response model for each pattern such that the observed data are a mixture of patterns weighted by their respective probabilities. Results are pooled over the various patterns for final inference.

It is hard to understand exactly how these methods treat missing data, especially for nonstatisticians. Therefore, as sensitivity analyses, especially for confirmatory trials in a regulatory setting, their utility is perhaps limited.

Delta-adjustment and reference-based imputations are transparent and easy to understand. These advantages are leading to a wider use of controlled imputations, especially as sensitivity analyses.

In reference-based imputation, deviations from MAR are typically created by assuming that drug-treated subjects after early discontinuation or initiation of rescue have outcomes similar to those in the reference group. In delta-adjustment, deviations from MAR are created by assuming that drug-treated patients after early discontinuation have outcomes worse than otherwise similar drug-treated patients who did not dropout by an amount equal to delta.

19

Methods for Incomplete Categorical Data

19.1 Introduction

19.1.1 Overview

In Chapter 10, it was noted that a number of issues in modeling categorical data could be handled in a similar manner as for continuous data. These similarities included modeling trends over time and accounting for within-subject correlations. In addition, the principles regarding analysis of incomplete data previously discussed for continuous outcomes also apply to categorical outcomes. For example, the missing data mechanisms (Chapter 12) apply to categorical data in essentially the same manner as for continuous data.

As such, the general methods of dealing with incomplete continuous outcomes can be considered for incomplete categorical outcomes. For the reasons detailed in Chapters 12 and 13, simple and ad hoc approaches to handling missing data are not appropriate for either continuous or categorical outcomes. Methods in the MNAR framework have an important place in the overall analysis plan, but that importance is primarily as sensitivity analyses. Therefore, as with continuous outcomes, analyses for incomplete categorical data center on likelihood-based approaches, multiple imputation and weighted generalized estimating equations (wGEE).

19.1.2 Likelihood-Based Methods

In continuous data, the linear mixed model provides a unifying analytic framework because the resulting estimates of fixed effect parameters have both a marginal and hierarchical model interpretation (Molenberghs and Kenward 2007). In other words, regardless of whether the scientific question is geared to marginal inference, where trial results are extended to the general patient population, or hierarchical inference, where trial results are conditional on the patients in the study, the same model can provide valid answers to both questions. However, this connection between the model families does not exist in nonnormal data. Therefore, analysis method must be tailored to the scientific question.

Likelihood-based methods are appealing for analyses of continuous data because of their flexible ignorability properties if missing data arise from an MAR mechanism (Chapter 14). However, Chapter 10 noted that the increased computational complexity inherent to categorical outcomes necessitate approximations. Although a full discussion of how these approximations influence results is beyond the present scope, the important implication is that the plausibility of being able to ignore the missing data in approximation-based likelihood-type analyses of categorical data is compromised over that seen with continuous data.

Therefore, analyses of incomplete categorical data may rely more on multiple imputation and wGEE than incomplete continuous data.

19.1.3 Multiple Imputation

As with continuous data, missing categorical data can be imputed by multiple imputation, followed by an analytic approach that would have been suitable had the data been complete (Schafer 2003). See Chapter 15 for details on and implementations of multiple imputation in continuous data.

Multiple imputation can be especially straightforward and useful for the analyses of dichotomized continuous variables. For example, assume, as was done in Chapter 10, that in the small example data set a change from baseline of 50% is used as the cut off to define clinically meaningful improvement. Each efficacy response on the original, continuous scale is categorized as clinically meaningful improvement: "yes"/"no."

Imputations could proceed to fill in the missing binary outcome. However, given the loss of information from dichotomizing continuous outcomes, it may be preferable to impute the missing values on the continuous scale and then categorize all outcomes, both observed and imputed, as meeting the criteria for response "yes" or "no."

19.1.4 Weighted Generalized Estimating Equations

Generalized estimating equations can circumvent the computational complexity of likelihood-based analyses of categorical data, and is therefore a viable alternative whenever interest is restricted to the mean parameters (treatment difference, time evolutions, effect of baseline covariates, etc.). In GEE, the missing data mechanism must be MCAR in order to be ignorable. Hence, similar to continuous data, weighted generalized estimating equations have been proposed to extend ignorability to both MCAR and MAR (see Chapter 16 for details of analyses in continuous data).

As detailed in Chapter 12, GEE is valid only under MCAR, and hence the interest in weighted GEE. With categorical data, as with continuous data, the idea is to weight each subject's contribution in the GEEs by the inverse probability that the subject does not drop out (i.e., remains on the assigned treatment) at a given time point (visit-wise weighting), or by the inverse probably of having observed the dropout pattern (subject level weighting).

Hence in practice, the only major modification needed for wGEE of categorical data compared with continuous data is to specify a link function for the means to account for nonlinearity and an appropriate distribution for the residuals. For binary data, the logit link is a common choice.

19.2 Examples

19.2.1 Multiple Imputation

This subsection illustrates two common analyses for categorical outcomes. The first example is a derived binary outcome (clinical response), and the second is an ordinal variable (PGI-Improvement). Similar examples were presented in Chapter 10 for analyses of complete data.

The derived binary outcome is defined as at least 50% improvement from baseline in HAMD depression score at the last scheduled evaluation. The MI analysis first imputes the underlying continuous scale data as illustrated in Code Fragment 15.1. Following imputation, the binary outcome is derived by applying the responder criterion to the observed and imputed values in each of the imputed (completed) data sets. Then, the primary analysis model is applied.

This primary analysis model is a logistic regression for responder status at Time 3, with treatment and baseline severity fitted as covariates. Finally, Rubin's combination rules are applied to produce a single estimate of treatment effect (converted to the odds ratio scale), along with the associated p-value and 95% confidence interval. A similar imputation strategy was evaluated by simulations and performed reasonably well (Lipkovich et al. 2005). The code to implement this analysis is presented in Code Fragment 19.1 (Section 19.3). Results are summarized in Table 19.1 and compared with the results from the complete data set using the same logistic model.

The second example is MI for the ordinal variable PGI Improvement (PGIIMP). To make the exercise more interesting, additional missing values resulting in nonmonotone missingness were created, similar to what was done in Section 15.3 when illustrating the MCMC method for multivariate normal data. Here, nonmonotone methods for imputing categorical data without easily specified joint distributions are illustrated. The SAS code to implement an approach using the so-called fully conditional specification (FCS) is presented in Code Fragment 19.2 (Section 19.3).

Once the completed data sets have been created, ordinal logistic regression is used to estimate the log odds ratio for the treatment effect and the associated standard errors. These results are passed to PROC MIANALYZE

TABLE 19.1

Treatment Contrasts and Least-Squares Means for Multiple Imputation of a Derived Binary Outcome Compared with Results from Complete Data Using a Logistic Model for Responder Status at Time 3[a]

Treatment	Complete Data (Logistic Model for Responder Status)		Incomplete Data (MI) (Imputing Underlying Continuous Score)	
	LSMEANS	CI (95%)	LSMEANS	CI (95%)
1	0.60	(0.38, 0.78)	0.49	(0.26, 0.71)
2	0.92	(0.72, 0.98)	0.86	(0.55, 0.97)
Endpoint Treatment Difference	7.83	(1.45, 42.3)	6.39	(1.01, 40.43)
		(p = 0.0167)		(p = 0.0487)

[a] LSMEANS are on probability scale, treatment difference = odds ratio.

TABLE 19.2

Treatment Contrasts and Least-Squares Means Estimated by Multiple Imputation and from Complete Data: Ordinal Logistic Model for PGI Improvement at Time 3[a]

Treatment	PGIIMP	Complete Data (Ordinal Logistic Model for PGIIMP Score)		Incomplete Data (MI) (Imputing PGIIMP Score Using FCS with Logistic Model)	
		LSMEANS	CI (95%)	LSMEANS	CI (95%)
1	≤ 1	0.10	(0.04, 0.25)	0.09	(0.025, 0.29)
1	≤ 2	0.55	(0.36, 0.73)	0.56	(0.34, 0.77)
1	≤ 3	0.74	(0.55, 0.87)	0.73	(0.49, 0.88)
2	≤ 1	0.30	(0.16, 0.49)	0.34	(0.17, 0.56)
2	≤ 2	0.82	(0.64, 0.92)	0.87	(0.66, 0.96)
2	≤ 3	0.91	(0.78, 0.97)	0.93	(0.76, 0.98)
Endpoint Treatment Difference		3.64	(1.18, 11.27) (p = 0.0249)	4.93	(1.17, 20.75) (p = 0.0298)

[a] LSMEANS are probabilities PGIIMP <= level, treatment difference are = odds ratios.

to conduct combined (pooled) inference. We also obtain MI inference for the probabilities of not exceeding each level of PGIIMP by treatment arm. The results are shown in Table 19.2.

19.2.2 Weighted Generalized Estimating Equation-Based Examples

Weighted generalized estimating equations can be applied to incomplete categorical data using the methods and principles outlined in Chapter 16 for analyses of continuous incomplete data, along with an appropriate link function and error distribution as described in Chapter 10.

19.3 Code Fragments

CODE FRAGMENT 19.1   SAS Code for Multiple Imputation Analysis of Derived Binary Outcome (Responder Analysis)

```
/* perform multiple imputation of monotone data from normal
distribution */
   proc MI data = all2_transp2 out = all2_miout nimpute
   =1000 seed =123;
   by trt;
   monotone method=reg;
   var basval Yobs1 Yobs2 Yobs3;
   run;
   /* compute responder status on imputed data set */
   data all2_miout;
   set all2_miout;
   responder=(Yobs3/basval <= - 0.5);
run;

/* apply analysis model to imputed data */
   proc sort data=all2_miout ; by _Imputation_; run;
       ods output Lsmeans=Bin_ls_imp
               Estimates =bin_est_imp;
       proc genmod data=all2_miout desc;
       by _Imputation_;
       class trt ;
       model responder=trt basval/error=bin link=logit;
       estimate "trt effect at vis 3" trt -1 1;
       lsmeans trt ;
       run;

/** combine estimates using Rubin's rules **/

ods output ParameterEstimates=es_logist_mi_final;
proc mianalyze data=bin_est_imp ;
 modeleffects LBetaEstimate;
 stderr StdErr;
run;
data es_logist_mi_final;
 set es_logist_mi_final;
 OR=exp(Estimate);
 OR_upper=exp(UCLMean);
 OR_lower=exp(LCLMean);
run;

proc sort data=Bin_ls_imp ; by trt; run;
 ods output ParameterEstimates=ls_logist_mi_final;
 proc mianalyze data=Bin_ls_imp ;
```

```
 by trt ;
 modeleffects Estimate;
 stderr StdErr;
run;

 data ls_logist_mi_final;
 set ls_logist_mi_final;
 prob_est=1/(1+exp(-1*Estimate));
 prob_upper=1/(1+exp(-1*UCLMean));
 prob_lower=1/(1+exp(-1*LCLMean));
run;
```

**CODE FRAGMENT 19.2   SAS Code for Multiple Imputation
Analysis of PGI Improvement as Categorical Outcome
Using Fully Conditional Specification Method**

```
proc mi data=all3_transpA out = all4_miout_fcs nimpute =1000
seed =123;
  class trt PGIIMPGR1 PGIIMPGR2 PGIIMPGR3;
  fcs logistic(PGIIMPGR2/details)
  logistic(PGIIMPGR3/details);
 var trt basval PGIIMPGR1 PGIIMPGR2 PGIIMPGR3;
/* imputation order is specified by var statement*/
run;

ods output Estimates =es_logit_imp
       Lsmeans=ls_logit_imp;

proc genmod data=all4_miout_fcs;
 by _Imputation_;
 class trt;
 model PGIIMPGR3 =trt basval/error=mult link=clogit;
 estimate "trt effect at vis 3" trt -1 1;
 lsmeans trt;
run;

 /* combine estimates using Rubin's rules */
 ods output ParameterEstimates=es_logist_mi_pooled;
 proc mianalyze data=es_logit_imp;
 modeleffects LBetaEstimate;
 stderr StdErr;
run;

 data es_logist_mi_pooled;
  set es_logist_mi_pooled;
  OR=exp(Estimate);
  OR_upper=exp(UCLMean);
  OR_lower=exp(LCLMean);
```

```
run;
  proc sort data=ls_logit_imp; by trt PGIIMPGR3; run;
  ods output ParameterEstimates=ls_logist_mi_pooled;
  proc mianalyze data=ls_logit_imp;
  by trt PGIIMPGR3;
  modeleffects Estimate;
  stderr StdErr;
run;

data ls_logist_mi_pooled;
  set ls_logist_mi_pooled;
  prob_est=1/(1+exp(- 1*Estimate));
  prob_upper=1/(1+exp(- 1*UCLMean));
  prob_lower=1/(1+exp(- 1*LCLMean));
run;
```

Section IV

A Comprehensive Approach to Study Development and Analyses

The intent of Section IV is *not* to provide specific guidance on analytic approaches for specific scenarios. Rather, the intent is to illustrate how the principles for analyses of longitudinal data discussed in earlier parts of this book can be generally applied. Two example data sets are used for illustration in Section IV. These data sets were described in Chapter 4 as large data sets, one with a high rate of dropout and one with a low rate of dropout. Although these data were somewhat contrived for convenience, they maintain most of the characteristics of the original data, and are therefore realistic and convenient examples.

20

Developing Statistical Analysis Plans

20.1 Guiding Principles

Recalling the process chart for study development introduced in Chapter 2, development of analysis plans begins with considering the objectives of the trial, which are determined from the decisions to be made from the trial. Estimands are chosen to address the objectives. A design is chosen to focus on the primary objective, and to also address key secondary objectives to the degree feasible. With clarity on objectives, estimands and design, analyses and sensitivity analyses can be chosen. It is important to appreciate the benefits from this being an iterative process, essentially then jointly considering all aspects of the process. Iteration can lead to objectives, estimands, and designs that are more relevant given the circumstances, and analyses that are aligned with the design, estimands, and objectives.

To illustrate, reconsider the example introduced in Section 2.6: a short-term, acute phase clinical trial is conducted where it is anticipated that the extensive efforts to maximize adherence will result in 95% of patients remaining on the initially assigned study medication. With this level of adherence, plausible departures from MAR are unlikely to overturn positive findings for a de jure estimand. Given this strong compliance and the highly-controlled study conditions, a de jure primary estimand may be most relevant. However, in a long-term trial in the same setting but with a design more similar to clinical practice, the more pragmatic nature of the trial and the inevitable loss of adherence over time may result in a de facto primary estimand being most relevant.

No single estimand is likely to meet the needs of all stakeholders. De jure and de facto estimands each have strengths and limitations, and more fully understanding a drug's effects requires understanding results from both families of estimands. Therefore, analysis plans need to address multiple estimands. Therefore, it is especially important that the analysis plans make clear which analyses address which estimands.

Choosing and specifying an analytic approach for a particular situation requires clarity on the data to be used, the method of estimation, and the model. A key aspect of choosing data is whether or not assessments after discontinuation of the initially randomized intervention and/or initiation of rescue medication should be included in the analysis. This is of course contingent on the estimand. However, including versus not including post-rescue data can have an important impact on results and therefore sample size implications must be considered.

For example, consider a scenario where estimand 1 from Table 2.1 (de facto estimand for effects of treatment regimen, post-rescue data is included) is of scientific interest. However, the medical condition addressed by the intervention is rare and patients are hard to enroll. Given that assessing pragmatic effectiveness via estimand 1 may require considerably more patients and therefore delay results of the trial for years, another estimand may be chosen as primary with estimand 1 evaluated secondarily.

Decisions regarding method of estimation are inherently tied to the model to be used. For continuous data, likelihood-based estimation in mixed-effect models provides a unifying framework for addressing marginal and random effect inference. With continuous data, the flexible ignorability property of likelihood-based estimation with regard to missing data is appealing. However, multiple imputation and weighted GEE analyses are very useful, especially for more inclusive modeling where additional covariates can be included to help account for missing data. Multiple imputation can also be useful when covariates are missing.

It is important to appreciate, however, that multiple imputation is, as the name denotes, an imputation technique, not a method of estimation. Even if the imputation step is valid and implemented via a principled likelihood-based model, the analysis model could be misspecified, resulting in invalid inference. The analyst must choose therefore also choose an appropriate method and model to analyze the data.

For categorical data, the elegant properties of the linear mixed-effects models with normal errors no longer hold and different analyses are needed for marginal inference versus hierarchical (random effects) inference. Often, interest in clinical trials will be more so on marginal inference that applies to the entire population as opposed to random effects inference that is specific to the subjects in the trial.

Moreover, the lack of simple specifications for multivariate distributions with categorical data leads to additional analytic complexity, which necessitates approximations for likelihood-based estimation. These approximations mean that missing data arising from an MAR mechanism are no longer ignorable and, as with GEE, the more restrictive requirement of MCAR is needed for ignorability. Therefore, for categorical data, multiple imputation and weighted GEE are particularly useful.

An overarching consideration regarding objectives is whether the study is considered exploratory (e.g., phase I or phase 2) or confirmatory (phase 3). The ICH E9 guidance (http://www.ich.org/fileadmin/Public_Web_Site/ICH_Products/Guidelines/Efficacy/E9/Step4/E9_Guideline.pdf) outlines the need for and benefit from pre-specification of statistical analyses.

These benefits include objectivity and avoidance of result-guided analytic choices that could bias inferences. Compared with confirmatory studies, analytic plans for exploratory studies can have greater flexibility, thereby relying more on methods and models developed from the data in the study. Confirmatory studies generally rely more on pre-specification of analyses. The basic idea is to exploit flexibility of exploratory studies to learn as much as possible, and then confirm those learnings in subsequent studies.

However, regardless of scenario, pre-specification of analyses to the degree appropriate is useful. The fundamental purpose of statistical analysis plans is to pre-specify analyses in order to provide the necessary scientific rigor and objectivity sought in the E9 guidance. Although pre-specification avoids bias from result-guided analyses, it also means that assumptions about the data must be made. It is therefore important to understand the characteristics of the anticipated data. Previous experience, especially results from earlier phase studies of the same intervention, can be extremely valuable in anticipating future data.

Consequently, exploratory phase analysis plans can be developed to help inform the decisions needed for pre-specification of analyses in confirmatory trials. To that end, there is a clear connection between exploratory and confirmatory analyses plans. Some of the same basic approaches to model building that are used in exploratory studies can be used to assess the appropriateness of pre-specified methods in confirmatory studies. Therefore, analysis plans will typically either employ several analytic approaches in order to test which one is best (exploratory studies), or use several analytic approaches to evaluate the validity of assumptions in the pre-specified primary analytic approach (confirmatory studies).

20.2 Choosing the Primary Analysis

20.2.1 Observed Data Considerations

In considering primary analyses it can be useful to divide the decision into two parts: how to model the observed data, and how to account for the missing data. Regarding the observed data, the general principles outlined in Part II of this book can be used to help inform choice of primary endpoint (change, percent change, etc.) along with how to model means over time, how to model the covariance between repeated measurements, and how to account for covariates.

Clinical trials typically have a pre-determined number of assessment times that are fixed within narrow intervals. The number of assessment times relative to the number of patients is typically small. These attributes suggest that unstructured modeling of mean trends over time (i.e., time is a categorical covariate) and unstructured modeling of within-patient covariance (the so-called full multivariate normal model) is possible. This is important, especially in confirmatory studies, because an unstructured model for the means requires no assumption about the time trend and models with fewer assumptions are preferred.

The number of parameters to describe the means over time from an unstructured model increases linearly with the number of assessment times. The number of parameters to be estimated for unstructured modeling of covariance increases by $n(n + 1)/2$, where n is the number of assessment times. Although convergence of the full multivariate normal model has been a consideration (Mallinckrodt et al. 2008), these models virtually always converge in practice. However, convergence should still be considered, especially if separate unstructured covariance matrices are fit by treatment or by some other demographic or prognostic factor.

Primary analyses in clinical trials typically have models with a few covariates at most. Additional covariates (subgroups) are assessed in secondary analyses. When a covariate is fit, including the covariate-by-time interaction should also be considered. Fitting just the main covariate effect imposes the restriction that the covariate has the same effect at all assessment times. If a covariate has many levels, such as investigative site, fitting the site-by-time interaction could require estimation of a large number of parameters, thereby inducing potential convergence issues. In exploratory studies that are often smaller and more limited in the number of parameters that can be estimated, analysis plans can specify methods for determining the model with the best fit.

Choice of the dependent variable, such as percent change versus actual change, and choice of the test statistic (endpoint contrast, main effect, etc.) are often driven by convention in confirmatory trials. However, analysts should always understand the alternatives and be willing to propose the most appropriate test and endpoint given the estimand and characteristics of the data.

20.2.2 Considerations for Missing Data

As noted in Chapter 2, choice of estimand influences what data are included in an analysis and whether or not data are considered missing. This section concerns those situations where some of the data that was intended to be collected to evaluate the particular estimand are indeed missing.

Fundamental issues exist in selecting a model and assessing its fit to incomplete data that do not apply to complete data. It was previously noted in Chapter 12 and elsewhere that the assumption of MCAR is unlikely to hold in most clinical trial scenarios. The validity of MCAR can be assessed using logistic regression analysis of probability of dropout. If the outcome variable being analyzed is associated with the probability of dropout, there is evidence to reject MCAR for that outcome. Tests for MCAR can also be based on comparing visit-wise means for patients that dropped out versus patients that continued. If means differ, there is evidence to reject MCAR (Mallinckrodt 2013).

These tests are geared toward assessing the association of observed outcomes with probability of dropout. Finding an association rejects MCAR. However, not finding an association isn't proof MCAR is valid. For MCAR to hold there must also be no association between the unobserved values and the probability of dropout, which as for testing validity of MAR, cannot be assessed from the observed data. Therefore, it is possible to prove MCAR doesn't hold, but it is not possible to prove MCAR is valid.

Given the implausibility of MCAR, analyses assuming MCAR are difficult to justify a priori and are therefore generally not appropriate choices for the primary analysis (Mallinckrodt et al. 2008; NRC 2010; Permutt 2015b). Ad hoc, single imputation methods, such as LOCF and BOCF, entail strong and restrictive assumptions that are unlikely to hold in practice. Therefore, these methods are also generally not suitable for the primary analysis in clinical trials (Molenberghs and Kenward 2007; Mallinckrodt et al. 2008; NRC 2010).

The assumption of MAR can never be confirmed in a clinical trial. However, MNAR methods also entail assumptions that cannot be verified. Both approaches are making assumptions about the missing data, which again cannot be verified (Verbeke and Molenberghs 2000). However, the difficulties in model selection and the consequences of model misspecification are generally greater for MNAR methods (Verbeke and Molenberghs 2000). In addition, departures from assumed distributions can be more problematic in MNAR models (Verbeke and Molenberghs 2000).

Therefore, assuming MAR in the primary analysis can be a reasonable starting point in many clinical trial scenarios. However, the possibility of MNAR can never be excluded. With an MAR primary analysis, sensitivity analyses are needed to understand how strongly inferences are influenced by departures from MAR (Verbeke and Molenberghs 2000; Molenberghs and Kenward 2007; Mallinckrodt et al. 2008; Siddiqui, Hong, and O'Neill 2009; Permutt 2015b). Sensitivity analyses are discussed in Section 20.4.

20.2.3 Choosing between MAR Approaches

When implemented in a similar fashion, likelihood-based, multiple imputation-based, and weighted GEE analyses tend to yield similar results, with the degree of similarity increasing with size of the data set, and in the case of MI, the number of imputations.

Likelihood-based methods tend to be more efficient. Hence, in situations where restrictive models that include only the design factors of the experiment are to be used, likelihood-based methods may be somewhat preferred. However, when more flexibility is desired in accounting for missingness, such as whenever inclusive modeling is used, MI and wGEE are generally preferred. When an appreciable number of covariate values are missing,

MI would be preferred over likelihood-based methods. When covariates to be included in the analysis are missing, wGEE and direct-likelihood exclude the entire record. However, multiple imputation can be used to impute the missing covariate values. A special case of the covariate considerations is for baseline severity. In this case baseline could be considered as part of the response vector for the likelihood analysis, as illustrated in Chapter 9. This avoids the need to discard the entire record, but entails further considerations.

20.3 Assessing Model Fit

20.3.1 Means

If an unstructured modeling of means over time is used, there are no assumptions to test. However, it may still be useful to evaluate more parsimonious models, especially in exploratory studies where the enhanced precision from a more parsimonious model could be especially beneficial. If a structured form of the mean trends is pre-specified, model fit should be compared with an unstructured model. Given that these models are nested (i.e., sub-models of each other), standard likelihood ratio tests can be used.

20.3.2 Covariances

Standard practice has evolved to use unstructured covariance/correlation matrices for modeling the within-subject errors. This helps avoid misspecification (Mallinckrodt et al. 2008). However, this approach does not guarantee validity. Structures more general than unstructured are possible, such as separate unstructured matrices by group (treatment).

Use of the sandwich estimator for standard errors in place of the model-based approach provides valid inference when the correlation structure is misspecified (Verbeke and Molenberghs 2000). Therefore, use of the sandwich estimator as the default approach would protect against correlation misspecification. However, when the sandwich estimator is used in SAS PROC MIXED, only the between-within method for estimating denominator degrees of freedom is available, an approach that is known to be biased, especially in small samples (SAS 2013). Moreover, the sandwich estimator assumes MCAR, which is difficult to justify a priori (Mallinckrodt 2013).

Therefore, a correlation structure deemed to be appropriate based on prior experience can be pre-specified as the primary analysis. Often this will be an unstructured covariance matrix. Model fit statistics and treatment contrasts from more general (separate unstructured matrices by treatment or other group) and more parsimonious structures can be compared to the primary analysis. If the primary analysis yields the best fit then the primary analysis can be considered appropriate. If the primary analysis does not provide the best fit but treatment contrasts or other relevant inferences do not differ between the primary analysis and the structure that yielded better fit, then the inferences from the primary analysis are robust to choice of covariance structure. Examples of fitting alternate covariance structures for the small example data sets were provided in Chapters 7 and 8. An example of assessing sensitivity to covariance assumptions is provided in Chapter 21.

20.3.3 Residual Diagnostics

Important assumptions required for valid regression-type analyses of continuous outcomes include linearity, normality, and independence (Wonnacott and Winacott 1981). These assumptions are in regards to the residuals (difference between observed and predicted values) not on the actual observations. An illustration of residual diagnostics from the small example data set was provided in Chapter 11 and an example from real clinical trial data is provided in Chapter 21. It is good practice to include residual diagnostics for the primary analysis in the clinical study report.

Diagnostics can reveal patterns in the residuals suggesting that the model is misspecified. Therefore, residual diagnostics can be an iterative process wherein residuals are rechecked after alterations to the model based on the first set of residual diagnostics. The focus of residual diagnostics is not as much on whether or not deviations from assumptions existed, but rather on how much departure from assumptions influenced results. For example, if the residuals were not normally distributed, but this lack of normality had a trivial impact on the primary treatment contrast, then the result would be useful, even if not entirely valid in the strictest sense, because inferences were not contingent on this assumption.

20.3.4 Influence Diagnostics

Influence diagnostics (and residual diagnostics) can be thought of conceptually as warning lights. These methods can flag data points or clusters of data that are unusual. Understanding to what degree study results are changed by the unusual data is important in understanding the overall robustness of results.

Although methods to test for the existence and impact of outlier (influential) observations have been around for decades, new methods have been developed for use in MNAR analyses. To this end, interest has grown in local influence approaches (Molenberghs et al. 2015, chapter 16). Local influence provides an objective approach to identifying and examining the impact of influential observations and clusters of observations on various aspects of the analysis, including the missing-data mechanisms and treatment effects (Mallinckrodt 2013).

However, given the newness and complexity of such methods, and that the methods are geared to the MNAR setting, the simpler influence diagnostics introduced in Chapter 11 are often appropriate. The basic idea is again not to simply identify whether or not influential observations or clusters (patients, investigative sites) were present, but rather to assess how the most influential observations affected the parameters of interest. It is good practice to include influence diagnostics for the primary analysis in the clinical study report.

20.4 Assessing Sensitivity to Missing Data Assumptions

20.4.1 Introduction

Assumptions about the missingness mechanism cannot be verified from the observed data, and therefore sensitivity analyses are needed to assess how departures from the assumed conditions influence inferences. In a broad sense, sensitivity analyses can be defined as several statistical models considered simultaneously, or further scrutiny of statistical models using specialized tools, such as diagnostic measures (NRC 2010).

One approach to assessing sensitivity is to fit a selected number of models, all of which are deemed plausible. A second approach is varying assumptions in a systematic manner within a particular analysis. This approach is often implemented by setting certain parameters, especially those that quantify the departure from MAR towards MNAR, at various levels within a plausible range. Unlike model parameters, sensitivity parameters by their very nature are not estimable from available data and represent the "untestable" portion of the model assumptions. The degree to which conclusions (inferences) are stable across such analyses provides an indication of the confidence that inferences are not contingent on assumptions.

The focus of sensitivity analyses, at least initially, should be more so on comparing the magnitude of the primary treatment contrast from the primary analysis with results from the sensitivity analysis (analyses). Initially, emphasis should not be placed too heavily on statistical significance. For example, if MAR was entirely valid and the primary result from an MAR analysis yielded a P value just under the pre-chosen significance level, sensitivity analyses may yield nonsignificant results despite the fact that estimated treatment contrasts would be similar to the primary result (Mallinckrodt 2013).

In addition, the focus of sensitivity analyses should be on sensitivity to assumptions, not sensitivity to methods. Many methods (e.g., likelihood-based mixed models, multiple imputation, EM algorithm, ...) rely on the same assumption that data are MAR. Therefore, comparing results from these methods does not assess sensitivity to the assumption of MAR and could lead to a misleadingly optimistic view of the robustness of the conclusions (Mallinckrodt 2013; Permutt 2015b).

20.4.2 Inference and Decision Making

In the previous section it was emphasized that the initial focus of sensitivity analyses is often based on estimation—how the magnitude of the treatment effect is influenced by departures from assumptions. However, ultimately the results of most trials are used to inform a "yes"/"no" decision as to whether the trial met its primary objective. In exploratory studies, this decision may be used to determine if development of the drug continues or is terminated. In confirmatory trials to be evaluated by regulatory agencies, the regulators must determine if the study provided confirmatory evidence of drug benefit. This need for a "yes/no" decision provides motivation for simple approaches to sensitivity analyses that focus on systematic changes to the primary analysis (Permutt 2015b).

Conducting a series of analyses that rely on different assumptions is useful for showing how much results are contingent on the assumptions, but this information is not all that useful in fostering the "yes"/"no" decisions made by regulators (Permutt 2015b). The problem is that if the results differ, it may be difficult to say why. Results could differ because the assumptions of one model are satisfied and the assumptions of the other are not. Alternatively, it could be that the assumptions of both models are satisfied and the difference is random. Finally, it could be that the assumptions of neither model are satisfied so that neither analysis is valid (Permutt 2015b).

Therefore, systematically varying the assumptions of the primary (often MAR-based) analysis may be more useful in supporting yes/no decisions than comparing results from a series of different analyses. To this end, the controlled imputation approaches described in Chapter 18 are particularly well-suited. Reference-based controlled imputation can be used to formulate a plausible worst-case scenario. The delta-adjustment approach can be used similarly by specifying a specific delta as the worst plausible cause, or deltas can be progressively increased as a stress test (Ratitch and O'Kelly 2014). This stress-testing format has been termed a tipping point analysis because it identifies the point at which results tip from significant to nonsignificant.

If a plausible worst-case scenario can be specified a priori, this can reduce the problem of sensitivity to a single analysis. If the results of the plausible worst case agree with the primary result, then inferences were not contingent on the assumptions. In cases where a plausible worst case cannot be identified, the delta-adjustment tipping point approach can be employed. However, the tipping point approach does not necessarily avoid the need to understand plausibility of departures from MAR. Inference from the tipping point approach is contingent upon whether or not the delta required to overturn the primary result is plausible or not. If the delta needed to overturn the primary result is not a plausible departure, then results are robust to plausible departures.

In providing specific advice on sensitivity analyses for confirmatory studies in a regulatory environment, Permutt (2015b) advocated the tipping point approach and noted that the decision problem then becomes a matter of judgment about the plausibility of values of delta. He suggested that protocols should address the question of what deviations might be considered plausible so that this may form the basis of discussion, and sometimes even of agreement, with regulatory agencies before results are known.

Such discussions and agreements can also inform planning of trials, especially with respect to sample size (Permutt 2015b). The crucial question is whether the plausible range of deviations from MAR lies entirely within the range of statistical significance. It is important to appreciate the regulator's perspective. In practice, an effect may confidently be considered significant only if it remains significant at the outer limit of a plausible range of deviations from MAR. The best estimates might be those based on MAR. However, binary decisions are needed in the regulatory setting. As a practical matter, regulators will need to act on the analyses at the unfavorable end of the plausible range, and applicants will need to anticipate and plan accordingly (Permutt 2015b).

For example, it might be best to power studies not on the anticipated magnitude of the treatment effect, but on the treatment effect minus the worst plausible departure from MAR. This regulatory perspective reinforces the need for the iterative study development process described in Chapter 2. It especially reinforces the benefits from minimizing missing data.

See Chapter 21 for examples of applying sensitivity analyses and drawing inference.

20.5 Other Considerations

20.5.1 Convergence

Failure of analytic algorithms to converge almost always results from improperly preparing the data (e.g., two observations on the same patient at the same time point) or from overspecified fixed effects models. Failure to converge almost never results from the pre-specified covariance matrix being too general. However, nonconvergence is possible with separate unstructured covariance matrices for groups, very high rates of dropout and/or need to estimate a large number of fixed effect parameters (such as when the time-by-site interaction is fit when there are many sites and frequent assessments).

If data are prepared correctly and the analysis fails to converge, convergence can be enhanced by using software features such as inputting starting values for parameter estimates, or the use in the initial round(s) (but not final rounds) of iteration algorithms such as Fisher's scoring rather than the Newton–Raphson algorithm, which is the default algorithm in many software packages.

Rescaling and/or centering of the data (e.g., using orthogonal polynomials to model time trends) are also options. If outcomes and covariates are made to fall in ranges in the order of magnitude of unity, interpretations and conclusions will not be changed; but, avoiding manipulation of large or small numbers from a numerical analysis perspective reduces the risk of ill-conditioned matrices, and ultimately, overflow or underflow (Mallinckrodt et al. 2008).

If all else fails, the protocol can envision one of several model-fitting approaches for determining the covariance structure. A set of structures can be specified. The structure converging to the best fit as assessed by standard model-fitting criteria is considered the primary analysis. Alternatively, a series of structures can be pre-specified in a fixed sequence, and the first correlation structure to yield convergence is considered the primary analysis. For example, unstructured could be specified as the structure for the primary analysis; but if it failed to converge, a series of ever more parsimonious structures appropriate to the situation at hand could be fit until one converges, which would then be considered the primary analysis.

Again, it is important to emphasize that in practical situations it is almost always possible to gain convergence from an unstructured covariance matrix. However, in instances when correctness of the covariance structure is a concern, standard errors and the associated inferences from maximum likelihood analyses can be based on the so-called sandwich estimator, which does not require correct specification of the correlation structure in order to yield valid inferences (Lu and Mehrotra 2009). However, as detailed in Section 20.3.2, the sandwich estimator requires MCAR. Therefore, specification of model-based standard errors as the primary approach is often preferable in likelihood-based analyses.

20.5.2 Computational Time

Mixed-effects models can be computationally intensive, and execution times can be long. Computational intensity stems from solving the mixed model equations and considerable CPU time is often required to compute the likelihood function and its derivatives. These latter computations are performed for each round of Newton–Raphson iteration (SAS 2013).

The following suggestions from the SAS on line documentation (SAS 2013) can be helpful when dealing with a model that has excessive compute time. Each of these factors could also be considered as means of aiding convergence:

- Examine the number of columns in the X and Z matrices. A large number of columns in either matrix can greatly increase computing time. Eliminating higher-order effects can markedly reduce the computational burden.
- In general, specify random effects with many levels in the REPEATED statement and those with a few levels in the RANDOM statement.

- Use the parms statement to specify plausible starting values for parameters.
- If the Z matrix has many columns (e.g., many subjects), consider using the between-within method to estimate denominator degrees of freedom in order to eliminate the time required for the containment method.
- If possible, "factor out" a common effect from the effects in the RANDOM statement and make it the SUBJECT = effect. This creates a block-diagonal G matrix and can often speed calculations.
- If possible, use the same or nested SUBJECT = effects in all RANDOM and REPEATED statements.
- The LOGNOTE option in the PROC MIXED statement writes periodic messages to the SAS log concerning the status of the calculations, which can help diagnose where the slowdown is occurring.

20.6 Specifying Analyses—Example Wording

20.6.1 Introduction

To fully specify an analysis, the method of estimation, the analytic model, and the choice of data must be made clear. Perhaps most importantly, it must also be clear what estimand the analysis is addressing.

A key principle of pre-specification is that analysts independently following the specifications arrive at the same results. For method of estimation, the primary options covered in this book include likelihood-based (maximum or restricted), generalized estimated equations, or least squares. Choice of data must include any imputation of missing data (e.g., multiple imputation) and whether or not data after discontinuation of initially randomized medication and/or initiation of rescue medication are to be included in the analysis.

All aspects of the analytic model should be pre-specified. Although there is no standard approach for model specification, a useful place to begin is in describing the dependent variable. Such specification should include the outcome variable and whether it is the actual values, change from baseline, percent change, etc., that is to be analyzed. In addition, any transformations or link functions that are utilized to account for nonnormality should be specified.

Concise and clear specification of covariates (independent variables) in the model is also essential. Such specification includes the variables themselves, interactions between variables, whether or not each variable is considered a categorical or continuous effect, and whether or not each variable is considered a fixed or random effect.

In addition, it is also necessary to specify what inferential tests will be the primary basis for evaluation (e.g., treatment main effect, endpoint contrast). In addition, it is also necessary to specify other details about the inferential test, such as the type of sums of squares (type I, type II, type III, etc.) and how denominator degrees of freedom are estimated.

20.6.2 Example Language for Direct Likelihood

The following example text illustrates one way to specify a priori all the details of a likelihood-based analysis such that independent analysts will arrive at exactly the same results. This particular wording specifies the full multivariate approach for an analysis of mean change from baseline with an unstructured modeling of treatment effects over time and within-patient error correlations.

Mean changes from baseline will be analyzed using a restricted maximum likelihood (REML)-based repeated measures approach. Analyses will include the fixed, categorical effects of treatment, investigative site, visit, and treatment-by-visit interaction, as well as the continuous, fixed covariates of baseline score and baseline score-by-visit-interaction. An unstructured (co)variance structure will be used to model the within-subject errors. The Kenward–Roger approximation will be used to estimate denominator degrees of freedom and adjust standard errors. Significance tests will be based on least-squares means using a two-sided $\alpha = 0.05$ (two-sided 95% confidence intervals). Analyses will be implemented using (insert software package). The primary treatment comparisons will be the contrast between treatments at the endpoint Visit.

20.6.3 Example Language for Multiple Imputation

The following example text is for an MI-based approach, assuming MAR, with sequential imputation for monotone missing data and multivariate Gaussian model/partial MCMC imputation for nonmonotone missing data. This model uses MCMC for partial imputation of nonmonotone data under MAR followed by sequential MI regression for monotone data. If desired, MCMC can be used for all missing data, both monotone and nonmonotone. Alternatively, a two-step process can be followed where only nonmonotone data is imputed first with the MCMC method, followed by a second step using the sequential MI regression to impute the remaining monotone missing data. This may be desirable if, for example, the primary outcome or other post-baseline auxiliary outcomes are categorical and would be better modeled with a logistic regression imputation model. In that case, sequential MI for monotone data can use regular regression models for continuous variables and logistic regression models for categorical variables that need to be imputed. In the example text that follows, measure1 is the dependent variable in the primary analysis.

Mean changes from baseline in measure1 will be analyzed based on data observed while the subject remains on study as well as data imputed using multiple imputation (MI) methodology for time points at which no value is observed. Multiple imputation will be performed under the assumption of missing-at-random (MAR) and will be implemented in two steps using {software, version}.

First, partial imputation will be carried out to impute intermittent (non-monotone) missing data based on a multivariate joint Gaussian imputation model using the Markov chain Monte Carlo (MCMC) method. A separate imputation model will be used for each treatment arm. The imputation models will include {list of baseline covariates}, measure1 assessments at each time point {Baseline, Visit x,...,y}. The MCMC method will be used with multiple chains, 200 burn-in iterations, and a noninformative prior. In case of nonconvergence or nonestimability issues, a ridge prior and a single model will be considered with treatment arm added as an explanatory variable to the model.

The remaining monotone missing data will be imputed using sequential regression multiple imputation, where a separate regression model is estimated for imputation of each variable (i.e., measurement at each time point). Each regression model will include explanatory variables for {list of baseline covariates}, treatment and all previous (Baseline, Visit x,...,y) values of measure1. No rounding or range restrictions will be applied to imputed continuous values.

Imputed data will consist of {MM} (e.g., 500) imputed data sets. The random seed number for partial imputation with the MCMC method will be {XXXXX}, and the random seed number for the sequential regression multiple imputation will be {YYYYYY}.

Each imputed data set will be analyzed using the following analysis method. Change in measure1 from baseline to each post-baseline visit will be based on observed and imputed data. {Insert description of analysis model/method, e.g., direct likelihood MMRM as described above, or ANCOVA.} Treatment group comparison at Visit T will be based on the least squares mean (LSM) difference between treatment groups in change from baseline in measure1 estimated by the analysis model in each of the imputed data sets. Results from analysis of each imputed data set, that is, LSM treatment differences and their standard errors, will be combined using Rubin's imputation rules to produce a pooled LSM estimate of treatment difference, its 95% confidence interval, and a pooled P-value for the test of null hypothesis of no treatment effect.

20.7 Power and Sample Size Considerations

Chapter 5 included a subsection illustrating how changes in variance components of a mixed-effects model influence parameter estimates and their uncertainty. A key implication of those illustrations was that variance components need to be considered when assessing power in planning longitudinal studies. Other key considerations in powering studies include the rate of missing data. It is intuitively easy to appreciate that the more missing data, the lower the power. Therefore, the impact to power and sample size from missing data should be considered in the protocol and some degree of protection against unexpectedly higher rates of dropout may be warranted.

Although a wide array of commercial software for power and sample size determination exist, simulation studies are fairly easy to conduct and often more useful. With fairly simple coding and reasonable compute times, flexible programs can be tailored to the specific circumstances at hand. The impact of correlation structure and missing data can be easily evaluated by changing the relevant input parameters. The need to maintain robustness to plausible departures from MAR could be addressed by including, for example, a delta-adjusted power/sample size. Results can be used to compare power for treatment main effects, interaction effects, or visit-wise contrasts. The impact of fitting versus not fitting a covariate can be assessed.

Clinical development in general relies increasingly on simulation studies to inform plans. Clinical trial simulation to inform power/sample size can be seen as simply one specific aspect of the general trend.

21

Example Analyses of Clinical Trial Data

21.1 Introduction

This chapter illustrates the analyses of longitudinal clinical trial data using the principles and recommendations outlined in previous chapters. The analyses conducted here are for illustration and should not be considered universal recommendations for similar situations. Data for these analyses are the so-called high and low dropout (large) data sets described in Chapter 4. Recall, these data are somewhat contrived for convenience, but were extracted from two real clinical trials and thus provide a useful illustration of analyses, model verification procedures, and sensitivity analyses. Parts of this example were previously reported in Molenberghs et al. (2015, chapter 22).

For this example, the primary objective was to compare treatment versus control in mean change from baseline to Week 8 on the Hamilton 17-item depression rating scale (Hamilton 1960). The primary analysis targeted a de jure (efficacy) estimand—the effects of the initially randomized medication if taken as directed; that is, estimand 3 described in Table 2.1. Effectiveness was assessed secondarily as the effects of the drug as actually taken; that is, estimand 2 described in Table 2.1. Post-rescue data were not collected in these studies. Therefore, it was not possible to assess the de facto treatment regimen estimand (estimand 1 in Table 2.1). Had post-rescue data been available, estimand 1 could have been evaluated using the same methods as for estimand 3. Additional details on descriptive, primary, and sensitivity analyses are provided below.

21.2 Descriptive Analyses

The number of observations by assessment time is summarized in Table 21.1.

Visit-wise mean changes for patients who completed the trials versus those who discontinued early were summarized by visit in Figures 4.1 and 4.2 for the low and high dropout data sets, respectively. In the high dropout

TABLE 21.1

Number of Observations by Week in the High and Low Dropout Data Sets

Week	High Dropout					Low Dropout				
	1	2	4	6	8	1	2	4	6	8
Placebo	100	92	85	73	60	100	98	98	95	92
Drug	100	91	85	75	70	100	98	95	93	92

data set, visit-wise mean changes for patients who discontinued early were less than for completers, suggesting that patients with poorer response were more likely to drop out; therefore, the missingness mechanism was unlikely MCAR. With only a few dropouts at each visit in the low dropout data set, trends were not readily identifiable.

21.3 Primary Analyses

To assess the primary de jure estimand, mean changes from baseline were analyzed using a restricted maximum likelihood (REML)-based repeated measures approach. The analysis included the fixed, categorical effects of treatment, investigative site (site), visit, treatment-by-visit interaction, and site-by-visit interaction, along with the continuous, fixed covariates of baseline score and baseline score-by-visit-interaction. An unstructured (co)variance structure was used to model the within-patient errors. The Kenward–Roger approximation was used to estimate denominator degrees of freedom. Significance tests were based on least-squares means using a two-sided $\alpha = 0.05$ (two-sided 95% confidence intervals). Analyses were implemented using SAS PROC MIXED (SAS 2013). The primary comparison was the contrast between treatments at Week 8.

Results from the primary analyses are summarized in Table 21.2. In the high dropout data set, the advantage of drug over placebo in mean change from baseline to Week 8 was 2.29 (SE = 1.00, P = 0.024). The corresponding results in the low dropout data set were 1.82 (SE = 0.70, P = 0.010). The standard error for the difference in lsmeans at Week 8 in the high dropout data set was nearly 50% larger than in the low dropout data set. This was partly due to the lower variability in the low dropout data set (see Table 21.4). The larger variability in the high dropout data set accounted for a 32% increase in standard error on its own. The additional increase in standard error in the high dropout data set came from the additional quantity of missing data.

The secondary, de facto estimand was assessed based on treatment success or failure. Treatment success was defined as improvement greater than or equal to 50% of the baseline severity and completion of the acute treatment phase. Any patient that discontinued study medication was considered

TABLE 21.2

Visit-Wise LSMEANS and Contrasts for $HAMD_{17}$ from the Primary
Analyses of the High and Low Dropout Data Sets

	LSMEANS		LSMEAN	Standard	
	Placebo	Drug	Difference[a]	Error	P
High Dropout					
Week 1	− 1.89	− 1.80	− 0.09	0.64	0.890
Week 2	− 3.55	− 4.07	0.52	0.81	0.518
Week 4	− 4.87	− 6.20	1.32	0.86	0.125
Week 6	− 5.51	− 7.73	2.22	0.93	0.019
Week 8	− 5.94	− 8.24	2.29	1.00	0.024
Low Dropout					
Week 1	− 2.22	− 1.76	− 0.45	0.38	0.235
Week 2	− 4.93	− 4.89	− 0.04	0.56	0.943
Week 6	− 7.79	− 8.31	0.52	0.61	0.392
Week 4	− 9.45	− 10.69	1.25	0.66	0.060
Week 8	− 10.57	− 12.39	1.82	0.70	0.010

[a] Advantage of drug over placebo. Negative values indicate an advantage for placebo.

TABLE 21.3

Percent Treatment Success for the De Facto Secondary Estimand in the
High and Low Dropout Data Sets

High Dropout Treatment Success (%)				Low Dropout Treatment Success (%)			
Placebo	Drug	Difference	P	Placebo	Drug	Difference	P
25	39	14	0.034	50	68	18	0.001

a treatment failure regardless of outcome. Treatment groups were compared
using Fisher's exact test. Results are summarized in Table 21.3.

Both trials yielded significant advantages of drug over control in percent
treatment success. The definition of the treatment success included completion, so there was no missing data and no need to assess sensitivity to missing data assumptions, per se. However, generalizability results should be
considered and it is still advisable to understand how changes in the rates of
dropout influence outcomes. The low dropout data set had greater within-
group mean changes in addition to greater adherence. It is unclear if or how
design differences may have influenced the within-group mean changes and
adherence. However, the two trials give different views of effectiveness. The
percent treatment success on placebo in the low dropout data set was twofold greater than in the high dropout data set.

21.4 Evaluating Testable Assumptions of the Primary Analysis

21.4.1 Sensitivity to Covariance Assumptions

Unstructured covariance matrices were used for the primary analyses. Correlations and (co)variances from the primary analyses of the high and low dropout data sets are summarized in Table 21.4.

Treatment contrasts from more general and more parsimonious covariance structures, with and without use of the sandwich estimator, are summarized in Table 21.5. In the high dropout data set, an unstructured matrix common to both treatment groups that was used as the primary analysis provided the best fit, thereby supporting results from the primary analysis as valid. However, the potential importance of choice of covariance structure with this high rate of dropout can be seen in the comparatively large range in treatment contrasts (1.69–2.29), standard errors and P-values across the covariance structures.

In the low dropout data set, the range in treatment contrasts across the covariance structures (1.76–1.85) was approximately six-fold smaller than in the high dropout data set, and all structures yielded a significant treatment contrast. Separate unstructured matrices by treatment group yielded the best fit, with the second best fit being from a single unstructured matrix that was specified as the primary analysis. The consistency of results across covariance structures indicates conclusions were not sensitive to correlation structure, thereby supporting validity of the primary analysis.

21.4.2 Residual and Influence Diagnostics—High Dropout Data Set

Given the comparatively small number of sites in these contrived data, influence of each site was investigated by removing sites one at a time and repeating the primary analysis on the data subsets. In scenarios with more sites, influence diagnostics as presented in Chapter 11 could be implemented to first identify influential sites and then repeat analyses deleting only the influential sites.

The influence option in the model statement of SAS PROC MIXED (SAS 2013) was used to determine which patients had the greatest influence on various aspects of the model. Results based on restricted likelihood distance (RLD) are discussed below. The RLD is a measure of influence on the objective function; that is, a measure of overall influence not specific to any particular model parameter. In addition, residual diagnostics were used to further identify unusual patients or individual observations.

Residual plots from the high dropout data set are shown in Figure 21.1. The upper left panel shows no association between magnitude of residual and magnitude of prediction, and no clear increase in variance across predicted values. The upper right and lower left panels suggest residuals satisfied normality assumptions.

Box plots of residuals for each treatment-by-time combination in the high dropout data set are shown in Figure 21.2. These plots suggest aberrant residuals

TABLE 21.4

Covariance and Correlation Matrices from the Primary Analyses of the High and Low Dropout Data Sets

	High Dropout					Low Dropout				
Week	1	2	4	6	8	1	2	4	6	8
(Co) variances										
1	20.16					7.22				
2	14.05	29.86				4.79	15.50			
4	11.55	19.74	32.09			3.87	11.54	18.07		
6	10.7	18.56	25.27	35.10		3.74	9.96	14.65	20.59	
8	11.51	17.67	22.57	30.88	39.55	2.23	7.03	10.73	16.61	22.82
Correlations										
1	1.000					1.000				
2	0.573	1.000				0.453	1.000			
4	0.454	0.638	1.000			0.339	0.689	1.000		
6	0.402	0.573	0.753	1.000		0.307	0.558	0.760	1.000	
8	0.408	0.514	0.634	0.829	1.000	0.174	0.374	0.528	0.766	1.000

TABLE 21.5

Treatment Contrasts from Alternative Covariance Matrices from the Primary Analyses

Structure[a]	AIC	Endpoint Contrasts	Standard Error	P
High Dropout				
UN	4679.82	2.29	1.00	0.024
UN EMPIRICAL	4679.82	2.29	0.97	0.020
TOEPH	4684.44	2.10	0.91	0.023
TOEPH EMPIRICAL	4684.44	2.10	0.92	0.023
TOEPH GROUP = TRT	4689.88	1.82	0.91	0.048
UN GROUP = TRT	4692.05	1.96	1.00	0.053
CSH	4735.81	1.86	0.93	0.047
CSH EMPIRICAL	4735.81	1.86	0.91	0.041
CSH GROUP = TRT	4739.34	1.69	0.93	0.070
Low Dropout				
UN GROUP = TRT	4861.70	1.85	0.703	0.009
UN	4867.68	1.82	0.699	0.010
UN EMPIRICAL	4867.68	1.82	0.666	0.007
TOEPH GROUP = TRT	4888.93	1.82	0.647	0.005
TOEPH	4897.89	1.79	0.649	0.006
TOEPH EMPIRICAL	4897.89	1.79	0.662	0.006
CSH	5030.40	1.76	0.705	0.013
CSH EMPIRICAL	5030.40	1.76	0.667	0.008
CSH GROUP = TRT	5031.92	1.80	0.708	0.011

[a] UN, unstructured; TOEPH, heterogeneous toeplitz; CSH, heterogeneous compound symmetric; GROUP = TRT means that separate structures were fit for each treatment group; Empirical means that empirical (sandwich-based) estimators of the standard error were used rather than the model-based standard errors.

were relatively rare compared to the total number of observations and that there was no systematic trend in the residuals, suggesting the model was appropriate.

RLDs for each patient in the high dropout data set are shown in Figure 21.3. The largest RLD values were approximately 2.0. Values of this magnitude generally suggest no individual patient had a large influence on the overall model.

Additional measures of influence (not presented here) include case deletion metrics based on Cook's D, as described in Chapter 11, to assess the influence of individual patients on each specific model parameter, including fixed effects and covariance parameters. No individual patient was found to have a large influence on any individual parameter.

21.4.3 Residual and Influence Diagnostics—Low Dropout Data Set

Residual and influence diagnostics for the low dropout data set were conducted as previously described for the high dropout data set. Residual plots

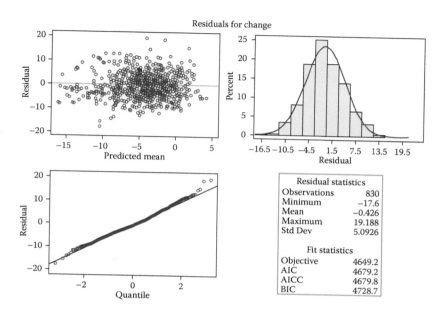

FIGURE 21.1
Residual plots for the high dropout data set.

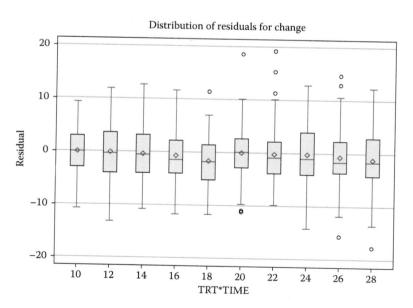

FIGURE 21.2
Box plots of residuals by treatment and time in the high dropout data set.

FIGURE 21.3
RLDs for influence of patients in the high dropout data set.

from the low dropout data set are shown in Figure 21.4. These figures show an unusual observation with a large residual. This value is seen in the upper left corner of the upper left panel, the residual–predicted value plot. This outlier is also seen in the far right tail of the residual histogram in the upper right panel, and in the upper right corner of the Q–Q plot in the lower left panel.

Box plots of residuals for each treatment-by-time combination in the low dropout data set are shown in Figure 21.5. These plots show the aberrant residual was in Treatment 2 at Week 8, an especially important finding because the primary analysis was the treatment contrast at Week 8. The magnitude of the aberrant residual was approximately twice that of the next largest residual.

RLDs for each patient in the low dropout data set are shown in Figure 21.6. The largest RLD value was, not surprisingly, from the same patient with the aberrant residual. This patient had an RLD of nearly 40, which was five-fold greater than the next largest RLD.

Additional measures of influence (not presented here) include case deletion metrics based on Cook's D, as described in Chapter 11, to assess the influence of individual patients on each specific model parameter, including fixed effects and covariance parameters. The influential patient identified above was influential on a number of fixed effect and covariance parameters, especially those involving Week 8.

The visit-wise data for the most influential patient is listed in Table 21.6. The data were unusual in several regards. The baseline HAMD score of 35

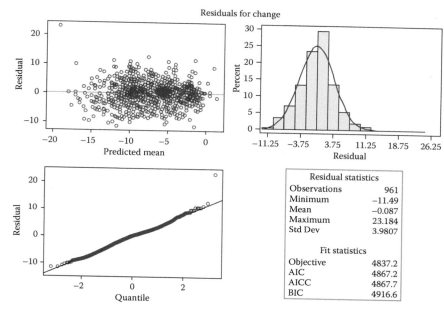

FIGURE 21.4
Residual plots for the low dropout data set.

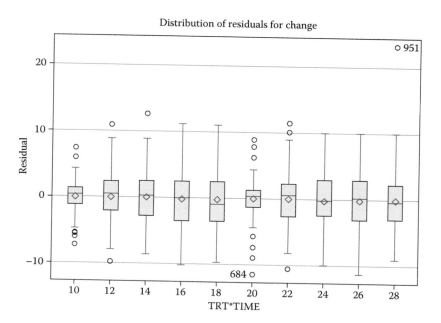

FIGURE 21.5
Box plots of residuals by treatment and time in the low drop out data set.

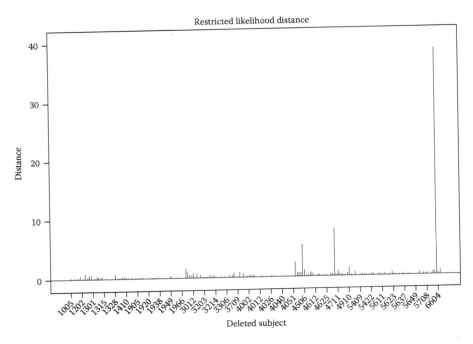

FIGURE 21.6
RLDs for the influence of each patient in the high dropout data set.

TABLE 21.6

Visit-Wise Data for the Most Influential Patient in the Low Dropout Data Set

Treatment	Site	Baseline HAMD	Time	HAMD Change	PGIIMP
2	141	35	1	−6	3
			2	− 7	5
			4	− 13	7
			6	− 18	7
			8	4	.

indicated this was one of the most severely ill patients. The patient had improvements at Weeks 1 through 6 that were greater than the group means. However, from Weeks 6 to 8 that patient had a marked worsening in condition, going from an improvement of 18 points to a worsening of 4 points. This 22-point change was the largest visit-to-visit change in the data set and was opposite in direction of other large changes. Interestingly, the patient-rated PGIIMP scores for this patient at Weeks 4 and 6 were 7, indicating a marked worsening; whereas, the corresponding clinician-rated HAMD scores showed improvement at those assessment times. At Week 8, the clinician-rated

HAMD scores reflected the worsening, and the PGIIMP score was missing. This unusual profile and the conflict between the clinician-rated HAMD scores and the patient-rated PGIIMP scores should trigger additional investigation. Entries in comment fields of case report forms and/or other site documentation could help lend insight into the situation.

21.4.4 Analyses with Influential Patients and Sites Removed

As previously noted, given the small number of sites, influence of each site was investigated by removing each site one at a time and repeating the primary analysis on the data subsets. In situations with more sites, influence diagnostics would be used to identify influential sites and the primary analysis repeated after removing each influential site. Emphasis was placed on the magnitude of change in the treatment contrasts rather than maintenance of statistical significance because of the markedly smaller sample size when a site was deleted. Results for this case deletion of sites are summarized in Table 21.7.

In the high dropout data set, deleting sites 003 and 028 decreased the treatment contrasts slightly. Deleting sites 005 and 001 increased the treatment contrasts slightly. Although statistical significance was lost when deleting site 003, this was due to the decreased sample size (nearly 300 observations removed) rather than a smaller treatment contrast. In the low dropout data set, deleting site 121 had the greatest effect on the treatment contrast. However, the treatment contrast remained significant. Therefore, statistical significance was not driven by a single site in either of these two data sets.

TABLE 21.7

Influence of Sites on Endpoint Contrasts in the High and Low Dropout Data Sets

Data Set	Numbers of		Endpoint Contrast	P
	Patients	Observations		
High Dropout				
All Data	200	830	2.37	0.021
Drop Site 005	175	723	2.96	0.008
Drop Site 001	165	684	2.78	0.013
Drop Site 028	159	677	2.18	0.049
Drop Site 003	132	536	2.27	0.079
Low Dropout				
All Data	200	961	1.85	0.008
Drop Site 121	167	801	1.56	0.047
Drop Site 131	145	694	1.82	0.028
Drop Site 141	147	710	2.10	0.005
Drop Site 101	141	678	1.77	0.044

The impact of influential patients was also assessed using a case deletion approach. However, all patients identified as influential were deleted by treatment group rather than one at a time, except for the most influential patient in the low dropout data set. In that instance results were repeated after removing just that one patient. Results from analyses of the primary outcome excluding influential patients are summarized in Table 21.8.

In the high dropout data set, the five most influential patients were investigated; two were randomized to the drug arm and three to placebo. Dropping placebo-treated influential patients decreased the endpoint contrast slightly. Dropping drug-treated influential patients increased the endpoint contrast slightly, as did dropping all influential patients.

In the low dropout data set, the six most influential patients were investigated; two were randomized to the drug arm and four to placebo. Dropping all placebo-treated influential patients decreased the endpoint contrast. Dropping all drug-treated influential patients increased the endpoint contrast, as did dropping all influential patients. Dropping only patient 6602, the most influential patient, resulted in a comparatively large increase in the treatment contrast and a decrease in the standard error. Patient 6602 had a very unusual response profile, which resulted in noticeable reductions in magnitude and precision of the estimated treatment contrast.

Observations with a studentized residual ≥ 2.0 or ≤ -2.0 were considered aberrant. The primary analysis was repeated with all observations from drug-treated patients having aberrant residuals removed, with all observations from placebo-treated patients having aberrant residuals removed, and deleting all the observations having aberrant residuals. Results are summarized in Table 21.9.

TABLE 21.8

Endpoint Contrasts for All Data and for Data with Influential Patients Removed from the High and Low Dropout Data Sets

Data Set	Numbers of Patients	Observations	Endpoint Contrast	P
High Dropout				
All Data	200	830	2.29	0.024
Drop All	195	808	2.50	0.015
Drop Drug	198	823	2.59	0.010
Drop Placebo	197	815	2.21	0.032
Low Dropout				
All Data	200	961	1.82	0.010
DROP 6602	199	956	2.07	0.002
Drop All	194	931	1.97	0.003
Drop Drug	196	941	1.97	0.003
Drop Placebo	198	951	1.80	0.011

TABLE 21.9

Endpoint Contrasts for All Data and Data with
Subjects Having Aberrant Residuals Removed
from the High and Low Dropout Data Sets

	Number of Observations	Endpoint Contrast	P
High Dropout			
All Data	830	2.29	0.024
Drop All	796	2.42	0.009
Drop Drug	809	2.57	0.006
Drop Placebo	817	2.13	0.035
Low Dropout			
All Data	961	1.82	0.010
Drop All	915	1.92	0.002
Drop Drug	938	2.16	0.001
Drop Placebo	938	1.59	0.019

In both the high dropout and low dropout data sets, excluding all placebo-treated patients with aberrant residuals decreased the endpoint contrast. Excluding drug-treated patients and all patients with aberrant residuals increased the endpoint contrast. However, changes in the treatment contrasts were small. Given the decrease in sample size due to excluding patients, influence on the treatment contrast is best judged by changes in magnitude rather than statistical significance. However, preservation of statistical significance for the treatment effect provided an extra level of assurance that outlier patients did not influence inferences.

21.5 Sensitivity to Missing Data Assumptions

21.5.1 Introduction

In this section, a variety of MNAR approaches are implemented to assess the sensitivity of results from the primary analysis to departures from MAR. In practice, not all these approaches would be needed. As illustrated in Chapter 18, controlled imputation approaches to sensitivity analyses are easy to understand and implement. For this reanalysis, the marginal delta-adjustment approach was chosen as the primary basis upon which sensitivity was assessed. Results from other MNAR approaches are included for illustration.

The intent is not to imply that delta adjustment is always the best choice for assessing sensitivity. Rather, the intent is to illustrate the general attributes of a variety in methods while also implementing a decision-making framework that would be useful in realistic scenarios.

21.5.2 Marginal Delta Adjustment

The marginal delta adjustment approach was implemented similar to the approach utilized in Code Fragment 18.1. In the present application, $m = 100$ imputations was shown to stabilize results and therefore each delta adjustment analysis used 100 imputed data sets. Results from applying marginal delta-adjustment to the high and low dropout data sets are summarized in Table 21.10. In the marginal approach, the delta adjustment at one visit does not influence imputed values at other visits. Results from using delta = 0 (i.e., no adjustment, the MAR result) are included for reference. The MAR (delta = 0) results differ slightly from the primary results in Table 21.2 because the primary result was generated using direct likelihood and the delta = 0 results in Table 21.10 are based on multiple imputation.

Deltas were progressively increased in the tipping-point format to identify the magnitude of delta needed to overturn the primary results. Delta = 2 was a particularly informative choice because that delta was approximately equal to the treatment effect and therefore is a useful reference point in gauging plausibility of a departure from MAR (Permutt 2015b). Specifically, a delta equal to the average treatment effect would typically be considered a plausible departure, but perhaps the largest plausible departure.

Using delta = 2, the endpoint contrast was significant in the low dropout data set, but significance was lost in the high dropout data set. In fact, delta = 1 was sufficient to overturn significance in the high dropout data set. In the low dropout data set, delta = 7 was required to overturn significance.

TABLE 21.10

Results from Marginal Delta-Adjustment Multiple Imputation—Delta Applied on Last Visit to Active Arm Only

	Low Dropout Data Set			High Dropout Data Set		
Value of Delta Adj	Endpoint Contrast	Standard Error	P	Endpoint Contrast	Standard Error	P
0	1.86	0.70	0.008	2.27	1.12	0.042
1	1.79	0.70	0.011	1.96	1.13	0.083
2	1.71	0.70	0.015	1.64	1.14	0.151
3	1.64	0.71	0.201			
4	1.57	0.71	0.027			
5	1.50	0.72	0.037			
6	1.42	0.72	0.049			
7	1.35	0.73	0.065			

Increasing the delta applied to the endpoint visit had a consistent and therefore predictable effect on the endpoint contrasts. For each 1-point increase in delta, the endpoint contrast was decreased by approximately 0.08 points in the low dropout data set and by approximately 0.30 points in the high dropout data set. As discussed in Chapter 18, this systematic change is intuitive in that 8% of the values were missing for Treatment 2 at endpoint in the low dropout data set, and 30% of the values were missing for Treatment 2 in the high dropout data set.

As discussed in Chapter 18, the effect of a marginal delta adjustment on the endpoint contrast can be analytically determined as follows:

$$\text{Change to the endpoint contrast} = \Delta \times \pi$$

where π = the percentage of missing values and Δ = the marginal delta adjustment

These results help reinforce the straightforward and easy to understand nature of marginal delta adjustment. First, there is a direct correspondence between the fraction of missing values and the sensitivity of results to departures from MAR. If π is cut in half, Δ will have half the effect on the endpoint contrast. In addition, progressively increasing delta results in predictable and easy to understand changes in the endpoint contrasts that make for a useful stress test to ascertain how severe departures from MAR must be in order to overturn inferences from the MAR result.

21.5.3 Conditional (Sequential) Delta Adjustment

Results from conditional (sequential) delta adjustment are summarized in Table 21.11. In conditional delta adjustment, imputations are done sequentially, visit-by-visit, with patients' delta-adjusted imputed data contributing to imputed values at subsequent visits. The net effect of sequential imputation is that when deltas are applied to each visit, they have an accumulating effect such that patients who drop out earlier have larger "net" deltas (indicating a more severe departure from MAR) than patients who drop out later.

TABLE 21.11

Results from Delta-Adjustment Multiple Imputation—Delta Applied on All Visits After Discontinuation to Active Arm Only

Value of Delta Adj	Low Dropout Data Set			High Dropout Data Set		
	Endpoint Contrast	Standard Error	P	Endpoint Contrast	Standard Error	P
0	1.85	0.71	0.009	2.31	1.02	0.024
0.5	1.77	0.71	0.013	2.00	1.03	0.051
2.0	1.52	0.73	0.037			
2.5	1.44	0.74	0.051			

In the high dropout data set, the delta = 0.5 points on the $HAMD_{17}$ overturned the primary result (P > 0.05). The endpoint contrast changed 0.62 for each 1-point change in delta. The corresponding tipping point in the low dropout data set was 2.5 points, with the endpoint contrast changing 0.16 for each 1-point change in delta.

In the conditional approach, the impact of delta for a patient in the drug group withdrawing at Week 2 was the accumulation of an increment of approximately delta × 1 + the sum of the correlations between Week 2 and subsequent visits. That is, delta × (1 + 0.51 + 0.63 + 0.83) = 2.97 in the high dropout data set. An early dropout therefore had a nearly threefold greater accumulation—and therefore larger impact—than missing data at the last visit only.

In the conditional approach, it is still possible to analytically derive the impact of a particular delta, but the calculations are more involved. The net effect of a conditional delta can be approximately explained using the accumulations described above, as applied to each assessment week, and the number of subjects discontinuing at each week, divided by the total number of subjects: $0.5 × (9 × 2.97 + 6 × 2.46 + 10 × 1.83 + 5 × 1)/100 = 0.32$. The corresponding tipping point in the low dropout data set was 2.5 points with a shift of 0.41, which is approximately explained as $2.5 × (2 × 2.66 + 3 × 2.29 + 2 × 1.77 + 1 × 1)/100 = 0.42$.

In marginal delta adjustment, each patient has the same impact on the endpoint contrast and it is therefore easier to understand the impact of any particular delta. In conditional delta adjustment, the impact on the endpoint contrast is not the same for each patient—it varies by time of dropout. If the same delta is applied at each visit in the conditional approach, patients dropping out earlier have a greater impact on the endpoint contrast because the "net" delta has a greater accumulation over visits.

21.5.4 Reference-Based Controlled Imputation

Results from reference-based imputation analyses are summarized in Table 21.12. Recall that the jump to reference approach (J2R) assumes the benefit of the drug immediately disappears after discontinuation or rescue; copy reference (CR) assumes a decaying benefit; and copy increment from reference (CIR) assumes a constant benefit. For these data, J2R is a reasonable worst plausible case sensitivity analysis. That is, if results from J2R were significant, then results from the primary analysis could be declared robust to plausible departures from MAR. Results were also assessed using CR and CIR for illustration. Analyses were conducted using the SAS macros made available freely to the public by the Drug Information Association's (DIA) Scientific Working Group for missing data at www. missingdata.org.uk.

As expected, treatment contrasts from J2R were smaller than from CR, and the treatment contrasts from CR were smaller than CIR. Also as expected, the J2R results closely mirror results from marginal delta-adjustment when delta is approximately equal to the mean difference between treatments.

TABLE 21.12

Results from Reference-Based Multiple Imputation of the High and Low Dropout Data Sets

	LSMEAN Changes		Endpoint Contrast	Standard Error	P
	Placebo	Drug			
High Dropout					
MAR	− 5.95	− 8.24	2.29	1.00	0.024
J2R	− 5.97	− 7.57	1.60	0.99	0.110
CR	− 5.96	− 7.71	1.75	0.98	0.075
CIR	− 5.95	− 7.78	1.83	0.97	0.040
Low Dropout					
MAR	− 10.56	− 12.40	1.84	0.70	0.009
J2R	− 10.55	− 12.26	1.71	0.70	0.016
CR	− 10.55	− 12.27	1.72	0.70	0.015
CIR	− 10.55	− 12.27	1.72	0.70	0.015

In the high dropout data set, the endpoint contrast from J2R was 1.60 (SE = 0.99, P = 0.110). In the low dropout data set, the endpoint contrast from J2R was 1.71 (SE = 0.70, P = 0.016). The difference from MAR was approximately sixfold smaller in the low dropout data set than in the high dropout data set. Statistical significance was preserved in the low dropout data set, but not for the high dropout data set.

21.5.5 Selection Model Analyses

A selection model was fit in which the parameters describing the MNAR part of the model were varied. The primary outcome was assessed using a repeated measures model similar to the primary analysis, and the probability of dropout was simultaneously modeled using a logistic regression that fit the log odds of dropout as a function of visit, separate intercepts (Ψ_1, Ψ_2) for each treatment group, and separate linear regression coefficients for previous (Ψ_3, Ψ_4) and current (possibly unobserved) efficacy outcomes (Ψ_5, Ψ_6). Hence, the outcome variable from the measurement model was a covariate in the dropout model. Fitting separate missingness models for each treatment allowed for different departures from MAR for drug and placebo groups. Analyses were implemented using macros made available freely to the public by the DIA Scientific Working Group for missing data at www. missingdata.org.uk.

The parameters Ψ_5 and Ψ_6 were of particular interest because they were the "MNAR" part of the model. These values assess the change in log odds for withdrawal per unit increase in the outcome measure. A value of 0.2 indicated that the odds of withdrawal increased by a factor 1.22 ($e^{0.2}$) for each 1-point change on the $HAMD_{17}$. Setting Ψ_5 and $\Psi_6 = 0$ was important

TABLE 21.13

Results from Selection Model Analyses of High Dropout Data Set

Input Values		Week 8 LSMEANS		Endpoint	Standard	
$\Psi_5{}^a$	$\Psi_6{}^a$	Placebo	Drug	Contrast	Error	P
0.2	0.2	4.87	7.33	2.46	1.09	0.023
0.0	0.2	5.60	7.38	1.78	1.05	0.091
−0.2	0.2	6.28	7.41	1.18	1.05	0.282
−0.4	0.2	6.76	7.42	0.66	1.06	0.527
0.2	0.0	4.94	7.97	3.03	1.07	0.005
0.0[b]	0.0	5.63	8.00	2.37	1.04	0.022
−0.2	0.0	6.29	8.04	1.75	1.02	0.087
−0.4	0.0	6.75	8.05	1.30	1.02	0.204
0.2	−0.2	4.97	8.57	3.60	1.06	0.001
0.0	−0.2	5.67	8.57	2.89	1.03	0.004
−0.2	−0.2	6.31	8.59	2.29	1.01	0.024
−0.4	−0.2	6.76	8.63	1.86	1.01	0.064
0.2	−0.4	4.97	8.97	4.01	1.07	<0.001
0.0	−0.4	5.68	8.96	3.28	1.03	0.002
−0.2	−0.4	6.33	8.98	2.64	1.01	0.009
−0.4	−0.4	6.78	9.01	2.22	1.01	0.027

[a] Ψ_5 and Ψ_6 are the regression coefficients (placebo and drug, respectively) for the association between the current, possibly missing efficacy scores and the logit for probability of dropout.

[b] Results differ from the primary result because the baseline value by site interaction was not fit in the selection model.

because the missingness and outcome models become independent and the model reduces to the MAR model in the primary analysis.

Results from selection model analyses of the high dropout data set with varying levels of both Ψ_5 and Ψ_6 are summarized in Table 21.13. These results are used to illustrate general aspects of selection model results. Subsequently, selection models are implemented in a tipping point approach for both the high dropout and low dropout data sets.

As expected, when $\Psi_5 = \Psi_6 = 0$, results matched results from the primary direct likelihood analysis. With negative values for Ψ_5 and Ψ_6, the within-group mean changes were greater than the mean changes when assuming MAR ($\Psi_5 = \Psi_6 = 0$). Conversely, positive values for Ψ_5 and Ψ_6 led to smaller within-group mean changes. A positive Ψ value implied that patients with negative residuals were more likely to drop out, leading to greater mean changes observed in the remaining data, with the selection model compensating for this by reducing the lsmean.

When there is more dropout in the placebo group and $\Psi_5 = \Psi_6 < 0$, the within-group mean change increased more in the placebo group than the drug group and the endpoint contrast was reduced. Conversely with $\Psi_5 = \Psi_6 > 0$, the endpoint contrast was increased. However, it is important to notice that whenever $\Psi_5 = \Psi_6$, that is, when the same MNAR model is assumed for both treatment arms, the impact of MNAR on the treatment contrast was fairly small.

When the input values for Ψ_5 and Ψ_6 differed, between-group differences (endpoint contrasts) followed a consistent pattern dictated by the within-group changes previously noted. Whenever Ψ_6 (the regression coefficient for the drug group) was less than Ψ_5 (the regression coefficient for the placebo group), the treatment contrast was greater than from the MAR primary analysis. When Ψ_5 was greater than Ψ_6, the treatment contrast was smaller than in MAR.

An understanding of these relationships can be used to systematically vary Ψ_5 and Ψ_6 in a selection model to generate departures from MAR in a tipping point approach. Results from a selection model tipping point sensitivity analyses are summarized in Table 21.14. A value of $\Psi_5 = 0$ was used to assume MAR for the placebo group. Recall that standard implementations of delta-adjustment and reference-based controlled imputations assume MAR for placebo. Values of Ψ_6 were progressively changed to create increasing departures from MAR that reduced the treatment contrasts. In the high dropout data set, $\Psi_6 = 0.2$ overturned the primary result. In the low dropout data set, $\Psi_6 > 1.0$ was required to overturn the primary result.

Although selection models can be used in a tipping point approach much the same way as delta-adjustment, judging the plausibility of departures from MAR is more complex in selection models. The regression coefficients (Ψ) in selection models are on the log odds scale. Judging plausibility therefore requires judging plausibility of changes in log odds per unit change in the (possibly unobserved) outcome measure.

TABLE 21.14

Results from Tipping Point Selection Model Analyses of High Dropout and Low Dropout Data Sets

Input Values		Low Dropout Data Set		High Dropout Data Set	
Ψ_5[a]	Ψ_6[a]	Endpoint Contrast	P	Endpoint Contrast	P
0	0.0	1.81	0.008	2.29	0.019
0	0.2	1.72	0.012	1.62	0.114
0	0.4	1.64	0.018	–	–
0	0.6	1.54	0.028	–	–
0	0.8	1.48	0.036	–	–
0	1.0	1.41	0.047	–	–

[a] Ψ_5 and Ψ_6 are the regression coefficients (placebo and drug, respectively) for the association between the current, possibly missing efficacy scores and the logit for probability of dropout.

For example, the value of Ψ that was sufficient to overturn the primary result in the high dropout data set was 0.2. This result indicated that if the odds of dropout increased by a factor 1.22 for each 1-point change on the current, possibly missing $HAMD_{17}$ score, the primary result would be overturned. The value of Ψ that was needed to overturn the primary result in the low dropout data set (>1.0) indicated that the odds of dropout had to increase approximately three-fold for each 1-point change in the current, possibly missing $HAMD_{17}$ in order to overturn the primary results.

With mean baseline scores of 20 and standard deviations >5, a 1-point change in HAMD is a small change. Therefore, the three-fold increase in odds of withdrawal per 1-point change in HAMD needed to overturn results in the low dropout data set doesn't seem plausible. Results in the low dropout data set appear to be robust to plausible departures from MAR.

In the high dropout data set, results are less clear. The key question is whether it is plausible that the odds of withdrawal could increase by a factor of 1.22 for each 1-point change in HAMD. This setup is less intuitive and transparent than in delta adjustment, where plausibility simply requires judging the magnitude of delta.

21.5.6 Pattern Mixture Model Analyses

Results from pattern-mixture model (PMM) analyses under various identifying restrictions are summarized in Table 21.15. Analyses were conducted using the macros made available freely to the public by the DIA Scientific Working Group for missing data at www.missingdata.org.uk.

Three identifying restrictions were implemented. The ACMV restriction assumed MAR, whereas CCMV and NCMV assumed MNAR. Therefore, comparing results from ACMV with those from other restrictions assessed the impact of departures from MAR.

Pattern mixture model analysis requires that all parameters are estimable in all patterns of dropouts. For analysis of the high dropout data set, sites had to be pooled into two grouped sites. Analysis of the low dropout data

TABLE 21.15

Results from Pattern-Mixture Model Analyses of High Dropout Data Set

Identifying Restriction	Endpoint Contrast	Standard Error	P
ACMV	2.67	1.17	0.022
CCMV	2.51	1.05	0.016
NCMV	2.87	1.69	0.089

Note: ACMV = available case missing values, CCMV = complete case missing values, NCMV = neighboring case missing values.

set was not feasible because, with so few missing observations, the treatment effect was not estimable in all dropout patterns.

Compared with ACMV, the endpoint contrast and standard error in the high dropout data set were slightly smaller in CCMV and larger in NCMV. Notice the large standard error for the NCMV result. Even with a high rate of dropout, the number of patients in certain patterns was limited, which in turn reduced precision of results, leading to a nonsignificant contrast even though the point estimate was larger than in ACMV.

21.6 Summary and Drawing Conclusions

21.6.1 Overview

The preceding examples from the high and low dropout data sets illustrated some fundamental points in analyzing longitudinal data. The primary analysis focused on a precisely defined estimand, in this instance a de jure estimand. Aspects of the model that could be evaluated from observed data were checked. Sensitivity analyses were used to aid understanding of the degree to which departures from MAR for the unobserved data could alter inferences from the primary analysis. A secondary estimand from the de facto family was also evaluated.

These illustrations were not intended to be general prescriptions or specific recommendations. The intent was to illustrate general approaches and considerations. Certainly, other approaches could be considered in these situations. And other situations could require different approaches.

Perhaps the most important aspect of these illustrations was the benefit from lower rates of missing data. Although this chapter in particular—and this book in general—focuses on analytic methods, the inescapable conclusion is that analyses can only assess sensitivity. Preventing missing data is the only way to improve sensitivity to missing data assumptions.

Importantly, the greater variability in results across various model assumptions from the high dropout data set was not limited to sensitivity analyses for plausible MNAR scenarios. Results from some of the standard diagnostics, such as choice of covariance structure, also showed greater variability with higher dropout.

21.6.2 Conclusions from the High Dropout Data Set

The primary analysis yielded a statistically significant result. Residual diagnostics showed no evidence that nonnormality or nonlinearity had an appreciable influence on results, thereby suggesting the model was appropriate. No patients or sites were found to have had a strong influence on results. The unstructured covariance specified in the primary analysis provided the best fit to the data.

However, the possibility of plausible departures from MAR overturning the primary result could not be entirely ruled out. Evidence for a treatment effect was supported by significance on the secondary de facto estimand.

The decision we would make from these analyses is that treatment was significantly better than placebo. However, we recognize the difficulty in making black and white decisions, and that others could come to a different decision. Again, the most important aspect of the illustration is not the decision itself, but rather the process for arriving at it.

21.6.3 Conclusions from the Low Dropout Data Set

The primary analysis yielded a statistically significant result. Residual diagnostics showed one clear outlier but no evidence that nonnormality or nonlinearity systematically influenced results, thereby suggesting the model was appropriate. Influence diagnostics also noted the aberrant patient with a very large residual. The RLD for this patient suggested it had an appreciable influence on results. However, that patient had an unfavorable outcome in the treatment group and therefore deleting data from that patient increased the magnitude and significance of the primary result. No one site had an undue influence on results. The unstructured covariance specified in the primary analysis provided one of the best fits to the data and significance of the primary result was insensitive to choice of covariance structure. Inferences from the primary analysis were robust to even the largest plausible departures from MAR.

Model diagnostics and sensitivity analyses, combined with a low rate of missing data, confirm the robustness of these results. Therefore, the decision we would make from these analyses is that treatment was significantly better than placebo.

References

Agresti A. (2002). *Categorical Data Analysis*. 2nd edition. New York: Wiley.

Alosh M, Kathleen F, Mohammad H, et al. (2015). Statistical considerations on subgroup analysis in clinical trials. *Statistics in Biopharmaceutical Research*, 7(4): 1–68. DOI: 10.1080/19466315.2015.1077726.

Ayele B, Lipkovich I, Molenberghs G, et al. (2014). A multiple-imputation-based approach to sensitivity analyses and effectiveness assessments in longitudinal clinical trials. *Journal of Biopharmaceutical Statistics*, 24(2):211–228.

Barnes SA, Carter K, Lindborg SR, et al. (2008). The impact of missing data and how it is handled on the rate of false positive results in drug development. *Pharmaceutical Statistics*, 7:215–225.

Buncher C. Ralph, Tsay J-Y. (2005). *Statistics in the Pharmaceutical Industry*. 3rd edition. New York: Chapman Hall.

Cao W, Tsiatis AA, Davidian M. (2009). Improving efficiency and robustness of the doubly robust estimator for a population mean with incomplete data. *Biometrika*, 96:723–734.

Carpenter JR, Kenward MG. (2007). Missing data in clinical trials|a practical guide. Birmingham: National Health Service Coordinating Centre for Research Methodology. Freely downloadable from http://www.pcpoh.bham.ac.uk/publichealth/methodology/projects/RM03 JH17 MK.shtml (accessed 28 May 2009).

Carpenter JR, Kenward MG, Vansteelandt S. (2006). A comparison of multiple imputation and doubly robust estimation for analyses with missing data. *Journal of the Royal Statistical Society, Series A*, 169:571–584.

Carpenter JR, Roger J, Kenward M. (2013). Analysis of longitudinal trials with protocol deviation: A framework for relevant, accessible assumptions, and inference via multiple imputation. *Journal of Biopharmaceutical Statistics*, 23(6):1352–1371.

Collins LM, Schafer JL, Kam CM. (2001). A comparison of inclusive and restrictive strategies in modern missing data procedures. *Psychological Methods*, 6(4):330–351.

Committee for Medicinal Products for Human Use (CHMP). (2010). Guideline on missing data in confirmatory clinical trials. EMA/CPMP/EWP/1776/99 Rev. 1.

Crowe B, Lipkovich I, Wang O. (2009). Comparison of several imputation methods for missing baseline data in propensity scores analysis of binary outcome. *Pharmaceutical Statistics*, 9:269–279.

Crump SL. (1947). *The Estimation of Variance in Multiple Classification*, PhD thesis, Department of Statistics, Iowa State University.

Daniel RM, Kenward MG. (2012). A method for increasing the robustness of multiple imputation. *Computational Statistics & Data Analysis*, 56(6):1624–1643. ISSN 0167-9473.

Detke MJ, Wiltse CG, Mallinckrodt CH, et al. (2004). Duloxetine in the acute and long-term treatment of major depressive disorder: A placebo- and paroxetine-controlled trial. *European Neuropsychopharmacology*, 14(6):457–470.

Diggle PD, Kenward MG. (1994). Informative dropout in longitudinal data analysis (with discussion). *Applied Statistics*, 43:49–93.

Diggle PJ, Heagerty P, Liang KY, et al. (2002). *The Analysis of Longitudinal Data.* 2nd edition. Oxford, England: Oxford University Press.

Efron B. (1994). Missing data, imputation, and the bootstrap. *Journal of the American Statistical Association*, 89(426):463–475.

Fedorov VV, Liu T. (2007). Enrichment Design, in *Wiley Encyclopedia of Clinical Trials*. Ralph D'Agostino, Lisa Sullivan, and Joe Massaro (eds.), Hoboken: John Wiley & Sons, Inc. pp. 1–8.

Firth D. (1993). Bias reduction of maximum likelihood estimates. *Biometrika*, 80:27–38.

Fisher RA. (1925). *Statistical Methods for Research Workers*. London: Oliver and Boyd. Gallant.

Fitzmaurice GM, Laird NM, Ware JH. (2004). *Applied Longitudinal Analysis*. Hoboken, NJ: Wiley Interscience.

Fitzmaurice GM, Molenberghs G, Lipsitz SR. (1995). Regression models for longitudinal binary responses with informative dropouts. *Journal of the Royal Statistical Society, Series B*, 57:691–704.

Flemming TR. (2011). Addressing missing data in clinical trials. *Annals of Internal Medicine*, 154:113–117.

Garrett A. (2015). Choosing appropriate estimands in clinical trials (Leuchs et al.): Letter to the editor. *Therapeutic Innovation & Regulatory Science*, 49(4):601.

Goldstein DJ, Lu Y, Detke MJ, et al. (2004). Duloxetine in the treatment of depression: A double-blind placebo-controlled comparison with paroxetine. *Journal of Clinical Psychopharmacology*, 24:389–399.

Graham JW, Olchowski AE, Gilreath TD. (2007). How many imputations are really needed? Some practical clarifications of multiple imputation theory. *Prevention Science*, 8:206–213.

Guy W. (1976). *ECDEU Assessment Manual for Psychopharmacology*. Rockville, MD: National Institute of Mental Health. pp. 217–222, 313–331.

Hamilton M. (1960). A rating scale for depression. *Journal of Neurology, Neurosurgery & Psychiatry*, 23:56–61.

Hartley HO, Rao JNK. (1967). Maximum-likelihood estimation for the mixed analysis of variance model. *Biometrika*, 54:93–108.

Harville DA. (1977). Maximum likelihood approaches to variance component estimation and to related problems. *Journal of the American Statistical Association*, 72:320–338.

Harville DA. (1988). Mixed-model methodology: Theoretical justifications and future directions, Proceedings of the Statistical Computing Section, American Statistical Association, New Orleans, 41–49.

Harville DA. (1990), BLUP (Best Linear Unbiased Prediction), and Beyond, in *Advances in Statistical Methods for Genetic Improvement of Livestock*, D. Gianola (eds.). Berlin: Heidelberg, Springer-Verlag. pp. 239–276.

Henderson CR. (1953). Estimation of variance and covariance components. *Biometrics*, 9:226–252.

Henderson CR. (1984). *Applications of Linear Models in Animal Breeding*. University of Guelph, Ont: University of Guelph.

Henning Z. (2011). Paracetamol and the placebo effect in osteoarthritis trials: A missing link? *Pain Research and Treatment*. Article ID 696791, 6, DOI: 10.1155/2011/696791.

Hogan JW, Laird NM. (1997). Mixture models for the joint distribution of repeated measures and event times. *Statistics in Medicine*, 16:239–258.

Holubkov R1, Dean JM, Berger J, et al. (2009). Is "rescue" therapy ethical in randomized controlled trials? *Pediatric Critical Care Medicine*, 10(4):431–438. DOI: 10.1097/PCC.0b013e318198bd13.

Horvitz DG, Thompson DJ. (1952). A generalization of sampling without replacement from a finite universe. *Journal of the American Statistical Association*, 47:663–685.

Hughes S, Harris J, Flack N, et al. (2012). The statistician's role in the prevention of missing data. *Pharmaceutical Statistics*, 11:410–416.

Hurvich CM, Tsai C-L. (1989), Regression and time series model selection in small samples. *Biometrika*, 76:297–307.

ICH guidelines. Available at: http://www.ich.org/fileadmin/Public_Web_Site/ICH_Products/Guidelines/Efficacy/E9/Step4/E9_Guideline.pdf, Accessed on July 14, 2015.

ICH guidelines. Available at: http://www.ich.org/fileadmin/Public_Web_Site/ICH_Products/Guidelines/Efficacy/E10/Step4/E10_Guideline.pdf, Accessed on July 14, 2015.

Jansen I, Beunckens C, Molenberghs G, et al. (2006). Analyzing incomplete binary longitudinal clinical trial data. *Statistical Science*, 21(1):52–69.

Jennrich RI, Schluchter MD. (1986). Unbalanced repeated measures models with structural covariance matrices. *Biometrics*, 42(4):805–820.

Kang DY, Schafer JL. (2007). Demystifying double robustness: A comparison of alternative strategies for estimating a population mean from incomplete data (with discussion and rejoinder). *Statistical Science*, 22:523–539.

Kenward MG, Molenberghs G. (2009). Last observation carried forward: A crystal ball? *Journal of Biopharmaceutical Statistics*, 19:872–888.

Laird NM. (1994). Discussion to Diggle PJ, Kenward MG. Informative dropout in longitudinal data analysis. *Applied Statistics*, 43:84.

Laird NM, Ware JH. (1982). Random-effects models for longitudinal data. *Biometrics*, 38:963–974.

Lane PW. (2007). Handling drop-out in longitudinal clinical trials: A comparison of the LOCF and MMRM approaches. *Pharmaceutical Statistics*, 7(2):93–106. (early view) DOI: 10.1002/pst.267.

Langley RG, Ellis CN. (2004). Evaluating psoriasis with Psoriasis area and severity index, Psoriasis Global Assessment, and Lattice System Physician's Global Assessment. *Journal of American Academy of Dermatology*, 51:563–569.

LaVange LM. Permutt T. (2015). A regulatory perspective on missing data in the aftermath of the NRC report. *Statistics in Medicine*, 35(17):2853–2864. DOI: 10.1002/sim.6840.

Leuchs AK, Zinserling J, Brandt A, et al. (2015). Choosing appropriate estimands in clinical trials. *Therapeutic Innovation and Regulatory Science*, 49(4):584–592.

Liang KY, Zeger SL. (1986). Longitudinal data analysis using generalized linear models. *Biometrika*, 73:13–22.

Liang KY, Zeger SL. (2000). Longitudinal data analysis of continuous and discrete responses for pre-post designs. *Sankhya: The Indian Journal of Statistics*, 62(Series B):134–148.

Lindstrom MJ, Bates DM. (1988). Newton–Raphson and EM algorithms for linear mixed-effects models for repeated-measures data. *Journal of the American Statistical Association*, 83:1014–1022.

Lipkovich I, Duan Y, Ahmed S. (2005). Multiple imputation compared with REPL and GEE for analysis of binary repeated measures in clinical studies. *Pharmaceutical Statistics*, 4:267–285.

Lipkovich I, Kadziola Z, Xu L, et al. (2014). Comparison of several multiple imputation strategies for repeated measures analysis of clinical scales: Truncate or not to? *Journal of Biopharmaceutical Statistics*, 24:924–943.

Lipkovich I, Ratitch B, O'Kelly M. (2016). Sensitivity to censored-at-random assumption in the analysis of time-to-event endpoints. *Pharmaceutical Statistics*, 15:216–229.

Little RJA. (1993). Pattern-mixture models for multivariate incomplete data. *Journal of American Statistical Association*, 88(421):125–134.

Little RJA. (1994). A class of pattern-mixture models for normal incomplete data. *Biometrika*, 81(3):471–483.

Little RJA. (1995). Modeling the drop-out mechanism in repeated measures studies. *Journal of American Statistical Association*, 90(431):1112–1121.

Little RJA, Rubin DB. (1987). *Statistical Analysis with Missing Data*. 1st edition. New York: Wiley.

Little RJA, Rubin DB. (2002). *Statistical Analysis with Missing Data*. 2nd edition. New York: Wiley.

Little R, Yau L. (1996). Intent-to-treat analysis for longitudinal studies with drop-outs. *Biometrics*, 52(4):1324–1333.

Liu GF, Kaifeng L, Robin M, et al. (2009). Mehrotra. Should baseline be a covariate or dependent variable in analyses of change from baseline in clinical trials? *Statistics in Medicine*, 28:2509–2530.

Mallinckrodt CH. (2013). *Preventing and Treating Missing Data in Longitudinal Clinical Trials: A Practical Guide*. New York: Cambridge University Press.

Mallinckrodt CH, Clark WS, Carroll RJ, et al. (2003). Assessing response profiles from incomplete longitudinal clinical trial data under regulatory conditions. *Journal of BioPharmaceutical Statistics*, 13(2):179–190.

Mallinckrodt CH, Kenward MG. (2009). Conceptual considerations regarding choice of endpoints, hypotheses, and analyses in longitudinal clinical trials. *Drug Information Journal*, 43(4):449–458.

Mallinckrodt CH, Lane PW, Schnell D, et al. (2008). Recommendations for the primary analysis of continuous endpoints in longitudinal clinical trials. *Drug Information Journal*, 42:305–319.

Mallinckrodt CH, Lin Q, Lipkovich I, et al. (2012). Structured approach to choosing estimands and estimators in longitudinal clinical trials. *Pharmaceutical Statistics*, 11:456–461.

Mallinckrodt CH, Rathmann S, Molenberghs G. (2016). Choosing estimands in clinical trials with missing data. *Pharmaceutical Statistics*. DOI: 10.1002/pst.

Mallinckrodt CH, Roger J, Chuang-Stein C, et al. (2014). Recent developments in the prevention and treatment of missing data. *Therapeutic Innovation and Regulatory Science*, 48(1):68–80.

McCullagh P, Nelder JA. (1989). *Generalized Linear Models*. 2nd edition. London: Chapman and Hall.

McLean RA, Sanders WL. (1988). Approximating degrees of freedom for standard errors in mixed linear models, Proceedings of the Statistical Computing Section, American Statistical Association, New Orleans, 50–59.

Meng XL. (1994). Multiple imputation with uncongenial sources of input (with discussions). *Statistical Science*, 9:538–574.

Molenberghs G, Fitzmaurice G, Kenward M, et al. (2015). *Handbook of Missing Data Methodology*. Boca Raton, FL: CRC Press.

Molenberghs G, Kenward MG. (2007). *Missing Data in Clinical Studies*. Chichester: Wiley.

Molenberghs G, Kenward MG, Lesaffre E. (1997). The analysis of longitudinal ordinal data with nonrandom dropout. *Biometrika*, 84(1):33–44.

Molenberghs G, Thijs H, Jansen I, et al. (2004). Analyzing incomplete longitudinal clinical trial data. *Biostatistics*, 5(3):445–464.

Molenberghs G, Verbeke G. (2005). *Models for Discrete Longitudinal Data*. New York: Springer.

National Research Council (2010). *The Prevention and Treatment of Missing Data in Clinical Trials*. Panel on Handling Missing Data in Clinical Trials. Committee on National Statistics, Division of Behavioural and Social Sciences and Education. Washington, DC: The National Academies Press.

O'Kelly M, Ratitch B. (2014). Clinical trials with missing data. Chichester: Wiley.

O'Neill RT, Temple R. (2012). The prevention and treatment of missing data in clinical trials: An FDA perspective on the importance of dealing with it. *Clinical Pharmacology and Therapeutics*, 91(3):550–554.

Patterson HD, Thompson R. (1971). Recovery of inter-block information when block sizes are unequal. *Biometrika*, 58:545–554.

Permutt T. (2015a). A taxonomy of estimands for regulatory clinical trials with discontinuations. *Statistics Med*. DOI: 10.1002/sim.6841.

Permutt T. (2015b). Sensitivity analysis for missing data in regulatory submissions. *Statistics Med*. DOI: 10.1002/sim.6753.

Phillips A, Abellan-Andres J, Andersen S. et al. (2016). Pharmaceutical Statistics, accepted. Estimands: Discussion Points from the PSI Estimands and Sensitivity Expert Group.

Piantadosi S. (2005). *Clinical Trials: A Methodologic Perspective*. New York: Wiley.

Prasad NGN, Rao JNK. (1990). The estimation of mean squared error of small-area estimators. *Journal of the American Statistical Association*, 85:163–171.

Ratitch B, O'Kelly M. (2011). Implementation of pattern-mixture models using standard SAS/STAT Procedures. PharmaSUG. Available at http://pharmasug.org/proceedings/2011/SP/PharmaSUG-2011-SP04.pdf, (accessed 4 October 2011).

Robins JM, Rotnitzky A. (1995). Semiparametric efficiency in multivariate regression models with missing data. *Journal of American Statistical Association*, 90:122–129.

Robins JM, Rotnitzky A, Zhao LP. (1995). Analysis of semiparametric regression models for repeated outcomes in the presence of missing data. *Journal of the American Statistical Association*, 90:106–121.

Robins JM, Wang N. (2000). Inference for imputation estimators. *Biometrika*, 87:113–124.

Robinson GK. (1991). That BLUP is a good thing: The estimation of random effects. *Statistical Science*, 6: 15–51.

Rubin DB. (1976). Inference and missing data. *Biometrika*, 63(3):581–592.

Rubin DB. (1978). Multiple imputations in sample surveys—a phenomenological Bayesian approach to nonresponse. In: *Imputation and Editing of Faulty or Missing Survey Data*. Washington, DC: U.S. Department of Commerce, pp. 1–2.

Rubin DB. (1987). *Multiple Imputation for Nonresponse in Surveys*. New York: Wiley.

SAS Institute Inc. 2013. *SAS/STAT® 9.4* User's Guide. Cary, NC: SAS Institute Inc.

Schafer JL. (1997). *Analysis of Incomplete Multivariate Data*. New York: Chapman & Hall.

Schafer JL. (2003). Multiple imputation in multivariate problems when the imputation and analysis models differ. *Statistica Neerlandica*, 57:19–35.

Seaman S, Copas A. (2009). Doubly robust generalized estimating equations for longitudinal data. *Statistics in Medicine*, 28:937–955.

Searle SR. (1971). *Linear Models*. New York: Wiley.

Siddiqui O, Hung HM, O'Neill RO. (2009). MMRM vs. LOCF: A comprehensive comparison based on simulation study and 25 NDA Datasets. *Journal of Biopharmaceutical Statistics*, 19(2):227–246.

Snedecor GW, Cochran WG. (1980). *Statistical Methods*. Ames, IO: Iowa State University Press.

Stroup WW. (1989). Predictable functions and prediction space in the mixed model procedure, in *Applications of Mixed Models in Agriculture and Related Disciplines*, Southern Cooperative Series Bulletin No. 343, Louisiana Agricultural Experiment Station, Baton Rouge, pp. 39–48.

Tanner MA, Wong WH. (1987). The calculation of posterior distributions by data augmentation. *Journal of the American Statistical Association*, 82:528–540.

Temple R. (2005). Enrichment designs: Efficiency in development of cancer treatments. *Journal of Clinical Oncology*, 23(22):4838–4839.

Thompson WA. (1962). The problem of negative estimates of variance components. *Annals of Mathematical Statistics*, 33:273–289.

Tsiatis AA. (2006). *Semiparametric Theory and Missing Data*. New York: Springer.

Tsiatis AA, Davidian M, Cao W. (2011). Improved doubly robust estimation when data are monotonely coarsened, with application to longitudinal studies with dropout. *Biometrics*, 67:536–545.

Van Buuren S. (2007). Multiple imputation of discrete and continuous data by fully conditional specification. *Statistical Methods in Medical Research*, 16:219–242.

Van Buuren S. (2012). *Flexible imputation of missing data*. Boca Raton, FL: CRC Press.

Van Buuren S, Groothuis-Oudshoorn K. (2011). mice: Multivariate imputation by chained equations in R. *Journal of Statistical Software*, 45(3):1–67.

Vansteelandt S, Carpenter J, Kenward MG. (2010). Analysis of incomplete data using inverse probability weighting and doubly robust estimators. *Methodology: European Journal of Research Methods for the Behavioral and Social Sciences*, 6(1):37–48.

Verbeke G, Molenberghs G. (2000). *Linear Mixed Models for Longitudinal Data*. New York: Springer.

Verbeke G, Molenberghs G, Thijs H, et al. (2001). Sensitivity analysis for nonrandom dropout: A local influence approach. *Biometrics*, 57(1):7–14.

Wang N, Robins JM. (1998). Large-sample theory for parametric multiple imputation procedures. *Biometrika*, 85:935–948.

Wonnacott TH, Wonnacott RJ. (1981). *Regression: A Second Course in Statistics*. New York: Wiley.

Wu MC, Bailey KR. (1989). Estimation and comparison of changes in the presence of informative right censoring: Conditional linear model. *Biometrics*, 45(3):939–955.

Wu MC, Carroll RJ. (1988). Estimation and comparison of changes in the presence of informative right censoring by modeling the censoring process. *Biometrics*, 44:175–188.

Index

Energy and Analytics

BIG DATA and
Building Technology Integration

John J. "Jack" Mc Gowan, CEM

River Publishers

Routledge
Taylor & Francis Group

LONDON AND NEW YORK

Energy and Analytics / John J. McGowan.

First published by Fairmont Press in 2015.

Published 2020 by River Publishers
River Publishers
Alsbjergvej 10, 9260 Gistrup, Denmark
www.riverpublishers.com

Distributed exclusively by Routledge
4 Park Square, Milton Park, Abingdon, Oxon OX14 4RN
605 Third Avenue, New York, NY 10017

First issued in paperback 2023

Routledge is an imprint of the Taylor & Francis Group, an informa business

Copyright © 2015 River Publishers.

Library of Congress Cataloging-in-Publication Data

McGowan, John J., 1950-
    Energy and analytics : BIG DATA and building technology integration / John J. "Jack" McGowan, CEM.
        pages cm
    Includes bibliographical references and index.
    ISBN 0-88173-744-5 (alk. paper) -- ISBN 978-8-7702-2325-6 (electronic) -- ISBN 978-1-4987-4429-4 (Taylor & Francis distribtion : alk. paper) 1. Buildings--Energy conservation. 2. Energy auditing--Data processing. 3. Buildings--Energy consumption--Data processing. 4. Big data. I. Title.

TJ163.5.B84M395 2015
696.0285'57--dc23

                                                                    2015015301

ISBN 13: 978-87-7022-933-3 (pbk)
ISBN 13: 978-1-4987-4429-4 (hbk)
ISBN 13: 978-1-00-315194-4 (ebk)

Dedicated

to
Judy
...with the love of a lifetime
and gratitude for your support in all things.

Table of Contents

Author's Note on How this Book is Organized

Given the complex nature of the energy and analytics topic, and the content provided here, it is appropriate to briefly discuss the format and use of this book. Energy management in the 21st century is being influenced by wide ranging policy, business and technology trends; none more significant than analytics and big data. Building owners, operators and Certified Energy Managers (CEM) can easily be daunted by the complexity of analytics implementations, as they entail a number of steps to fully leverage the opportunity. An important factor is that energy and analytics technology cannot produce optimum results, unless it can access an underlying fabric of building/energy technology, and that technology must be fully interoperable and operational. This simple fact explains a great deal about the organization of this book.

This book is organized in three sections. Section I is an introduction to and thorough treatment of the energy and analytics market opportunity. Chapters 1 through 7 define analytics and related technology available in the market today, as well as how they may be leveraged for optimum economic value. Equally important, it articulates the energy context, which primarily involves electricity. Electricity is the highest quality form of energy because it offers the cleanest and most diverse use. It is essential to business, education and entertainment, and the buildings in which all of these industries operate. This is because electricity is the primary energy source for the information economy, powering smart phones, tablets, computers, the "Cloud" and everything in between. In other words, electricity is central to the 21st century lifestyle, and Section I also describes changes in the way electricity is purchased and sold, which demands analytics technology. An important note for this section, and those that follow, is that every effort was made to arrange content in the best order possible, so that more general topics are covered prior to more complex. The idea is to start with a high-level view of the market, industry and technology, and then progress to discussions of how this technology may be used for critical applications.

Section II of the book focuses on the fabric of underlying building and energy technology that is critical for analytics to drive maximum value. Because these topics are both interdependent with, and essential to, energy and analytics, they warrant an introduction from one of the most influential people in building systems, Ken Sinclair, founder of www.automatedbuildings.com. His knowledge of building automation systems (BAS) and energy engineering is unparalleled, making him uniquely qualified to introduce Chapters 8 through 18. He can also provide insight on how these technologies are interconnected and interoperable, and what that can mean for energy and analytics. These underlying systems must exist to capture enough data for meaningful analytics. In many cases they are also required to execute the changes in building operations and energy consumption recommended by analytics engines. Chapters in this section discuss the full range of technologies that are critical to effective implementation of energy and analytics, as well as related topics including the Internet of Things (IoT), financing for energy projects, and measurement and verification.

Section III of the book offers case studies in energy and analytics, to provide a glimpse of what success looks like. James M. Lee, CEO of Cimetrics, Inc., has decades of real world experience with analytics, as it is discussed here. No one is better able, than Mr. Lee to write an introduction to the topic of analytics success. These chapters present readers with real examples of how this technology is producing dramatic results in a wide range of building and campus types. Mr. Lee has perhaps the longest and most technically diverse tenure in this industry, while also being one of its most successful business leaders. Under Mr. Lee's leadership Cimetrics, Inc., has deployed, and been an industry leader, in energy and analytics solutions. These projects span a wide range of applications including: large campuses with a who's who of higher education, public and private hospitals, industrial/pharmaceutical facilities, and a wide range of buildings. The stories in these chapters also come from all types of buildings and campuses, and show what is possible with energy and analytics. These are but a glimpse of the operations and business value of this technology, and the breadth of applications to which it's been applied.

PROFESSIONAL ACKNOWLEDGEMENTS

Over nearly four decades working with energy, buildings and technology is has been my sincere honor to meet and work with thought leaders, visionaries and exceptional professionals from across multiple industries.

There are a number of these people without whom this book could not have been written. Particular thanks are due to:

John Petze for writing the Book Foreword, and for making contributions to my work based on his knowledge and business acumen in the form of; written material, edits and an unparalleled industry perspective. **Jim Lee** for writing the Case Study Foreword and for his amazing industry insights, as well as his contribution of written material, and for sharing his incomparable perspective on the far reaching impacts that this technology is having on many industries. Thanks also to Jim's team at Cimetrics including **Mary Ellen Cantabene, Karim Bibawi** and **David Landman** for their contributions. **Ken Sinclair** for writing the Technology Section Foreword and for making the most significant advancement to the automation industry in decades, through creation of www.automatedbuildings.com. This book drew from his writings on automatedbuildings, as well as from articles published there by Anno Scholten, Jim Sinopoli and Nirosha Munasinghe. **Anno Scholten,** in particular is a true visionary and serial entrepreneur in the building intelligence and energy space. Ken Sinclair has attracted a host of gifted writers such as those above to www.automatedbuildings.com. His vision in starting an Internet-based magazine, industry portal and worldwide gathering place nearly twenty years ago is a marvel. **Glen Allmendinger** for sharing a wealth of business and technology knowledge in his excellent chapter on the Internet of Things. **Leighton Wolffe** for allowing the ESCO 2.0 work to be incorporated with the finance chapter, and to Leighton and **Peter Kelly-Detwiler** for sharing their vision for the future of electricity that influenced the chapter on that topic. **Professor Jim Lee** and his team at the University of Louisiana at Lafayette for the Six Sigma chapter. **Kurt Yeager** for introducing me to **Bob Galvin** and for giving me the opportunity to work with them for three years. Their passion for excellence, and for the transformation of the electricity business, provided major inspiration for this book. Their selfless sharing of that vision for the future was critical to forming this view of a 21st Century Electric System. **Tom Shircliff** for sharing what the future for Smart Cities can be, in his chapter on Envision Charlotte. **Darell Smith** for taking that Smart City view to the next level, by showing how corporations and cities could join forces to change the world, in the chapter on Microsoft 88 acres. **Ron Rajecki and Contracting business** for inclusion of the Smart Grid Smart People story that is so illustrative of success for these ideas and technologies. **Pat**

Gibson and Luanne Garcia, partners and friends who made it possible for me to pursue excellence, and create projects that exemplified my vision for the future, in the form of projects, business and technology. **Dave Flood, John Christensen, Andy Watson, Bobbie Gutierrez, Leslie Carpenter, Lisa Randall, Don Swick and Andrea Mammoli, PhD** are also important to thank as visionary executives and building managers, who embraced the leading edge in energy management and sustainability, and who I had the great honor to serve with exciting projects. **Brian Goodchild, John Nicholls, Scot Stickle, Jay Garbarino and Drew Perrin** at Delta Controls Inc. and Coppertree Analytics for sharing content and industry perspectives selflessly to improve this book. **Nick Michaels** for his vision, courage and singular business skill. **Jim Young and Howard Berger** for creating the premier industry venue for building intelligence, in Realcomm and IBcon, allowing professionals to share insight and success. **Anto Budiarjo** for vision and fortitude in setting the bar for what a truly excellent industry event should be, and for continuing that work with www.PointView.com. **Bob Graves** of the Governing Institute for inviting me to speak and participate with them in Energy Roundtables around the country, that made it possible to interact with cities pursuing excellence in energy initiatives. **Julia Burrows,** Director of the Governing Institute for continuing to include me with Big Data programs and as an advisor on the Institutes work in the pursuit of infrastructure renewal. **Jim Heath** for his vision and exceptional business and finance acumen in creating a solar business model like no other. **Santa Fe Mayor Javier Gonzales** for his vision, resolve and leadership in creating a ground breaking initiative, called the Climate Action Task Force, to create an unparalleled vision for the future, and for giving me the incomparable opportunity to work on energy and sustainability at the community level. The Mayor-appointed Co-Chairs; **City Councilor Peter Ives and Former Mayor David Coss,** who working together with **Director of Utilities Nick Schiavo and Renewable Energy Planner John Alejandro** assembled an unparalleled team including: **Randy Grissom, Beth Beloff, David Van Winkle, Kathleen Holian, Glenn Schiffbauer, Rob Hirsch, Regina Wheeler, David Breeker, Harold Trujillo, Craig O'Hare and Linda Smith. Eric Lightner,** visionary leader of the U.S. Department of Energy (DOE) Smart Grid task force. **Steve Widergren, Rik Drummond, Lynne Kiesling, Tracy Markie, Wade Troxell, Alison Silverstein, Richard Schomberg, Nora Mead Brownell, Erich Gunther, Dave Cohen, Ron Ambrosio, Ward Camp, Tracy Markie** for their leadership and contributions as members of the DOE GridWise Architecture Council. **Dave Frederick** for his dedication and taking on the leadership of Energy Control. **Bruce Cantrell** for founding a business in ECI that was ideally positioned for growth, and infusion of new leadership, but never lost sight of the customer. **Rob Masinter** for his tenacity in pursuing a deal and his insatiable appetite to understand businesses and markets. **Barney Capehart** for graciously allowing me to use John Petze's chapter from his book. **Mahesh Ramanujam** and **Brendan Owens** at USGBC for the vision to see the next frontier for green buildings in PEER and acquiring **John Kelly** and his team from the Galvin Electricity Initiative to lead the effort. **Marc Petock** for being the distinguished gentleman of building technology and for generously sharing his knowledge of the industry. **Terry Swope** and his team at LynxSpring including **Bob Mealey**. **Greg Dixon** of EnerNOC for sharing industry insight and allowing me to speak and participate in EnergySmart events. **B. Scott Muench** for his amazing technical prowess and having the unique combination of tech smarts with sales and marketing skill.

Part I— Foreword

By John Petze

There can be no turning back. The age of data has arrived and not a moment too soon for the buildings that provide the environment for our modern lives.

For decades now we have witnessed the development of building systems that attempt to exploit the power of the microprocessor to deliver better performance. Analog controls became digital, sensors became more precise, controllers became networked and connected to computer screens so we could "see" what our systems were doing—in 32 million colors no less. Each technological advance promised the potential to improve the operation of our facilities and reduce energy costs, yet the consistency of those results has never met our expectations.

Throughout this digital evolution, however, I think it is fair to say that few of us saw the impact that the data produced by these systems would have. That is changing. The growing realization of the value of the data produced by building equipment systems is creating growing interest from owners and operators, along with the hype and confusion attendant to all new technologies. Its especially fitting then that one of the most respected energy engineers of our times is now tackling the topic to bring clarity and understanding to the people responsible for designing, constructing, operating and maintaining the facilities we live, work, learn and play in.

The reality is that the people responsible for managing buildings rarely have the time to be expert in all of the systems and technologies that populate their buildings. And they shouldn't have to. Instead, they need to be able to rely on trusted experts to guide and advise them and insure that all of this promising technology operates effectively. Those experts in turn have a responsibility to use good engineering principles to insure their recommendations and counsel are correct. Fundamental to achieving that goal is the need to use data to continuously validate and verify the results of their designs, control strategies and recommendations. In short, we have an obligation to use data effectively. While it could be argued that this obligation isn't new, what is new is that technology has given us the tools to do that effectively and consistently.

1

The explosion of data available from the myriad "smart devices" found in today's buildings demands a convergence—bringing together, or perhaps forcing together, professionals with different knowledge, training, experiences and responsibilities—a shotgun marriage of IT, mechanical, control, and financial disciplines. Only through the combined efforts of all parties involved in the process of designing, building and operating buildings can we achieve the efficiency and sustainability that investors, operators, occupants and society deserve. It is a fundamental responsibility that requires we effectively use this new data resource.

Buildings are complex. No one knows it all—although Jack does come close. Enjoy the read. You will profit greatly from it.

John Petze, C.E.M., is a partner at SkyFoundry, the developers of SkySpark®, analytics for building, energy and equipment data. John has over 30 years of experience in building automation, energy management and the Internet of Things, having served in senior positions for manufacturers of hardware and software products including: President & CEO of Tridium, VP Product Development for Andover Controls, and Global Director of Sales for Cisco Systems Smart and Connected Buildings group. At SkyFoundry he helps owners take advantage of advanced operational analytics to create truly intelligent buildings.

Chapter 1

The 21st Century
Energy Marketplace and Facilities

The energy marketplace has seen dramatic changes over the last three decades. A combination of market and business developments have occurred, but these have been complimented by explosive growth in technology. Information technology (IT) has been at the center of many of these changes, and in particular web services, but those developments are only part of the story. Focal points for this book will be around energy, particularly electricity, and the impact that the deregulation of electricity had on nearly half of the United States, and on the internet with web enablement of nearly every piece of building equipment, especially with the internet of things. Completely intertwined with that discussion of web services and the internet for the world wide web, is coverage of data communication standards for all of the equipment inside the building, and the opportunities that these developments present for building managers as well as business managers. Standards covered here, in particular BACnet for BAS and web services for nearly everything, have made it possible to both communicate with, and extract data from, any piece of equipment or building. The focus here is on deriving value from this data-rich environment through analytics, which is the latest technology development taking advantage of IT and the internet for energy management. The term "big data" has received huge attention across many domains in recent years. Most consumers seem to understand the notion of using information to track buying preferences, similar to the way companies like Amazon.com™ do, and then using those data to enhance the buying process. Most people have had the experience of searching for a book online, and then being contacted later with a recommendation for a book they might like. With energy, a similar set of opportunities exists to improve value, but analytics is much more than a trend, it is actually a crescendo of technological development that has unified systems throughout the energy and buildings landscape, with

3

particular emphasize on electricity. Recovery from the great economic downturn that began in 2008 was slow and arduous. This affected building managers trying to get approval for capital renewal, and it affected businesses alike. Analytics has been a great opportunity to bring value in an environment where managers wanted to do more with less, and it appealed to both groups. The idea of managing and measuring buildings to a set of key performance indicators (KPIs) has also been very appealing to building owners and operators.

Analytics brought value to owners in many ways, but in general there have been four predominant applications for the technology:

- Energy management,
- Fault detection and diagnostics (FD&D),
- Regulatory compliance, and
- Meeting organizational objectives

This book focuses primarily on the energy application for analytics, but that topic closely aligns with FD&D because equipment, whether mechanical or electrical, accounts for the vast majority of energy consumption in buildings.

Energy management is a primary use for analytics technology, and will be covered in great detail throughout the book, beginning with the next chapter. That chapter, entitled 4^{Plex} Energy™, begins to define the complexity that is found in the 21st century energy marketplace, and the value that analytics technology can offer. This topic is the next generation of enterprise energy management, and is being integrated into a wide range of energy services. The goal of this book is to open the reader's eyes to the significant opportunity that this technology can offer.

Analytics for fault diagnostics and detection (FD&D) may be the first topic readers think of when energy and analytics is mentioned. FD&D is an excellent application for analytics, especially relating to heating ventilation and air conditioning (HVAC), because of the complexity associated with equipment control and operation, as well as the environmental control of buildings for comfort, indoor air quality and cost.

Analytics for regulatory compliance is another related topic, particularly with FD&D. Perhaps the best example of this would be joint commission compliance requirements for hospitals. Joint commission evaluates hospitals for accreditation and certification based upon meeting certain performance standards. There are numerous examples of buildings that must meet a performance standard to be licensed, to meet health or other codes, and for many other reasons. Analytics is a highly effective way to establish performance and to document it over time, when regulatory compliance is required. In many respects this process is similar to energy or FD&D, and in many cases compliance means operating equipment to meet certain environmental or other conditions. In that way, using analytics for regulatory compliance is not unlike the above. However, since the focus here is on energy, details relating to the use of analytics to meet compliance are not be covered in this book.

Meeting organizational objectives and key performance indicators (KPIs) is the last common use of analytics. The objectives may relate to measurement of certain aspects of a facility such as sustainability. Tracking carbon emissions, etc. can be done very easily using analytics. This is because energy consumption units for customer facilities are already in the database, so it is a simple calculation to assess carbon. This creates real synergy between energy analytics and sustainability. Another example of organizational objective is vendor performance. Many managers have realized that it is possible to develop a vendor oversight program using analytics. Consider the example of an HVAC service contractor that the owner wanted to evaluate. Measurable data are already being captured by analytics regarding environmental quality, equipment runtime, energy consumption or repair intervals. It is possible to develop rules that can be evaluated based on operational data and very quickly indicate how well the vendor is performing. There are any number of similar organizational objectives that may lend themselves to analytics. Again, since the focus here is on energy, details relating to the use of analytics to meet compliance will not be covered in this book.

Dashboards are a final related topic to energy and analytics. A dashboard of some type is typically integrated with energy and analytics technology, and these will be discussed further throughout the book.

To simplify discussion of the complex array of systems deployed as analytics systems, a blanket term, *"energy and analytics,"* will be used here. Energy and analytics will be the lens through which technology and operational discussions unfold throughout the book. Electricity is the highest quality form of energy, which makes it most essential for a 21st century quality of life, including technology for education, business and entertainment. At the heart of this discussion is a new marketplace that reflects human lifestyle changes, but equally important, it also reflects major changes in how electricity is used and where it is generated. The key technology to unlocking the economic value presented by this new market is analytics, coupled with an understanding of both building technology and electricity markets.

As a founding member and chairman emeritus of the U.S. Department of Energy GridWise Architecture Council, the author had the opportunity to play a role in shaping the evolution of this new electricity market and the technology that has come to make up the smart grid. As an energy manager for more than three decades, participating in development of BAS, open systems, energy management and data standards, the author also saw the evolution in those disciplines and was able to apply this knowledge to the smart grid. This combination of experiences has been ideal for positioning the author to understand this rich landscape of opportunity and share it with the reader. However the landscape is even more complex because the energy, automation and smart grid evolutions occurred during a time of huge growth in two other areas—electricity and the internet. With electricity, onsite electric generation from renewables and conventional sources has grown dramatically. The onsite generation trend was driven by a series of factors, like climate change and energy resiliency after a series of "super storms." Starting with the massive power outage on the eastern seaboard of the U.S. in 2003 and continuing with climate change and resiliency issues, these issues with electricity resulted in wide ranging new government policy that shaped the development of this new electricity marketplace. Without effective access to and use of information, or analytics, it is not possible for managers to leverage the full economic value of technology-enabled building/energy management and onsite generation that are the hallmarks of this new electricity marketplace. Understanding how to capitalize on this new marketplace requires fluency with the technology, which is the purpose of this book. More importantly, this book is about the power of the information that resides in buildings, all of the new electricity technology, and how that information can be manipulated in an automated fashion to enhance operations and optimize the economics associated with running an enterprise.

This chapter introduces the overarching topic of buildings and energy/electricity management along with the power of analytics. The evolution of the technologies, systems, and business rules that govern the marketplace presents both opportunities and challenges for managers. These managers realize that it is critical to integrate systems for seamless facility operation, but also to provide access to lucrative utility markets that offer significant cost savings for smart buyers. Part one of this book will begin to outline the new *electric reality* that will be referred to as 4^{plex} *energy systems*. Energy, building and campus managers are among those professionals who face daunting challenges as they work to operate increasingly complex facility energy systems.

The author coined the term *"4^{plex} Energy Systems"* to describe the new electricity environment, and analytics is a key topic because effective systems operation requires sophisticated analysis. Managing these systems orchestrates power and energy use from four sources:

1. Power from local utility,
2. Power purchased from electric retailer,
3. Onsite generation from solar and other systems,
4. Efficiency *PLUS* demand response and market participation including bidding in synchronized, day-ahead, and real time markets.

Chapter 2 will provide a more detailed discussion of 4^{plex} energy systems.

With regard to the new energy marketplace, the reader might ask what are analytics and why should we care. These topics will be explored in detail, but quite simply, analytics are software systems that perform analyses on operational information, in the form of electronic data from many sources. The analyses compare actual operating data to "rules," which indicate ideal operating conditions. The result of these analyses is that analytics change data into knowledge. This knowledge allows a system manager to evaluate performance and to take action to improve performance, creating economic value. The energy and analytics payday is one reason this topic is so important. This payday comes from efficiency cost savings that are achieved through optimization of energy use, but it can also come from the cost benefits available from participation in the deregulated electricity market. In this market, legislative and regulatory policy has been enacted that requires utilities to pay energy users for changing electricity usage patterns through demand response (DR) and to buy electric capacity that is offered to the grid. Building and Certified Energy Managers (CEMs) can utilize sophisticated building automation systems (BAS) to participate in these programs. They can also use power from onsite generation to operate more cost effectively, and to sell power back to the grid.

To truly leverage the power of analytics, readers must develop a good working knowledge of a significant number of technology topics that are covered in this book. With the advent of smart grid and the growing predominance of high-speed data communications in most homes, much of this technology is being deployed residentially as well. That is why Part II of this book will provide a thorough treatise on these technologies. Among these technologies are building automation systems, data communications and networking, and "Middleware." Pervasive standards for data communications, such as BACnet, are the price of entry for buildings to be active participants in new energy markets. Middleware involves a new class of technology products, which allows owners to "integrate" legacy BAS systems with new standard systems, but also opens access to a host of other system integrations.

The reader may already be aware that building systems are made of a set of complex technologies which in many cases operate independently. The movement toward integrated, or smart connected, systems via middleware and web access presents that opportunity for a wealth of building information. Yes, this information is disparate, coming from many independent systems, and it comprises huge volumes of data that can be daunting as well. The first task is to distill the volumes of data into knowledge. For example, 15-minute-interval data on electric demand from a utility revenue meter just looks like an array of numbers. An energy manager's skilled eye can make sense of those data, but these professionals don't have time if it is necessary to review tens or hundreds of meters, each with 35,000 interval data points per year (4-15 minute reading per hour x 24 hours x 365 days). Analytics software, on the other hand, can analyze those data to determine when peak consumption occurs and whether those times are appropriate electronically. With this information it is possible for the energy manager to focus on anomalies that may be pointed out by the analytics. Energy and analytics tools have been developed to sit at a higher level of the architecture, above the building systems, to access data from those systems, and to perform analyses. Again the volume of data is daunting, so these systems can identify problems and see opportunities that the manager cannot identify in any other way.

In the past, a major obstacle to deploying this type of building analysis has been the cost associated with implementing instrumentation at every piece of equipment, deploying data communication networks to transport those data, and finally deploying a highly sophisticating processing engine to conduct analysis. All of those factors translated to very high cost. Energy and analytics as discussed in this book sit at a nexus of technology development that has made it possible to overcome all of those past challenges and to unlock the value that the technology can offer. Cloud computing, the internet, data communication standards, and web services are among the 21st century technologies that have removed the obstacles to implementation of analytics. Through this book analytic architecture will be discussed in detail to clarify systems technology options. This is particularly important as managers consider integration using middleware, web services and software as a service (SaaS)—alternatives that are common in the world of analytics. All of these options create specific requirements for analytics technology, making it essential for this book to discuss them along with the evolution of standards for networking and the internet.

Case studies highlighting successful analytics applications will be covered in Part III of this book. Common applications for this technology were discussed earlier in this chapter, and this book focuses on energy and analytics. Professionals are demanding tools and technology to drive positive energy results in this complex business and technology environment for buildings and campuses. In the face of that demand, the market has responded with a barrage of evolving hardware, software, and web services, making decisions about which analytics tools are best challenging. This book will address that topic under the chapter on analytics tools, but will also provide case studies showing successful implementation of the technology. Managers want to achieve optimal energy efficiency and also get the maximum useful life from current equipment and technology investments. There is no better alternative to achieve such goals in today's market than energy and analytics.

Chapter 2

4PLEX Energy

The energy commodity business (sale of units of any type of energy) has seen a number of technology waves and engineering evolutions over the decades. Whether the reader is a building operator, Certified Energy Manager (CEM), engineer or other professional dealing with a single building/campus, overseeing multiple buildings, or a consultant keeping pace with technology that is barraging the industry is a *resource* challenge.

As discussed in Chapter 1, energy and analytics encompasses a wide range of technology; however, the focus for technologies to be discussed here is on energy and buildings. Energy and analytics offer a wide range of application functionality, and these technologies typically include the analytics algorithms, as well as dashboards to visualize reports. This overarching topic of energy and analytics is a monster trend impacting energy, buildings and large-scale energy management across one or many facilities. Considering that approximately ±70% of the energy consumption in buildings is electricity begs the question, how can energy and analytics technology support managing and reducing that consumption? The answer to that question may become clear if that discussion emphasizes the *"EcoImprint" (EI)* of buildings and campuses. EI is more than a carbon footprint, which implies local impact only. EI takes into account the far reaching impact of electricity. The imprint for electricity, as an energy resource is unique, because it leaves very little imprint where it is used, rather it leaves an imprint tens or hundreds of miles away where it is generated, transmitted and distributed. The imprint also extends to where the source energy (i.e., coal) for the generation is extracted as well. A major driver for President Obama's Clean Energy Plan, which was announced by the Environmental Protection Agency (EPA) in June of 2014, was the realization that coal-fired power plants have a significant carbon footprint. This is therefore about a far reaching resource impact, but eco in this case has two meanings. First it refers to the <u>eco</u>logical (environmental and climate) impact that the full electricity system has on land, air and water, but it also refers to the economic impact of electricity. Electricity is a commodity for which the cost can vary from pennies a unit, to thousands of dollars per unit, depending on customer use at different times of the day, month or year. Highlighting the ecological and economic impact of electricity is critical. However it is equally important to also understand that this energy source is essential to quality of life, business vitality and the economy as a whole in the 21st century. Leveraging technology to maximize the output for every unit of electricity consumed (resource efficiency) and minimizing the ecoimprint of every unit consumed (economic efficiency) must be the cornerstone of planning the future. The technology tools provided by energy and analytics, and visualized by dashboards, are ideally suited to fulfilling those tasks.

Technologies in the form of numerous energy and analytics tools, which may include software and services or solutions, are being presented to CEMs, building managers and consultants on what seems like a daily basis. These technologies could be called "disruptive" because they are changing the way energy management is carried out. It is also worthwhile to note that analytics is not new technology looking for a market; on the contrary, there is growing demand for solutions. The demand is from CEMs and a range of building and campus managers facing real energy challenges, as they work to operate increasingly more complex facility energy systems. Beyond system complexity, these managers are also striving to control energy cost in an ever more complex marketplace. Energy management given these challenges has become more challenging, but there is another new dilemma, energy resiliency or "keeping the lights on." In the face of "super storms," attributed by many as a real indication of climatic impacts from climate change, essential facilities of all types are grappling with the effects of long-term power outages and looking for ways to protect themselves.

The wave of emerging technology for energy and analytics is still very new to energy and building professionals. The intent of this chapter, and this book, is to provide an introduction to next generation energy technology and to describe how it is being used. Some examples of past building system technology evolutions that required energy engineers to embrace new technology were: the move from mini-computer based building automation systems (BAS) to microprocessors for BAS with distributed direct digital control (DDC), sometimes called energy management systems (EMS); BAS legacy systems and proprietary protocols migrating to data communications standards like BACnet™; and then middleware (i.e. Tridium), Convergence, Web Services, the cloud and now analytics and dashboards. These evolutions occurred over four decades, and the same managers were also dealing with a host of other technology evolutions at the same time including distributed generation technology ranging from solar or combined heat and power (CHP) to microgrids, advanced energy metering, deregulation of natural gas and electricity leading to energy procurement, demand response and much more.

The notion of 4^{PLEX} Energy™ takes into account the full range of complexities outlined above, with a focus on technology that can assist managers in addressing energy challenges in today's market and beyond. In fact, this nexus of energy and technology may have motivated the reader to pick up this book. The reality is that energy markets and technology are in a continual state of flux, so this chapter cannot anticipate every evolution that might occur over the years. Yet within the context of the 4^{PLEX} energy segments covered here, it is the author's belief that this material will remain timely well into the future. This discussion, by defining the concept of 4^{PLEX} Energy™, and describing how each aspect of it relates to energy and analytics technologies, as well as visualization tools or dashboards. Dashboard will be discussed in some detail in a later chapter. This book has several chapters devoted to the use of analytics for energy management, building operations and managing electricity, but prior to discussing 4^{PLEX} Energy™, it may be helpful to begin with a brief treatment of energy and analytics.

ENERGY AND ANALYTICS

The technology discussed here might be called *"Big Data for Buildings,"* or *"Big Data for Energy,"* but this effort has elected to focus on *"Energy and Analytics."* This is because the author believes that emergence of this technology could not have been more timely, in light of the significant opportunity for improvement that it offers for energy, building and campus management. For CEMs, building owners, and managers there is a critical need to optimize performance, to control cost, and to find new ways to leverage greater value from buildings as assets. For the buildings community, energy and analytics is exciting because it is a technology-rich discipline, which requires professionals who understand every aspect of building operations, as well as the complex technology deployed. Building technologies and activities that can find value in analytics include; commissioning, metering, building automation systems (BAS), dashboards, middleware, web services tools for buildings, energy services. Of equal value is that each of those technologies and activities is also a source of data for energy and analytics. With content knowledge in all of these areas, the reader will be better positioned for analytics success than anyone else in the building space. This is combined with an understanding of energy management programs like United States Green Building Council (USGBC) LEED™/PEER™ and EPA Energy Star™, as well as utility efficiency rebates, continuous commissioning, meters, etc. Figure 2-1 is a bit busy, but it should provide insight into how these technologies, combined with the 21st century electricity market offer exciting opportunities for integrators and building owners.

Readers might associate analytics with "continuous commissioning or "fault, diagnostics and detection" for HVAC, but as outlined in Chapter 1, that is just one of the applications for this technology. Analytics, again focusing on energy in this book, are generally combined with visualization tools, or dashboards, to provide an essential management tool. This tool can unleash value by optimizing building operations and energy management, particularly electricity, use and cost. It has been noted here that electricity is the highest quality form of energy, and it is essential for a 21st century quality of life, including education, business and entertainment technology. Yet electric energy cost represents the largest *controllable* operation expense in commercial buildings, and the U.S. Department of Energy (DOE) has predicted that these buildings will make up 80 percent of projected growth in energy consumption between now and 2040—a good reason to leverage energy and analytics technology for energy management.

ENERGY MANAGEMENT APPLICATIONS FOR ANALYTICS

Analytics present exciting technologies to enable energy managers to participate in an electricity marketplace, which offers huge savings opportunity through ecoimprint reduction. The author calls this new market 4PLEX Energy, and it is a central "application" for analytics. Analytics is the brain that enables both participation in and value genera-

Figure 2-1. Analytics are the Brains of 21st Century Building/Energy Management

tion from this market. A simple explanation of how analytics tools work is:

- Analytics contain "rules," which define an ideal performance metric for equipment, etc.

- Analytics are deployed with data communication technology that enables them to access current operating data from equipment, etc. and

- Analytics execute algorithm-based analyses to compare current operating data against rules, thus determining current performance.

Based upon the analytics applications discussed in Chapter 1, this process can determine performance for a wide variety of processes. At times the term key performance indicator (KPI) will be used to refer to the performance metric of interest. In this book, performance metrics will primarily focus on energy management, but as discussed in Chapter 1, the basic analytics process is somewhat universal. Electricity is a complex and data rich environment that the book will cover in detail, because understanding these concepts is necessary to achieve energy and cost savings. As the reader considers the analytics process outlined here, and the real time, fast-paced, business of buying, using and managing electricity, these savings benefits should become more evident.

With an introduction to electricity and analytics, this discussion will now focus on the concept of 4^{PLEX} *Energy.* As the name implies, this concept highlights four types of energy. The first 4^{PLEX} *Energy* type has been around for more than 100 years—electricity purchased from the local utility. It has often been said that the utility system was designed for *energy to go one way* and *money to go the other,* when the bill is paid. The electric meter is generally seen as the demarcation point between "supply side" (generation, transmission and distribution of electricity) and "demand side" (the customer's use of electricity). It may appear at first look that there is little new in this plex-segment of electricity, but look closer. The supply side of this segment is dramatically different in deregulated states and, with implementation of the President's Clean Energy Plan, it could become even more diverse. Many of these changes will be discussed under the fourth plex segment below, but it is clear that the electricity business is diverse, complex and in a state of change. One of the most complicated factors about this business is that it is regulated independently in each state. The Federal Energy Regulatory Commission (FERC) regulates the wholesale electricity business, and in recent years has had a major impact on retail markets in deregulated states, but the retail electric business is still regulated, for the most part, by each state public utility commission. This adds complexity for building owners who operate in multiple states because they must analyze the business rules independently in each state before applying energy and analytics technology.

The second 4^{PLEX} *Energy* type exists because electricity is deregulated in approximately half of the U.S. states, and natural gas is deregulated nationally, so either fuel may be purchased from a retail energy provider (REP). The basic transaction looks the same to a customer, and again energy goes one way and money the other. The premise is that "unit cost" for a kilowatt hour of electricity is lower when purchased from a retailer, but it still must be delivered over the local utility's distribution system, often call "wires." Therefore the customer pays both an energy unit cost and a transportation or wires charge for use of the utility system. Buying electricity this way will make sense for a customer if the net cost of energy and distribution from the REP creates a savings compared to buying from the local utility. It is also worth noting that the distribution fee is an added cost, and generally the customer will still get a utility bill for that fee. These fees are established as part of "rate cases" held before the state public utility commission (PUC). When rates are approved by the PUC, a utility has a fee structure that it may use to bill customers for energy and for fees, such as distribution charges. State PUCs establish distribution charges that the utility may assess on electricity units purchased from retailers (where deregulation exists) and for distribution of natural gas energy. Analytics offer an excellent tool to analyze energy consumption profiles and create metrics that can help managers negotiate the best pricing on energy procurement.

The metrics available from energy and analytics tools also enable managers to use the energy consumption profiles to identify efficiency opportunities, and to better understand how to plan for 4^{PLEX} *Energy* types 3 and 4. The reader should note that if this content is not completely clear, the purpose of this book is to offer further discussion that should provide clarity on all of these topics. Energy profiling can be approached in a variety of ways, from simple spreadsheets that track consumption, demand and also summarize costs for each as well as service charges, etc. Utilities can be very helpful in this area by providing online tools to access billing histories, and for a nominal fee, they will install an interface to allow the building owner to connect the meter to a building automation system (BAS). These data are very helpful in tracking managing and rectifying bills, and to understanding electricity consumption profiles. The most sophisticated systems will enhance this capability by capturing "interval data," which captures and tracks information at 15- and 30-minute intervals. This is particularly valuable to understand peak demand and correlate equipment operation with consumption profiles to determine whether cost savings can be achieved. These data can also be very helpful in negotiating final cost proposals from electricity retailers.

The third 4^{PLEX} *Energy* type is distributed generation (DG). Generating electricity onsite can be a highly effective way to reduce cost, improve sustainability and electricity "resiliency" or reliability and much more. It is not the intent of this discussion to review design criteria for sizing the right amount of onsite generation. However it is important to utilize interval data and analytics to ensure that DG has been deployed effectively, and that the overall operation of the facility is driving the greatest benefit. This type of 4^{PLEX} *Energy* has seen significant growth over the past two decades, because there has been extensive implementation of DG from solar photovoltaics (PV). PV has been deployed at utility scale, but has also become very popular for installation onsite by customers. Solar caught the national consciousness and has been installed at all sorts of commercial and residential facilities. The popularity has been stimulated by federal and state subsidies and a variety of business models like power purchase agreements. Dramatic decline in the cost of solar technology has further stimulated installation of renewable electric generation. That is all good news for the energy consumer, but utilities feel very differently. Their big problem is that consumers who generate power onsite are taking money out of their pockets, and they also complain that the output in electricity from solar systems is variable. The utilities say that they still need to build power plants to ensure that power is available when the output from the solar system varies downward because a cloud blocks the sun. This is a complex topic that is beyond the scope of this section, and it remains to be seen if these issues will result in market changes that reduce adoption of solar technology. Readers who are interested should pay particular attention to what is happening in the local market. Yet renewables are not the only form of DG. There are still many buildings, often campuses, with combined heat and power systems (CHP), traditionally called cogeneration. With deregulation, and the ever increasing number of "super storms," cogeneration has seen resurgence. In many cases, these systems are now being operated through "microgrids" that are capable of interaction and trading of power with the local utility. After Super Storm Sandy, for instance, large parts of the eastern seaboard were without power for days. Notable exceptions included places like Princeton University, which was able to insulate its facilities from the outage that occurred after Sandy because it had distributed generation and operated a campus microgrid.

Energy resiliency has already been mentioned as a term that is used to describe actions that facility operators are taking to protect themselves from long power outages after major storms. Of course, utilities are taking action to make the grid more reliable and resilient, but with growing demand and the potential that supply-side assets like coal-fired and nuclear power plants may be taken offline, this issue is creating more concern among electric consumers. Actions by consumers typically involve distributed generation, though there is growing viability in new forms of electricity storage. While motivation for most renewable energy installations focuses on sustainability, customers who build other types of DG are usually more interested in creating resiliency by building a microgrid. These DG systems are more likely to use conventional energy sources like natural gas. The author expects to see more and more hybrid systems in coming years, which combine renewable energy and conventionally fueled electric generation technology. In any case it is typical to size these systems to provide part, not all, of a building's energy needs. Analytics are essential to the design of these systems for several reasons. First, the analytics tool maintains energy profile data, based upon utility bills, that are ideal for determining the right balance between utility-supplied power and onsite generation. Second, it is common for analytics tools to use "middleware technology" to access "interval data" from meters, BAS and other sources, which provide even more meaningful data on energy profiles that include energy (kilowatt hour) and demand (kilowatt). Even more valuable in this process is that the analytics tool can use the same middleware to develop reports that inform the customer what loads (equipment using electricity) are operating during peaks throughout an entire year. The resulting value this energy and analytics process offers to the manager is unparalleled to achieve optimal system sizing. Even more exciting is that the manager can use this information to develop truly 21st century energy management programs that leverage building automation system (BAS) technology, energy procurement from the utility and the REP, DG and programs that will be described under the fourth type of 4^{Plex} Energy. Developing these robust energy profiles is extremely important during a major electricity outage, because it enables the managers to use the BAS to shut down non-essential equipment, so that they can operate on less power. During all other times though, managers can operate this equipment to save money through efficiency and to reduce utility cost. The building and energy manager should recognize that this may sound simple, but it is a completely new discipline for many operators. Traditionally, building operators have focused on equipment operations, and maintaining a building to ensure that occupants have ideal conditions to carry out their activities. For example a hospital surgical suite has a different profile for temperature, humidity, etc. than an elementary school classroom. Fulfilling these tasks was already daunting for building operators. Now asking a building operator/manager to take on the added responsibility of understanding and managing the use of all building equipment to meet energy/electricity consumption levels is a new and complex task. That is why analytics tools bring tremendous value to the operator and those who ultimately benefit from the savings that result from these new complex tasks.

The fourth 4^{PLEX} *Energy* type is really about monetizing the value of energy, particularly electricity units, which the building does not consume. With effective analytics tools, at certain times managers can actually sell back to the grid power that they do not use. This means that electricity and money can both go two ways. This process is governed by a variety of programs, and when the building/manager participates, they can get a revenue stream from selling power (that they do not use or that they generate onsite and send to the grid) back to the utility.

The term "monetizing energy" may seem foreign to the reader, but it is worth learning about. Again, these programs are for electricity, and the benefits may apply in both regulated and deregulated electric markets (states). The basis for this idea is that electricity is a unique commodity because it is generated and consumed almost instantaneously. As the reader knows, electricity cannot be stored in a warehouse for use later. For that reason, the value fluctuates dramatically over time, based upon how much electric demand there is from customers at any specific time. Many may say, "Wait, my energy bill each month shows a number of units or kilowatt hours (kWh) consumed, and every unit is charged the same unit cost." That is true but the nature of the monopoly, regulation business model makes it possible for utilities to make up the cost volatility in various ways. One way is for utilities to add demand charges for large users, which assess an added penalty to those who consume more during high use periods. Other charges may be assessed as well. The real point is that the information on the utility bill can be confusing and only tells part of the story. Again, electricity is a regulated monopoly business and rate structures (prices) are established to insulate the consumer from short-term fluctuations in the market. At the same time these rate structures also allow the utility to recover its cost of operations, as well as the cost it incurs from building new electricity infrastructure (generation, transmission, distribution, etc.). The intent of this text is not to provide a treatise on utility rate analysis, but to point out a simple fact: The cost of electricity is changing continuously. At the state level, retail pricing is regulated by public utility commissions, but utilities invest tremendous legal and staff resources to ensure that all of their costs are recovered, plus a profit margin, through that single "rate" or price per kWh. The more important point here is that the US electric grid is under more pressure almost daily to keep the lights on in the face of ever growing demand for this precious commodity. Many of the appliances, devices, etc. that we associate with business excellence, and quality of life at home, are completely reliant on electricity. The net result is that utilities have had to develop a whole series of options (programs) that enable them to balance supply-side resources with demand from all of its customers. In the old days, utilities forecasted future demand at regular intervals and requested rate increases from the PUC to cover the cost of building more and more new infrastructure. In the 21st century, a host of factors that have been discussed obstruct this old approach to doing business. Utilities will still build new infrastructure, but under pressure from customers and regulators they are also developing programs to use demand from customers. Again customers who participate in these programs are rewarded monetarily for changing consumption profiles. Changing those profiles relieves demand from the grid and makes sense as a strategy to reduce the ecoimprint of the utility and to hedge against the rate at which new infrastructure must be built. The program rewards customers for changing behavior/electricity consumption, and in many cases these payments provide the incentive for customers to invest in efficiency and renewable energy projects. This is what has been called monetizing electricity. Critical to this discussion is that commercial buildings cannot monetize value from such changes in behavior on a repeatable basis without building intelligence systems and analytics.

This fourth type of *4Plex Energy* includes a rich ecosystem of programs and strategies that will pay customers to change behavior and consumption patterns in return for payment. Again analytics are the price of entry to maximize the benefits of such programs, however, and a robust system of building intelligence technology is ideal as well. A great example of these utility programs, which excel with BAS and analytics technology, is demand response (DR). It is also exciting that the same technology, which enables DR, can also be used with capacity, reliability, bidding and other programs in deregulated electricity markets that allow customers to sell power back to the grid. Again this may be power that the customer agrees not to use for a period of time, or DG power that is put back onto the grid through an "interconnect" agreement. All of these programs are based upon the time value of electricity, and customers must contract with the utility through an enrollment process of some type. Concurrent with the enrollment, customers will also install technology to enable these strategies, which will be discussed later in this book. These strategies allow consumers to be paid for changing electricity consumption patterns, and for implementing methods to sell power back to the grid. Blending these strategies with microgrid DG creates even greater opportunity for monetization.

In a 4^{PLEX} *Energy* market, energy managers and all professionals will benefit from both understanding and leveraging the technology discussed here. Electricity markets and programs offer real economic value, but applying analytics is the ideal way to unlock those benefits for building owners. There are also requirements in many markets to implement automated demand response (ADR) technology to execute the sequences. Taking this a step further to also couple BAS technology with the power of analytics software (i.e. Skyspark™ or Analytika™) can create even more value.

Readers may want to avail themselves of the many opportunities that exist to gain knowledge in this area. Local utilities usually offer training for many of these programs. Trade associations like the Association of Energy Engineers, *www.aeecenter.org*, are great sources of training and information provided through conferences and seminars. The reader should also pay attention to opportunities for seminars and articles in industry periodicals as well. Project-Haystack is a relatively new organization that focuses on helping drive standard approaches for sharing device data among applications, such as analytics and visualization tools. The open source community hosts an event called HaystackConnect on a bi-annual basis—*www.haystackconnect.org*. These are just a few of the great places to learn more about this exciting area.

4^{PLEX} *Energy* is an indicator of how dramatically energy management is changing. Taking advantage of the technology, strategies, programs, etc. outlined in this chapter can drive huge value for managers. Further, the author believes that a voracious appetite for information about energy and analytics, as well as electricity markets, will pay off with exciting opportunities for buildings and businesses.

Chapter 3
Dashboards and
Visualization Tools

In 2001 this author introduced the term "dashboard" to the energy and buildings community. It was not a flash of insight, but rather the awareness that a trend, and a term, which was already established in the information technology (IT) world was appropriate for this space. This chapter will focus on the topic of dashboards as a "web-based interface" for building systems including building automation systems (BAS) and myriad technologies from analytics to metering, onsite generation via renewables and cogeneration, special systems such as security and life safety, digital signage and a host of other computer-based equipment.

The focus here is on visualization and dashboards, but it may be helpful to revisit energy and building technology network standards, and the underlying basis for enabling internet-based interface. An entire chapter is devoted to this subject later in this book to provide detailed content for the reader. In the late 1990s and early 2000s, BACnet and LON were vying to become the data communication and networking standards for building automation systems (BAS). By that time it was already clear that building and energy managers wanted technology to unify the interface to these systems. In fact, they were demanding a single-user interface to all BAS, and this group vocalized that demand starting in the mid-eighties. It was not uncommon then, and even today, for building operators to have a room, or a countertop, with multiple computers, each running different BAS and building systems software interfaces. What this author, and others, started to write about and to demand in articles, papers, etc. beginning in the early 1980s, ultimately became known as "open systems." A standard and/or unified BAS interface was considered one of the primary goals of open systems. As early as the mid to late 1970s there were companies offering aftermarket systems for unified BAS interface, but the technology was immature. A secondary demand from owners began to take shape in the late 1980s and early 1990s, and this was for an open systems approach to BAS expansions and would allow them to "integrate" BAS from multiple manufacturers. As a matter of practicality, the standards committees ultimately made a decision that this latter need for "integration" was the highest priority for open systems. As a result, the open systems standards development process became focused on the data communications networking for BAS systems, and the services that have to be addressed to operate a distributed direct digital control system. The reasons for this were many, but at its heart was the belief that the cost for systems is in hardware and software that provide the automation, and the best way to control system cost was to make it easier to integrate existing systems with new ones. The key complaint from customers and operators was that they were "locked in" to a system because the automation technology, including the equipment and the data network, was proprietary. The interface was also proprietary, but it represented less cost. Fast forward three decades and that decision looks like pure genius. Why? Because of the internet and ubiquitous web interfaces.

Merging these web interfaces, or dashboards, with analytics, even embedding the dashboard within the analytics, is the next monster trend that will impact energy, buildings and BAS. At one time, the computer interface was a differentiator for BAS manufacturers, but now many of these companies are integrating third-party dashboards with their systems. A variety of products utilizing variations on these technologies are being presented to energy engineers, building managers and consultants on a daily basis. These technologies might even be considered "disruptive" because they are changing the way building and energy management is carried out. There is actually great demand for solutions to a host of day-to-day energy management challenges, which these tools are targeted to meet. However, this wave of technology is new to many energy engineers. The intent here is to provide an introduction to this next generation dashboard technology, and describe how it is being used. This technology is evolving rapidly and no book can keep pace with all of those developments as a buyer's guide, but it is possible to introduce fundamentals of the technology that will assist buyers in asking the right questions. Dashboards and analytics will be somewhat disruptive in the way that they impact energy and building management, making it critical to include these issues in any long-term operations plan.

DASHBOARDS

Since being introduced to the energy and buildings community, the term "dashboard" has reached "buzzword" status. Yet a dashboard is nothing more than a software visualization tool to provide system information about a facility. The IT industry was already applying dashboards to all kinds of applications decades ago. Consider how Amazon.com tracks buying preferences and offers up the kinds of products a consumer is likely to buy. With the proliferation of BACnet™ systems, and the advent of web services, it became possible to explore new visualization technology in this space. As mentioned above, prior to this dashboard explosion, building and energy managers often had multiple computers, each running different BAS software interfaces. This is still the case for many users today because dashboards may be available today, but the technology is new and intimidating to some managers. As a result, one purpose of this book is to assist those professionals with understanding and making good purchasing decisions regarding this technology.

The genesis for dashboard technology in energy and buildings may have been demand for a unified BAS interface, but in fruition these systems are unifying more functions than just BAS. These functions or systems include those mentioned in Chapters 1 and 2, which in the past required independent computer infrastructure, data communication networks and ancillary gear for visualizations. Among these systems may be: computerized maintenance management systems (CMMS) or continuous commissioning technology, metering, and many more. In this chapter, a sampling of implementations will be discussed, but what is even more exciting is that integrating these previously disparate systems also opens up the true power of big data for energy and analytics. For example, integrating BAS and metering systems for interval data, along with a utility interface dashboard, makes it possible to achieve efficiency and electric demand savings on the customer side of the meter. This concept was covered under 4^{PLEX} *Energy* and presented exciting opportunities for energy management.

In the 21st century, almost all BAS manufacturers offer some form of web-based interface, or dashboard, for their systems, but a robust aftermarket of dashboards exists as well. These dashboards have been widely accepted, and a robust web services market has developed from companies that are offering customized dashboards to the BAS manufacturers. This means that BAS manufacturers have come full circle, from using the software interface as a differentiator to accepting that they are now ancillary products sold to the automation industry by many suppliers. Quite simply, these dashboard tools are truly "interfaces," meaning that they may be used to monitor the BAS, but not to configure or program the BAS components or networks. This is a fact that energy/building managers have accepted, along with the understanding that a separate software tool is needed, and must be purchased from the BAS manufacturer, to complete configuration of systems and to program sequences of operations on any control device. There are also a growing number of "workbench" tools being introduced to the market, which provide non-manufacturer developed configuration and programming tools. The viability of such tools, however, is limited by the accessibility of operating systems, data communication networks and programming tools to external developers. Of course technical viability is not the only issue; the greater concern is whether or not there is a market for programming tools. As with all products, a market opportunity would only exist if the tools offer unique features that deliver real value to customers. It remains to be seen whether such features will be offered, but what is clear today is that dashboard interfaces are generating tremendous interest and creation of a whole new eco-system of companies in the industry.

The fact that dashboards cannot configure and program the BAS, or other building systems, is not necessarily a limitation, because the true value is in using these tools for energy and building management. All of the tasks outlined in the last three chapters for equipment operation and energy management require dashboards. The dashboard is also critical as an interface to the analytics tool allowing managers to develop and track consumption profiles, conduct FD&D, etc. Given this distinction between programming tools for initial BAS setup and dashboards for day-to-day operations and energy management, managers can decide whether to have in-house programming expertise on both types of systems or to outsource one of these functions. After initial startup, there is limited need for the programming tool, except when it is necessary to replace a controller or tweak program sequences as necessary.

The term "dashboard" now encompasses much more than BAS web interfaces, but these interfaces are critical to successful long-term energy management. Coupling the dashboard with analytics to evaluate specific KPIs is one way that managers can trump the single greatest cause of BAS failure. That happens when minor changes and "overrides" to equipment program sequences occur little by little over time, until the systems are completely ineffective. Normally no one at the building even notices that systems are being circumvented, but the *analytics tool* will notice. This chapter will provide a situation analysis on the dashboard technology, as well as on the dashboard applications.

DASHBOARD TECHNOLOGY SITUATION ANALYSIS

Dashboard technologies will be classified in two broad categories for this discussion: 1) operational tools for energy/building managers, and 2) kiosk tools for building occupants and visitors. In fact, both are primarily software tools that leverage data from a host of systems onsite and online. The earliest incarnations of operator tools did not see widespread implementation because they required a hardware system like a computer, along with an extensive network of ancillary components, which had to be hardwired back to a BAS computer. The first cost was prohibitive and few facilities, other than universities and industrial applications, had the staff sophistication to use them, as well as the energy and operating costs to justify the investment. Today, operational tools are lower in cost to implement and much more user friendly. Implementation costs have been reduced due to web-based data communications standards, beginning with BACnet™ but including many others, and these systems have incorporated web services compatibility.

Communication standards, and web services, combined with expert system integrators who can create (program) drivers to access data from "legacy" or proprietary BAS, and other equipment, have launched an independent world of "middleware" products. Capable integrators can buy these products and program or purchase "after-market" drivers that make it possible to communicate with, and extend the useful life of, legacy BAS equipment. This is because the equipment can be maintained in operable condition at the building, or even application, level so that the manager can develop "migration paths" to allow phased upgrade of legacy to standard systems over time. The take-away for dashboards is that all of this technology can extract the data needed to provide an interface to almost any building system. The Ethernet LAN, VPN or other network that already exists in most buildings, and on most campuses, is able to move those data, and they can be housed on a local computer, or a server accessible via wide-area network or "the cloud." This marriage of technology and need has opened up a new world of functionality and dramatically reduced the cost of the systems. That means that almost any managers' requirements for access to energy and building data can be met by today's dashboards.

Given this complex building level, data intranet, a dashboard can provide BAS interface to get status information about a building or campus. Dashboards combined with analytics can then be expanded to provide the features of enterprise energy management or continuous commissioning. These latter features are disciplines within themselves, and will not be discussed in detail here. Twenty-first century energy management, discussed in Chapter 2 as 4^{PLEX} $Energy$™ highlights some of the ways these technologies can bring value. Dashboards discussed thus far are software driven tools, used by operators, typically for two reasons. First to optimize building performance and operating cost, and second to ensure that the building is maintained in a way that serves the mission. Building occupants pay no attention to the complex equipment that maintains the environment, but if a surgical suite must be maintained at a specific temperature, or an office building is uncomfortable, major issues develop very quickly. So the building operator's job is to manage to a set of requirements that defines the optimal building environment, and work continuously to meet those requirements. Cost is an ongoing factor in any operation, so the true value of a dashboard is to give an operator one tool to use for monitoring the building and the output of the analytics tool. In this case monitoring is a real-time activity that operators carry out attempting to address issues that arise, and to ensure that the building is operated within specific tolerances. Those tolerances may be comfort or process, but the management process must also control cost and energy consumption. With the growing emphasis on sustainability there are mandates and policies that require buildings to be operated to a number of indices. To be successful these activities must be integrated management activities combining the power of the BAS, analytics and dashboard with the content knowledge of the manager. Operators are only capable of conducting so many tasks at one time, and particularly when conditions and variables are in a state of continual change. It is not possible to do this work with a dashboard alone, rather analytics become essential. Determining the optimum role for dashboard interface becomes very important to the energy/building manager, and these tasks will become clear when we discuss analytics.

The second type of dashboard will be called a "kiosk." In recent years it has become very popular to summarize high level building data on a screen that is available for any building visitor to see, or available to managers and others within an organization. Providing this sort of user friendly interface is a great way to share sustainability accomplishments with building and campus users. Often a kiosk or touch screen is provided in a building entrance or other central area to summarize high-level information about sustainability and efficiency goals, as well as current or real-time performance against those goals. This same level of data may also be duplicated on a "cloud" based website, or as a link from the organization's website to make the information available to a very large audience. The data provided on a physical screen or kiosk, typically are produced by a server, or operator dashboard, that resides elsewhere on a network. The data are then "pushed" to a computer/computer screen for display to the visitor.

Kiosk dashboards are usually graphically driven, much like a PowerPoint presentation, and may incorporate other information for visitors like an office directory, electricity output from an on-site solar array or fire evacuation plans. These are sometimes also referred to as digital signage and can include the day's events or even advertising. Ultimately the primary value of dashboards is awareness about current status and performance of the building or campus, which is easy to visualize and understand. There is very little analysis provided by the tools other than perhaps some averaging of information points, etc.

This was a high level discussion of dashboard technology and the reader may want more technical detail. To address that need, this book has been separated into two parts. Here in Part I the trends, business reality and overarching technology topics related to energy and analytics are covered. To better understand the underlying technology, Part II of the book will dive more deeply into the technologies themselves. A curious fact however, is that the underlying technology requires study of multiple related topics. Those topics include: BAS and other systems technologies, data communications and networking technology, middleware and more. This book cannot provide detailed training on computers, or information technology, so the author will assume that readers come to the topic with enough basic knowledge in that area, or pursue study elsewhere, as a foundation for discussion of these topics. With that introduction to dashboard technology it is now possible to talk about the applications for which the technology is intended.

DASHBOARD APPLICATION SITUATION ANALYSIS

Under the heading of dashboard applications, there is a wealth of new control products, technologies, and buzzwords. As noted above, due to the evolution toward data communication standards, middleware and web services, it is now possible to develop products faster and easier. For that reason, and due to the market growth in energy services, technology products of many types are being developed and launched. This chapter cannot cover all of the various product types, but it can provide a good foundation for future discussion. An obvious first application to discuss is building automation systems (BAS) interface and related applications, which in the past consisted of a very small number of manufacturer developed offerings. The BAS industry now includes dozens of companies offering many types of software and hardware, including dashboard interfaces, and equally importantly those that offer web services and analytics technology to expand the power of these systems. Under the in-depth discussion of analytics, another important development is the creation of a new organization, Project Haystack, -which was discussed in the last chapter and has an entire chapter devoted to it later in the book.

Market demand and reduced technology development barriers to entry and data standards have created a perfect storm of opportunity for dashboard products. As a result, many different players, not just name brand BAS manufacturers, may introduce new advances in BAS interface. This becomes more common as the lines blur between traditional BAS manufacturers and heating, ventilation and air conditioning (HVAC) manufacturers. As these companies continue to merge, grow and expand their product families, it becomes less likely that the traditional BAS manufacturers will be technology leaders. A strong argument could be made that these companies have not been technology leaders for some time. The real leaders today are part of this new ecosystem of software/technology companies developing products including dashboard and analytics tools. In many ways standards are "the price of admission" to leverage off-the-shelf technology and web services in integrated system projects. This is particularly true in the 21st century.

During the first wave of web-based products, the energy and buildings industry was inundated by IT developers who thought that building systems were like email or any other web service. Today however, the energy systems industry is much more IT savvy and the developers are coming from the energy and buildings world. This means visualization tools and other web based products are much better conceived and deployed than before. The stage is now set to go beyond seeing the dashboard as a BAS interface only, but seeing it an integration tool for the applications described in Chapter 1 as well as building commissioning, facility management including maintenance and operations, video surveillance, electronic access control, digital signage and much more. Dashboards are valuable tools to simplify interface and save time by unifying daily operations tasks associated with monitoring these systems. They become even more valuable when the act of interfacing makes it possible to achieve system integration. An example would be integrating fire and security with HVAC control for energy management. Since integration requires data and system level interface, it goes beyond dashboard monitoring. True integration will be more relevant as we discuss analytics. However, dashboards can be used for troubleshooting and diagnostics to ensure that integration sequences are operating properly.

The dashboard becomes a tool that brings together information so that mangers can make effective decisions. It is a portal that allows the manager to get access to real-time information about building operations, and to link to other systems, like building automation or access security, for interrogation and update. It can also provide access to other websites, such as the local utility site, or to internal software like the budget. This makes it possible to access data from the analytics tool and view current energy consumption and costing data from the local utility and retail energy providers. The dashboard can also report on sustainability metrics and provide interface to onsite generation from renewable energy or cogeneration.

This opportunity for dashboards is not without challenges however, and there are risks that must be managed. Cyber security is an ongoing concern, but the benefit of combining automation and information systems is that integrators can leverage existing firewalls and other security measures. In early 2012 an investigative report was published in the *Washington Post* about the "middleware" technology that was installed at sensitive government facilities. The article implied that hackers, and others prone toward terrorist activities, could gain access to the computer networks in these facilities through the middleware systems. The reporter asserted that the password security for these systems was not robust enough, and that a hacker could gain access to a password that would open the system. There were several flaws in this argument, but nonetheless extensive work was done to enhance the integrity of the system for the future. There were also upgrades to these technologies to protect password security within the systems. Data reliability could be another concern, particularly if the control information is completely reliant upon the web. Improving middleware security from cyber threats also addresses data reliability issues, but adding storage at the building level and uploading data more frequently to cloud storage addresses most of these issues. Of course all such obstacles can be overcome with these and other strategies as they have in other industries like online banking.

In light of the previous discussion about cyber threats, there is value in briefly addressing the topic of data communications and cyber security. Managers should engage experts to develop approaches and take precautions in using these systems, as they would with any IT technology. Anyone living in the 21st century is well aware of the threats that information based computer systems may face from unsavory characters. This is a major focus for the smart grid interoperability panel (SGIP). SGIP started life as an entity operated by the National Institute of Standards and Technology of the Department of Commerce, under a direct mandate from Congress in the Energy Independence and Security Act. Its charter was to identify standards for interoperability, both data communications and functionality, between the grid and buildings as well as all other electricity users. The reason SGIP is relevant here is that it has focused very specifically on cyber security. Through the SGIP's work the bar has been raised for internet and data communication security between any piece of equipment in a building and the grid.

Without question, integrators and astute managers will succeed in creating cost effective building environments by synthesizing industry information to leverage technology and optimize system control and facility management. Dashboards are the windows that will make information about those efforts easily accessible for a wide range of people and in user friendly formats.

Chapter 4
Introduction to Analytics

Thus far in this book the goal has been to frame the dramatic market opportunity that exists for energy and analytics. In Chapter 4, John Petze, Partner in SkyFoundry, LLC, co-founder of Project Haystack and author of the foreword to this book, shares a high-level view of what the technology offers. Mr. Petze is both a serial entrepreneur and a serial technology visionary, and initially developed this content for an industry technical paper. The content was then expanded for inclusion as a chapter in Barney Capehart's book, *Automated Diagnostics and Analytics for Buildings*, also published by The Fairmont Press. This very informative introduction to the emerging technology and business practice being deployed with analytics should be valuable to the reader. Of equal importance is that Mr. Petze also dispels some of the confusion regarding analytics and helps to highlight the differences between some technology-driven solutions that exist in the marketplace.

Analytics, Alarms, Analysis, Fault Detection and Diagnostics
Making Sense of the Data-oriented Tools Available to Facility Managers
John Petze, Partner, SkyFoundry, LLC

Using data from smart devices such as building automation systems, smart meters, smart sensors, etc., is one of the hottest topics in the industry. The goal is to use these data to better understand the operation of building systems and identify ways to improve that operation.

Facility managers are confronted with a wide range of products and features that can contribute to improved facility performance. From alarms to fault detection and diagnosis (FD&D) and analysis tools, to automated analytics, each has their place and offers specific capabilities and benefits. Systems integrators and owners, however, are often faced with comparing "apples and oranges" as they try to evaluate the different tools.

Comparing the technologies with sets of criteria can help facility managers better understand the roles, capabilities and benefits of these tools so they can assess the best fit for their needs. This chapter explores the range of tools from the perspective of:

- Time and location of implementation (when they are defined and where they run)

- Data scope—the range of data items being analyzed

- Time range of analysis

- Expressiveness of the tool—the tools available to describe the issue to be detected

ALARMS

Alarms are one of the fundamental tools that have been available in BAS systems since the early 1980s and remain an important tool. Often, when first introduced to advanced analytic tools, people compare them with alarms. After all, doesn't an alarm programmed in a BAS tell the operator something is wrong? On a very basic level there is a similarity, but if the reader looks a little bit deeper they see that there are fundamental differences between alarms and more advanced analytic tools.

First of all, alarms require an understanding of what you wanted to look for at the time you programmed the system. In other words, you knew exactly what you wanted to look for and took the time to program that specific alarm definition into the system. This is fine for simple issues like a temperature going outside of a limit. However, there are many inter-relationships between equipment systems that may not be known at the time the control system is installed and commissioned.

One of the great benefits of analytics is that it enables you to find patterns and issues you weren't aware of at the outset of a project—providing results that show how your building systems are really operating vs. how you thought they were operating.

Given that alarms require you to define the specific condition ahead of time, *time of implementation* is typically during the initial programming of the control system. This requirement fits a wide range of conditions that we want to identify in our control systems, but is also a limiting factor.

Data Scope

Alarms usually evaluate a sensor value vs. a limit. They may also include a time delay—i.e., the condition must be true for 5 minutes before an alarm is generated. Alarms are most often associated with a specific point. For example, one of the most common approaches is to set alarm limits for each individual point when it is configured. The data scope of alarms is also typically limited to the data in the local controller or other devices within the control system. Alarms do not typically evaluate enterprise data or data from other external sources.

Time Range

Alarms are typically evaluated "now." By this we mean the real time condition of the sensor vs. the alarm limit. This is a key point—very different techniques are needed to look back over months or years of data to identify conditions patterns and correlations.

Describing What Matters

The next difference to consider is the flexibility of expressing what you want to find. Alarms don't typically allow for sophisticated logic that interrelates multiple data items, conditions, data sources, etc. For example, an alarm definition might be: "Is the value of the room temp sensor above 76 degrees F right now?" An analytic evaluation on the other hand might be: "show me all the times when any room temperature was above 76 degrees in the last year for more than 5 minutes at a time during occupied hours, and total the number of hours by site."

Processing Location

Adding new alarms typically means modifying control logic or parameters in controllers. This means you need to have access rights to modify the controller logic to change or create alarms. This can be very limiting if you just want to "find things" in the data or are trying to analyze data from a system installed and managed by others.

The need to "reach into the controller" makes alarms "expensive" when trying to use them as an analysis tool. For example, could we justify reprogramming controllers in 500 remote sites because we have an idea of a data relationship we want to look for? Most likely this would be cost prohibitive. We might also ask whether the "analyst" should even have access rights to the configuration tools in an automation system. The important point is that there is significant "friction" involved in using basic alarm techniques for anything beyond limit-based relationships of individual points.

FD&D—FAULT DETECTION & DIAGNOSIS

FD&D techniques are typically equipment centric and characterized by pre-defined rules that are based on an engineering model of a piece of equipment—for example, FD&D rules for a type of packaged AHU.

Time of Implementation

There are two "implementation time" components to consider with FD&D. Generally FD&D requires that an engineering model of the equipment be developed beforehand. In this respect they require significant pre-knowledge of the system. As such, FD&D rules are often not flexible for use on custom, built-up central systems, etc. The fact that no two buildings are alike can further limit where FD&D techniques can be applied.

Because of the dependence on predefined equipment models FD&D is typically not a good fit for *ad hoc* analysis—e.g., "I have this idea about a behavior I want to detect." In addition, FD&D rules can often be developed only by the software/service provider. The rules are "part of the product" versus being programmable on a project-specific basis.

Processing Location

FD&D solutions are typically applied as a separate software application that pulls data from the BAS system. The software may be installed locally or hosted in the cloud. Some FD&D solutions can be programmed into BAS controllers. In this case they require "touching" the control system. As previously discussed, this can be a limiting factor in their application.

Data Scope

FD&D rules are typically focused on the predefined points associated with a known piece of equipment. They may include data such as weather, but do not typically encompass external data, like age of building, historical energy consumption, type of facility, square footage, type of equipment, etc. or provide the ability to roll up and correlate data from hundreds of pieces of equipment.

Time Range

FD&D rules typically look at real time conditions, but some have the ability to look at data from a sliding window of time—such as the last hour or day of operational data. *Ad hoc* analysis of random time periods (i.e., last August vs. this June) may not be available.

Analysis Tools

Most often discussed in relation to energy meter data, analysis tools provide an experienced user with the ability to look at data with a range of charting tools and "slice and dice" that data with a range of tools to identify peaks, and other anomalies. Analysis tools typically include the ability to perform normalization against weather, building size, and other factors, etc.

The most significant characteristic of analysis tools is that they require a knowledgeable user to be sitting in front of a screen to interpret charts and graphs that identify the important issues—in other words, "wetware" is a key part of the issue identification process.

Data Scope

Most commercially available analysis tools focus on a specific type of data and application, for example, energy meter data. They integrate weather data (degree days as a minimum), occupancy schedules and building size, but do not integrate the full set of equipment data such as temperatures, pressures, speeds or rate of operation, equipment status, etc.

Time Range

From a time perspective, analysis tools provide the ability to analyze across a wide time range. As for "real time" data they can typically handle data "up to the last reading"—often a 15-minute sample—but are much less likely to be connected to a data feed that updates values every minute or second. They also support batch loads of historical data from meters, utility sources etc.

Processing Location

Analysis tools can be applied on top of existing systems as long as

the data are available in some open format. They do not need to be part
of the initial installation and typically do not require any changes to BAS
programming. Analysis software can be hosted in the cloud or installed
on-premise.

Analytics

In many ways, analytics can be thought of as a superset of the other
categories we have described. For example, analytics can be applied to
"real-time" alarming situations and offer the ability to define more sophisticated alarm conditions to create "enhanced alarming."

FD&D rules that diagnose equipment performance issues are a
type of analytics as well. While most FD&D solutions employ pre-writ-
ten rules based on known models of equipment, programmable analytic
tools enable experienced engineers to implement rules based on their
knowledge—they are not limited to rules defined by the software provider.

In comparison to the other technologies analytics have the following characteristics:

Automated Processing

An analytics engine continuously processes data to look for the issues that an experienced engineer would normally look for manually.
This ability to automatically process rules to identify important patterns
and correlations is the hallmark of modern analytics solutions.

Time of Implementation

Analytic solutions can be implemented anytime, during initial
installation or years after. They do not require reaching back into the
control system to make programming changes for analysis. They do
of course require that data be accessible (we will talk more about data
availability in a moment).

Expressiveness—Flexibility to Define Rules for
Conditions to be Detected

While a typical alarm might evaluate a single item against a limit
at a single point in time—analytic rules crunch through large volumes of
time-series historical data to find patterns that are difficult or impossible
to see when looking only at real-time data.

For example, while an alarm might tell us our building is above a specific kW limit right now, analytics tells us things like how many hours in the last 6 months we exceeded the electrical demand target. How long were each of those periods of time, what time of the day did they occur, and how were those events related to the operation of specific equipment systems, the weather or building usage patterns?

Analytic rule languages should enable sophisticated data transformations beyond limit checks. Examples include: Rollups across time periods, calculation of max, min, average, interpolation across missing data entries, linear regression, correlation of data sets to find patterns such as intersections (or lack thereof), etc.

One of the key characteristics of analytics is that they expose things you were not necessarily looking for, or even knew to look for. Analytic data presentations expose data relationships and correlations even without writing rules. And systems that offer user programmability enable new rules to be implemented as findings illuminate actual operating characteristics, and new priorities emerge due to changing energy costs, operating requirements or building usage patterns. In fact, the successful application of analytics is a journey with one discovery providing insight for additional analytic rules. More on this later.

A Wide Data Scope

Analytics enable multiple data sets from different sources, in different formats and with different time sampling frequencies. They are not limited to data within a controller or a control system. Examples might include:

- Energy, weather, and control system data

- Size of facility (sq ft/sq m)

- Age of building

- Type of building and systems (packaged HVAC vs. built-up central systems)

- Equipment brand

- Service company

In many cases the analytics process starts with data available without establishing live connections to control systems, meters of other devices. More on this topic shortly.

Analytic tools can be applied on top of existing systems as long as the data are available in some open format. They do not require changes to the control system and do not need to be part of the initial installation. This is a key benefit, as it allows analysts to apply rules to the data without disturbing underlying systems.

Analytic software can be hosted in the cloud or installed on-premise. Each approach offers tradeoffs. For example, hosted solutions allow the software to be managed centrally, but require that the customer accept an external connection to their network for continuous access to data.

SOME EXAMPLES HELP TO HIGHLIGHT THE DISTINCTIONS

An Alarm
Detect zone temperatures above 76 deg F when occupied.

An Analytic Rule
Look at signature of data associated with all sensors to indentify "broken" sensors or sensors out of calibration. See Figure 4-1.

Alarm
Detect kW above a specified limit in real time. See Figure 4-2.

Analytic Rule
Identify periods of time when demand is above a specified kW limit (see Figure 4-3), calculate cost impact, make reports available showing duration and even cost across any selected time frame, and provide continuous real time processing of the rule as new data are received.

An Analysis
Generate a graph of energy consumption across a specific time.

Analytics
Automatically correlate equipment operating status with energy consumption across a specific period of time. See Figure 4-4.

Figure 4-1

Figure 4-2

Figure 4-3

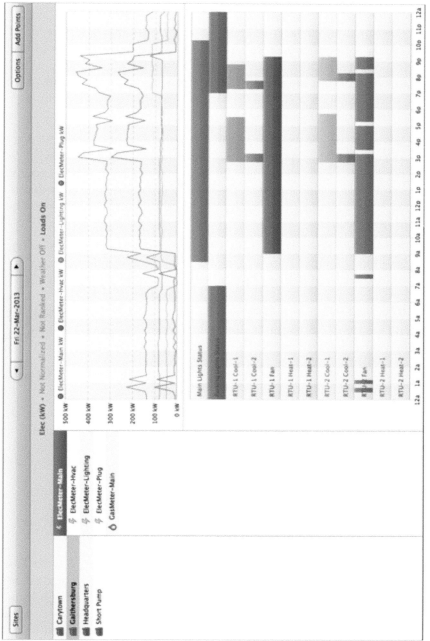

Figure 4-4

CAN ANALYTICS EFFECT CONTROL ACTIONS?

Once analytics detects a pattern of interest can the system act on it? The answer is yes, analytics can be used to issue commands to control systems, but it's important not to overestimate the applicability of this feature. Many issues found using analytics will not lend themselves to being corrected with a simple "command" to the control system. Two quick examples are illustrative:

1.   Errors in control strategies. If an analytic rule detects conditions resulting from defects in a control sequence, the logic will need to be modified. An example might be simultaneous heating and cooling. While you could command the heating or cooling off when detected, the correction of the problem will require actual changes to the control sequence.

2.   Physical equipment issues. If a damper linkage is broken or stuck, or a valve won't fully close, or a sensor is out of calibration or not reading correctly, there is no command to "fix" these issues.

This doesn't mean there is no use case for automated response to analytic results. Two examples of an automated response to analytic findings are:

1.   Automatic generation of more intelligent work orders by the integration of analytics and CMMS tools.

2.   Automated demand response. Demand response actions can be executed in response to energy use patterns detected (or predicted) using analytics. This provides more intelligence than simple limit-based demand response control.

DATA ACCESS—A KEY REQUIREMENT FOR
ALL DATA-ORIENTED TOOLS

All of these tools are dependent on being able to access relevant data. Because alarms are processed locally in the control system, data access is not an issue—the data "is there." In order to take advantage of the other tools, however, we need to assess the process to gain access to the data. A good way to start an assessment is by answering the following:

1. What data do you have? Examples: Energy meter data, facility data (size, location, type, year of construction, etc.), equipment operation data such as on/off status, sensor data, etc.

2. Where are the data located? Examples: BAS system, SQL database, utility company website, Excel spreadsheets, etc.

3. What method will be used to access them? Examples: Live collection of data via BACnet™ or oBix™, Haystack™, Modbus™, etc., data download from utility website via xml (perhaps Green Button™ data), CSV file import, SQL queries processed on a daily, weekly, hourly or minute basis. The answers to these questions will vary dramatically based on characteristics of the specific project and customer's needs.

ANALYTICS AS AN EXPLORATORY PROCESS

Analytics needs to be viewed as an exploratory process. Analytics show you how your buildings really operate, identifying where opportunities for savings exist, which assumptions are correct and which are not. Results from one rule or algorithm often identify behaviors that provide insight into other rules that should be implemented.

Because of this, the analytic process is best applied incrementally, driving value to the owner with each step. We have a tendency to think of any energy conservation measure as a big capital expense project. Unlike energy conservation measures that involve the installation of major capital equipment, you can start small with analytics and generate returns in a very short period of time—you don't have to "do it all" at once to get value from analytics. The results from initial analytics generate the savings to go deeper into your operational data. This is a great advantage to building owners, in that it's possible to start with a limited amount of data, and a low-risk, low-cost initial evaluation, to produce short-term financial results.

An Example of a Shallow and Wide Approach

Basic interval energy data, combined with building occupancy, and weather data are a great place to start as shown below. Let's say the only data I can easily access are my interval meter data (kW demand), which are provided once per day by my utility company, and a list of occupancy schedule times in an Excel™ spreadsheet (see Figure 4-5). We can gain any valuable insight from that limited amount of data. With just that limited amount of data SkySpark can identify:

- Buildings starting early,
- Buildings running late,
- Buildings that operate continuously,
- Demand peaks that occur outside of occupied times,
- Peak load, annual and monthly, and short load durations. See Figure 4-6.

Here's how: Using conventional energy analysis tools I can easily identify my kW demand pattern for each day. By looking at it manually I can determine whether the pattern follows occupancy times.

If I have a large number of buildings this type of manual review would be prohibitive. With analytics I can automate the process and have the software find these patterns for me. A rule can look for a percentage change in kW demand at the transition to and from occupancy. The rule generates "notifications" whenever the demand does not change by the expected amount within a defined period of time around the occupancy transition. In this way the system automatically identifies when buildings run late, and start early. A weekly (or monthly) view shows how many times the issue has occurred and the total cost. There's no need to hunt through the data manually.

Do They Have to be Live Data?

Another common misconception is that you can't derive value from data unless they're live and continuously updating in real time. This simply isn't true. Live data are great, but by no means essential to getting started with analytics. You can get tremendous value from running analytics on a snapshot of historic data. One of the benefits of using snapshot data is that you can avoid the costs and delays associated with gaining IT approval for network access to live systems. A great example is an initial portfolio assessment, but you can also do deep equipment analytics with historic data.

It's worth digging into the topic of "real time" data a bit more. We have found that there is a significant variation in what people mean when they use the term real time data. A few definitions can help clarify the topic and enable a clear understanding of how analytic tools can be used with "real time" and historic data.

Figure 4-5

Figure 4-6

A Definition

Real time means fast enough for the application. So if we are controlling a piece of industrial manufacturing equipment, that might mean we need a control loop response time of 10 milliseconds to meet the real time needs of the process. Many processes require even faster real time requirements—perhaps on the order of microseconds.

For a VAV box controlling temperature of a room, the control response time of the temperature control loop might be 30 seconds, a minute or longer. On that same VAV box, though, the control loop responsible for managing the airflow volume to maintain an airflow setpoint might have a response time requirement of 1 second.

At the other end of the spectrum, in energy metering applications real time often means 15-minute interval data. When we are looking at applying analytics to data there are a few facets of "time" to consider.

Resolution of Data—The Sampling Rate

One aspect of "real time" we need to consider is the resolution of the sensor data. By this we mean how frequently a system senses (and records) data values. For example, many BAS controllers can store data values on the second. In this case the data-sampling rate would be once per second.

The sampling rate of sensor data has a major impact on the volume of data created. For example a history record of zone temperatures once per minute will generate 1,440 values per day. That same sensor recorded on a sampling rate of 1 second will generate 86,400 sensor values—sixty times as much data!

In most systems it's common that the control response capability and sampling rate are equal. For example, a controller capable of providing 1-second control response will often allow sensor values to be recorded once per second. One major limiting factor, however, is that most controllers will typically run out of storage space if you choose to record sensor values every second. So in reality they are often set to record values once per minute or longer, or need to upload the history data to a repository on a frequent basis.

Freshness of Data

The next concept to consider when discussing real time applications is the "freshness" of data or frequency of the updates to the software application consuming the data. A common example of this would be the update frequency of sensor data on an operator screen such as a graphic representation of an air handler. The capability of a system to deliver updates to the user is affected by a variety of factors including:

- Bandwidth and speed of the communication network,

- Computing resources of the controller that can be dedicated to communicating data to the UI application,

- Efficiency of the software that presents that data to the user,

- Computing resources of the computer that is displaying the data.

Different systems vary considerably in this area and it's not uncommon for screen updates of 10 seconds to be considered "real time" updates. Going back to our definition of real time, the "application" here can be described as the ability (or need) of the human operator to read and respond to changing values he sees on the screen. Based on this definition a 10-second update frequency may be considered adequate.

The data source—the controller—may be operating its local control loops with a response time of 1 second or 100 milliseconds, but the fastest that new data will appear on the screen might be once every 10 seconds or longer. In some building automation systems it's not uncommon to see screen update times be much longer. That might be perfectly acceptable for the "application" of the human user (although most people find that a bit frustrating).

Application of These Principles with Analytics

When planning the application of an analytics solution, all of these factors need to be considered. For example, knowing the sampling rate of the data will enable us to understand the richness that analytic rules will be able to work with—think about the different level of insight provided by 15-minute-interval meter data versus monthly energy data. The sampling rate will also tell us about the volume of data we will need to store and manage. In many applications there will be different data sources, each with its own sampling rate. The analytics application must be designed to handle the challenge of aligning and analyzing data with different sampling rates.

Next there is the question of how frequently data can be pulled from the source. Here again different data sources may have different update frequencies. Data freshness is related to the application. The frequency with which you pull new data into the analytics database varies based on the needs of your application and limitations of your communication infrastructure. For example, you might have an application where you can only upload data from a site once per night at midnight (we've seen these restrictions placed on systems by IT departments). At that time, however, you might be pulling in data that has 1-second resolution. So in this case, the data freshness would be once every 24 hours, but the data sampling rate would be once per second. The sampling rate and the freshness are "decoupled." Then there is the question of the frequency of the rule processing. Ideally, rule processing is decoupled from the sampling rate and freshness of the data.

Next consider the user of the analytics application. Using the same example, we might have a situation where building operators want to see their analytic results (sparks) every morning. They could subscribe to a daily digest notification, which will provide a daily summary email. When they view their sparks they will be seeing all of the issues detected in the last 24 hours of data. Their "response time" would be on the order of a day (about the same time frame as the data freshness).

Too slow you say? It depends on the application and needs of the user—there is no one-size-fits-all answer. For example, we have seen some examples where the data sampling rate is once per minute, the data freshness is once per 15 minutes, and yet the update provided to the user (the building operator) is once per week or once per month. That's right, building operators are informed of sparks once per week! Why might an operator find this level of "freshness" in sparks acceptable or even desirable?

It could be because the types of issues they are looking for can't really be addressed more quickly. Perhaps they need to be planned into their facility maintenance schedule, which is set on a weekly basis. Or it could be because they have so many issues requiring attention that they simply can't do anything with issues presented on a more frequent basis.

It could also be because the issues they are tracking take time to form—the patterns appear over a period of time. Some patterns form in a minute, some take hours, some take days and some might take a season or a year to form. This is a key point where people often confuse analytics with alarms. For example, the pattern that represents a defective sensor might require 12 or 24 hours of operation to detect. It can't be detected at any specific second in time—it is detected by interpreting a pattern in data that appears after some period of time has elapsed.

All of this leads us to appreciate that there is yet another "decoupled" response loop involved in the use of analytics—that of the corrective action response time. The limiting factor here is typically the human systems that will respond to analytic results. An issue detected by analytics might not be able to be addressed until the next planned service call to the facility.

A Fast Moving Field

None of the examples presented is meant to be absolute, rather they are offered to help systems integrators and facility managers gain an understanding of these tools, their requirements and potential benefits. With the rapid advances in data-oriented facility management tools, there is some overlap between them, and the lines blur as vendors advance their technology.

As we stated in the introduction, each of these tools plays an important role in achieving an efficient building. Analysis tools help us gain insight into operating characteristics, which then support automated analytics to provide continuous detection of important issues relating to equipment operation and energy use.

Chapter 5

Analytics for Energy Management in Buildings and on Campuses

In Chapter 1, the four essential applications for analytics were introduced. Energy was one of those applications for analytics, and has been highlighted as the focus for this book. Optimizing energy consumption is central to addressing the complex challenges facing business, government, institutions, the economy and the planet, and it is required to achieve the high standard of living that is sought by every nation in the world. These aspects of life on the planet are all reliant upon energy, and energy is also highly interdependent with the other three applications for analytics. Moreover it is essential to mention the old adage "one cannot manage what one cannot measure." It will be cited more than once in this book, and this statement is particularly true for energy. The emphasis in this book will also turn heavily to electricity, because it is the highest quality form of energy, but more importantly because the electricity market creates unparalleled challenges and opportunities to leverage analytics for significant financial, operational and mission (work done in the building) benefits. The preceding chapters have provided clear justification for engaging in a robust and persistent analytics program. This one will reinforce that justification with a focus on energy.

This chapter and the two that follow will begin to provide more specific content about deploying analytics for targeted applications and opportunities. In the author's mind, electricity holds some of the most significant opportunity of any form of energy, but the interruption of electricity flow also presents a significant risk. The number-one reason for any manager to engage in energy and analytics is to keep these two dynamics, opportunity and risk, in balance. The opportunity will be explored further here. At the same time, electricity resiliency, already defined as the reliable and continuous flow of power, is essential to this topic of analytics for building owners and managers. Some may say that there is nothing a building manager can do to support energy resiliency, but this author would disagree. This book is about the full spectrum of opportunity that analytics can offer to aide building owners/operators and Certified Energy Managers (CEMs) in maximizing the use and cost of energy, as well as strategies that can improve the environments created within the building. The resiliency of energy, especially electricity, to support the mission, or the work that is being done in that facility, offers the opportunity to forge a true 21st century energy management program.

Management professionals, in the building community today, must oversee enterprise infrastructure to address a wide range of short- and long-term objectives. Many of these objectives are in some amount of conflict; such as creating the optimal balance of occupant comfort with energy cost reduction. Some might ask, how does energy and analytics technology fit an overall program for building operations and energy management? Lawrence Berkeley National Laboratories (LBNL) is among the national labs that has established leadership in this area. LBNL's Electricity Markets and Policy Group has conducted technical, economic, and policy analysis of energy topics centered on the U.S. electricity sector. Much of this research is intended to aide in public and private decision-making, by managers, on issues related to energy efficiency and demand response, renewable energy, electricity resource and transmission planning, and electricity reliability. One report is cited here, but the reader is encouraged to research the wealth of information available from LBNL, Pacific Northwest National Labs, the Office of Energy Efficiency and Renewable Energy within the U.S. Department of Energy (DOE) as well as state and local agencies and resources. The bottom line is summarized in a 2008 DOE report called Energy Efficiency Trends in Residential and Commercial Buildings http://apps1.eere.energy.gov/buildings/publications/pdfs/corporate/bt_stateindustry.pdf. That report points out that buildings account for 40% of all energy used annually in the United States. By energy type, buildings account for 72% of U.S. electricity use and 36% of U.S. natural gas use. Given the significance of building energy use, it should come as no surprise why measurement, and active management, are so important, and why there is a growing market for energy analytics.

HISTORY AND PROCESS

History is a big topic and cannot be covered in detail, but there are some important topics that must be touched upon. First and foremost, management of energy requires measurement of how energy is consumed. In fact the overarching term that is used to refer to the discipline is "measurement and verification" (M&V). Many people think of M&V as the process to evaluate energy investments, and it is, but before the investments it is critical to develop a thorough understanding of energy consumption baseline measurement. It is only reasonable to assume that most readers are well versed in these topics, however the author will ask your indulgence to provide some perspective for those who may not be knowledgeable in this area. Equally important, this section will be extended somewhat because it is also logical to describe the process of energy analysis, and how some of these historical evolutions added to what has become a very robust discipline. The formation of this discipline that we now call *"Energy Analytics"* is based on work done by the DOE, Association of Energy Engineers and many other thought leaders in the energy management world, and it begins with a simple mantra: You must baseline. Baseline means capturing a history of energy consumption including electricity, natural gas, oil, gasoline, propane, etc., and summarizing that history in a tabulated energy profile reporting on monthly and annual utility cost for at least two years. The best place to start is with the "baseline," which could be called measuring the building energy intensity. In fact some have referred to the baseline as an energy intensity index. Developing the baseline typically begins with gathering utility bills for a building, and in the beginning this was done by contacting each utility, requesting copies of the bills and then summarizing the information with pencil, paper and calculator. Today most utilities make this information available on line. Of critical importance, especially for managers of multiple facilities in different geographies, utility territories, etc. is that it is important to "normalize" the baseline.

Normalizing means that all of the energy consumption is translated to a standard form of unit, typically a British thermal unit (Btu). Most readers will know that 1 Btu represents the amount of heat that is created by one match burning, and that there are Btu equivalents for all units of energy—kWh, Therm, etc. Normalizing will also include a way to compare facilities, so it usually includes a square footage calculation and a weather calculation. The universal standard for weather is a degree day; heating degree days count each degree of average outside temperature during 24 hours that is below 65 degrees Fahrenheit, and cooling degree days count each degree of average outside temperature for 24 hours that is above 65 degrees Fahrenheit. To calculate the heating degree days for a particular day, find the day's average temperature by adding the day's high and low temperatures and dividing by two. If the number is above 65, there are no heating degree days that day. If the number is less than 65, subtract it from 65 to find the number of heating degree days. For example, if the day's high temperature is 60 and the low is 40, the average temperature is 50 degrees. Sixty-five minus 50 is 15 heating degree days. Cooling degree days are also based on the day's average minus 65. For example, if the day's high is 90 and the day's low is 70, the day's average is 80. Eighty minus 65 is 15 cooling degree days. Degree day information is available from a number of sources including the National Oceanic and Atmospheric Administration (NOAA) www.noaa.gov. So step one in analysis is to create a baseline of annual energy consumption by month and year that is normalized to arrive at Btus per square foot per degree day per year. This process is sometimes called developing a "building energy profile."

The next step is to use this information to understand how the building is performing, and a good way to do that is to compare it with other buildings. The holy grail for building energy performance data is the Energy Star for Buildings and Plants (Energy Star) program of the U.S. Environmental Protection Agency (EPA), and its ENERGY STAR Portfolio Manager® software. Portfolio Manager is an online tool you can use to measure and track energy and water consumption, as well as greenhouse gas emissions. Sustainability was mentioned in Chapter 1, because carbon is an organizational performance metric that has been established for many buildings. Analytics can be very valuable in tracking sustainability metrics, but it will not be discussed a great deal in this book. Most readers are already aware that greenhouse gas emissions and energy consumption are inextricably linked. This was underscored by the EPA ruling targeting greenhouse gas emissions from power plants, which is discussed more in Chapter 7 and emphasizes the alignment of these topics. The EPA discusses this in its report "Regulatory Impact Analysis for the Proposed Carbon Pollution Guidelines for Existing Power Plants and Emission Standards for Modified and Reconstructed Power Plants," June 2014. In that report the EPA states that carbon dioxide (CO_2) is the primary greenhouse gas pollutant, and it accounts for 84% of U.S. greenhouse gas emissions. According to the report, the single largest emitters of greenhouse gas, primarily in the form of CO_2, are fossil fuel fired electric generating units or power plants. At the building and campus level, it seems that most organizations have developed sustainability plans to address "carbon" and to add this factor to the analysis that is conducted for the building. Again sustainability will not be covered in great deal in this book, however the energy and analytics tools discussed here, such as Portfolio Manager, are often used to measure and track carbon emissions as well as energy consumption.

Of particular significance in tracking, measuring and understanding how buildings consume energy is being able to have a frame of reference for how the building performs. Clearly there is value in developing a building energy profile and comparing the building to itself over time, but it is even more valuable to compare the building baseline to other similar buildings. The process of comparing buildings to one another based on performance is called "benchmarking." Again the EPA Energy Star program offers significant help with this task, because it has published a database of such information including consumption profiles by building type. This allows building owners to benchmark their buildings against similar buildings, and truly understand how they are performing. Most readers will also know that it is not useful to compare a hospital to a church, because the equipment installed, consumption patterns and hours of operation are completely different. For this reason Energy Star provides information to allow energy managers to compare similar buildings, normalizing for square footage and weather.

This section is about the history and process of energy analysis, and how energy and analytics are revolutionizing this discipline, but it can't explain every approach in technical detail. Therefore the focus will be on what energy analysis entails and why, rather than on how specific software developers, etc. complete the task. This author was a corporate energy manager for a retail chain with 20 million square feet of buildings in 23 states, purchasing electricity and natural gas from dozens of utilities. At that time, VisiCalc was the tool of choice for spreadsheet/paper and pencil analysis, but the predominant tool today is, of course, Microsoft Excel™. The point is that tracking energy in this way is a manual process, and the size/complexity of the dataset make it difficult to do this without errors. A few decades ago some very forward thinking professionals launched what became known as the "Enterprise Energy Management" (EEM) industry. These products performed all of the history and normalization functions of paper and pencil or spreadsheet, but purportedly with many fewer errors. Spreadsheets are wonderful, but many, many times they become works in progress and undergo continuous changes that open up the potential for errors and flawed reports. EEM tools on the other hand were developed by software engineers who conducted bug correction, with the intent of eliminating errors. Equally important was that these tools could calculate energy performance metrics on an ongoing basis and present reports that included graphic visualization charts depicting energy profiles. This visualization allows managers to see how energy profiles change by time of year or season, by differing periods when occupancy changes (think K-12 school or university) and based on various other factors. Another development that was introduced during the EEM era was software that maintained history and energy profiles, but these tools also made it possible to enter utility rate structures as well. Including the rate structure in the software made it easier for the analysis to determine several important things. First, comparing billing data to the rate structure makes it possible to verify that the building is on the right rate. It is not uncommon for some anomalies in energy consumption, particularly with electricity, to cause a building to be put on a rate structure, in error, that is more costly. Whether the building belongs on that rate structure should be the subject of ongoing analysis. At the same time, efficiency projects and active energy management programs may also qualify a building to be put on a different rate that is more advantageous. So re-evaluating rates is important, but it is time consuming, and software analysis can be very valuable. A very sophisticated tool may even be able to look for billing errors that can also be costly, and are rarely picked up by the energy consumer. From a historical perspective, the EEM market gained a certain amount of traction, but initially these were stand-alone packages, and required dedicated staff time to operate and use. They were particularly appealing to large users with campuses of buildings or multiple buildings in different geographies, and were of particular value to those who had buildings in many utility service territories. To a great degree, EEM has evolved to become part of the energy and analytics tools that are the focus of this book.

Energy measurement and profiles based upon billing data are very useful in getting a high level understanding of the buildings' performance. This brings even greater value when benchmarking is done. As discussed, baselines can be developed for any commodity (electric, natural gas, propane, oil, water, sewer, steam, refuse, recycling, telecom, etc.) and any number of accounts, meters, bills, and bill details. Baselines allow the manager to view each account's cost and consumption history in graphical or tabular format, and easily compare fiscal year, monthly, or annual summaries. Armed with this baseline data it is then possible to benchmark any building or account against others with information such as that available from Energy Star.

Benchmarking is extremely valuable, but for electricity more information is required. Electricity is a very unique commodity that requires more than a billing-based analysis. That is because of the impact that electric kilowatt (kW) demand fees introduce to the billing process. Even more importantly, kW demand is integral to how utilities create rate structures and to how the owner should manage electric use. The term that has become common when discussing kW demand is "interval data." Throughout this book the topic of 21st century energy, most importantly electricity, and systems will be discussed, and no topic is more important to that discussion than interval data. Interval data in this book will be concerned with kW demand. It is possible to capture interval data for kilowatt hours as well, but the opportunity discussed here is more focused on demand. Tracking interval data for kW is essential to optimizing energy use through demand management. Demand management can include demand limiting, as well as optimizing cash flow through demand response. Further demand management is essential to sizing for every type of distributed generation from solar photovoltaics to combined heat and power. The term "interval data" most likely comes from the fact that kW demand is measured on an "interval of time," typically 15 or 30 minutes. At some point in the history of electric regulatory policy, utilities were able to convince state commissions that energy charges alone ($0.00 per kilowatt hour consumed) were not sufficient to maintain the electricity system. Maintaining that system, or grid, requires utilities to cover all of the costs associated with operating existing electricity infrastructure, but it also requires that utilities cover the capital cost of building new infrastructure (generation, transmission and distribution systems). One of the ways that utilities are able to support that capital cost is to assess demand charges. This creates challenges for the building owner because electricity demand varies over time, and reality for the electricity business is that utilities must be able to meet that changing demand. For this reason, utilities must build enough power plants, transmission and distribution systems to meet the peak demand. An alarming fact is that as much as 25% of the U.S., and even worldwide, electricity infrastructure is in place to meet the demand for electricity for about 100 hours per year. Peak demand occurs for relatively short periods of time over a handful of days each year, typically driven by air conditioning demand on the hottest summer days. So the baseline electric analysis for buildings must include the energy consumption charge in kilowatt hours and the demand charge in kilowatts. It is critical to also add a record of interval demand data over the year as well. Of particular interest to the consumer is that the utility bill only contains one peak demand reading, the highest reading for any interval during the billing month. To get all of the interval kW data over an entire year, the owner must request special metering equipment that allows them to capture and record every interval during that billing month, so that they can analyze their demand peaks. The patterns (or profiles) of energy usage contained within this interval energy data are great for discovering how and when the building consumes energy, and can be very informative in identifying where savings can be achieved. The fine-grained detail of interval data (such as 15-minute or 30-minute data) is key—daily, weekly or monthly data don't carry nearly as much information about how energy is being used. EEM and most modern analytics programs will evaluate interval data.

Initially EEM functionality resided in stand-alone software, which was typically "shrink-wrapped," "licensed" and sold to the consumer. The database would therefore reside on the local computer. Today it is more common for this functionality and the data to reside on services in a cloud computing environment, and they often sold via software as a service (SaaS) rather than shrink-wrapped. Today's systems therefore may incorporate EEM, as an added module, and combine it with analytics for other applications. These cloud based analytics systems may be built around any number of applications, such as dashboards for visualization. Again the focus here is energy, and the author firmly believes functionality should not be sacrificed because it has been incorporated into other types of software. The goal here is simply to restate the importance of establishing requirements and carefully evaluating functionality before choosing a solution. The growth of the analytics market has resulted in the integration of this functionality into many offerings that go to market in a variety of ways. The balance of this book will cover this content from a variety of perspectives. Approaches to analytics tools will be discussed further in Section II. The topics of baselines, benchmarks and interval data will not be elaborated further here, but they are essential topics to energy and analytics. Readers who need to understand these topics further are encouraged to refer to the reports, etc. highlighted here and to explore training and further information from the Association of Energy Engineers, as well as state and federal agencies.

Bringing the Building into Focus

The value of developing baselines and benchmarks for a building, campus or entire large portfolio of properties is significant. However, it becomes evident quickly that a more detailed understanding of the building, and the work being done in that building, is critical to making meaningful change. This is why the author discussed the four applications for analytics in Chapter 1, and emphasized the importance of an overall energy management program. Bringing the building into focus means having a team of content experts conduct a thorough and detailed building inventory and analysis. In some circles this might be called an "investment grade audit," but the goal is not to jump to identifying improvement measures, rather to develop a granular understanding of what makes up the energy baseline. There have been numerous articles and texts written on the topic of conducting a detailed building analysis. The emphasis here will not be on the steps to complete that analysis, but on the importance of this work and what to do with the information. At the end of the day, bringing the building into focus is about conducting a "forensic energy analysis." This process evaluates the energy consumption history and the interval data for electricity to identify what "equipment" and "occupancy/operational patterns" are causing the energy profile to look the way it does.

This building analysis must consider three important topics: 1) building type and characteristics, 2) baseline utility data and alignment with mechanical/electric equipment loads and 3) whether a building automation system (BAS) and metering technology are installed. The building type and energy history have been discussed already, but in summary these are topics that should be evaluated:

• Type of building (office, retail, university, hospital, etc.)

- Number of buildings and their locations
- Building size(s) in square feet
- Hours of operation
- Critical areas of the facility (data centers, operating rooms, laboratories, etc.)
- Sensitivity to environmental changes (HVAC and lighting)

Once these key factors about a building are understood, the equipment inventory is the next essential step in this process, and it should be conducted by Certified Energy Managers (CEM) who understand the use of that building. CEM is the term being used here because CEMs are usually highly diverse professionals with content expertise in engineering, equipment, systems, energy management and applications. The team may be made up of CEMs, mechanical or electrical professional engineers and/or facility management professionals. The CEM should develop a load profile that is validated against actual electrical usage data from utility bills. Elements of this analysis include:

- Electric Utility Accounts
  — Number of meters/accounts
  — Are interval meters installed? If so, what interval (hourly, 15-minute, etc.)
  — Utility rate program (standard commercial, interruptible, time-of-use, etc.)

- Load Profile Align with Energy Baseline
  — Annual consumption (kWh)
  — Summer and winter peak demand (kW) and what time of day does the peak typically occur?
  — Primary loads that impact the load profile (HVAC, lighting, process, etc.)

- Equipment
  — Significant electrical loads (process loads, large equipment, etc.)
  — What operations program could be implemented with this equipment/load?
  — Is there any on-site backup generation?

— How is cooling and heating supplied, and by what energy source?

In the end it is equally critical to understand both the equipment and the application (building function/use) of the building to do this job well. A thorough inventory of mechanical and electrical equipment will allow the team to begin to understand what makes up the kW peaks in the interval data. In most cases it will then take a content expert on the application (i.e., hospital, school, etc.) to analyze how the building is operated. There are still buildings that are operated inappropriately because staff are trying to avoid conflict, keep the maintenance office phone line from ringing, etc. There are also buildings that are operated inappropriately because of design errors, installation errors and changes in the building that have not been mirrored by changes in equipment configuration, sizing, operations, etc. Whether caused by one of these conditions, or any number of other issues, the forensic analysis process is the same. Using the inventory, the CEM can then look at electrical loads, occupancy and operations patterns and operational effectiveness of the building, individual pieces of equipment and systems (i.e., central plant, variable air volume air handlers and boxes, etc.) to understand what causes the interval data profile. The final element of this analysis is to determine what systems are in place that may be utilized. This technology provides a foundation for operational programs, and first cost for participation may be lowered by leveraging existing technology and systems in the building:

- BAS manufacturer, type, and vintage

- Centralized control of multiple locations; internet accessibility

- Communication type (Ethernet, proprietary, phone line, etc.)

- Electric metering through the BAS or dedicated energy information system

- Lighting control or automatic dimming through the BAS or stand-alone

The forensic energy analysis combined with the baseline and interval data history for electricity, and other energy sources, is the foundation for implementing an effective analytics program. This program can then be tuned to drive high performance energy management programs. As stated, this book is focused on the energy applications of analytics, but more importantly on electricity. This is because electricity is a highly transient energy source, which can experience significant price volatility, but also because it is the most essential fuel for every aspect of business and quality of life in the modern world. Some may ask what is meant by price volatility, because the prices have traditionally been regulated. This will be touched on in more detail throughout the book, but the simple fact is that electricity is one of the largest controllable costs for any building, and effective operations are the logical result of effectively applied analytics. Legislative and regulatory policy that defines the rules by which the electricity business operates will be touched on elsewhere in this book; the primary goal in this chapter is to discuss how analytics can be used as a tool to drive high performance building operations.

One last comment on this topic regards energy procurement, which was discussed as part of 4^{Plex} *Energy* but won't be covered more in this book. There are many sources for content on this topic including Association of Energy Engineers conferences and seminars. The emphasis here will be on using energy and analytics to effectively and efficiently manage the building, rather than on procurement. However, it is important to note that these tools will arm the manager with very effective information to use in negotiating the best energy procurement agreements. Particularly if the manager is able to use interval data to drive a better understanding of how their consumption and demand patterns have traditionally manifested, this will be very helpful in creating a solicitation and defining needs. Beyond that it should also be possible to negotiate with retail energy providers on terms that make the manager a better electricity customer. For example, the manager could demonstrate through the history that the building can operate within certain thresholds. A well operated building with effective analytics can operate under certain consumption/demand thresholds, even during peak period, and this will allow managers to provide the seller with a high degree of confidence on power to be provided. This is the basis for many of the operational programs run by utilities that will now be discussed. Electric utilities must serve all of the load (electricity) use on their systems to ensure that they can keep the customers' lights on and that they don't make unnecessary investments in new infrastructure. This requires that enough generation, transmission and distribution infrastructure is in place to serve customer demand. They may need to buy capacity from other utilities who have excess, are able to provide power onto the utility's grid and are willing to sell. The option is to operate programs that help them to balance bringing peaking generation units on line and orchestrated electric demand reduction. As the same time many utilities incentivize actions the customer may take that will help them in balancing load on the systems and managing demand with "base load" generation that typically runs full-time and peaking plants that can come on line quickly to meet peak demand.

Energy Analytics in Operations
     With energy and analytics the next critical topic has to do with ensuring that the right analysis is conducted, based upon the needs and goals of the organization. As part of this analysis, the manager should pay careful attention to internal needs, as well as to programs from utilities and others. At the end of the day the goal should always be to meet organizational goals, with the minimum level of capital and operational resources, while ideally finding programs that provide ongoing funding or "electricity income." Therefore it is worthwhile to consider the programs that leverage energy and analytics data, and that also use these tools to evaluate taking actions that can improve overall building performance. Table 5-1 provides background on energy management operations, many of which that are aligned with programs that provide funding. It should be clear how valuable the energy and analytics data are in determining operations that can be implemented in a building. The table outlines four categories of operational activities for buildings, and the first column lists factors for consideration. The factors include what motivates action, what design considerations are necessary to implement the action, what the operational processes are that must be implemented, and where the action is initiated? Demand response is the only measure shown as initiated remotely, and this will be discussed further below.
     There are five types of energy management operations in Table 5-1. Efficiency and conservation applies to any type of energy resource—electricity, natural gas, etc., as well as water. The other four operational types however apply specifically to electricity, and will begin to make it clear why energy and analytics technology is so important for the future.

Table 5-1. Energy management terminology and building operations

Factors	Efficiency and Conservation (Daily)	Peak Load Management (Daily)	Distributed Generation (DG) (Daily)	Demand Response (Dynamic Event Driven)	Electric Market Participation (Analytics Based)
Motivation	Economic Environmental protection Resource availability	TOU savings Peak demand charges Grid peak	Energy Resiliency Cost Savings Optimization Carbon reduction with Solar PV	Price (economic) Reliability Emergency supply	Manage and reduce cost
Design	Efficient shell, equipment, systems, and control strategies	Low power design	Many options: -Solar PV -Micro-turbines -Combined heat & power	Dynamic control capability	Evaluate electric use, DG, interval data profile and building need to identify capability
Operations	Integrated system operations	Demand limiting Demand shifting	Balance utility purchase with on-site generation, and also may supplement heat	Demand shedding Demand shifting Demand limiting	Integrated system operations
Initiation	Local	Local	Local	Remote	Local

ENERGY EFFICIENCY AND CONSERVATION

The definition of energy efficiency is the percentage of total energy "input" that is required to achieve useful "work." So the efficiency percentage increases as less energy is required to perform work. This could be the result of installing a high efficiency motor, or a variable frequency drive on an air handler, which achieve the same work; moving air, with less energy (in this case electricity) input. Efficiency focuses on insulating the work from the energy reduction, so that the process is not impacted by the diminished energy input. Energy conservation, on the other hand, reduces unnecessary energy use. Among the first steps that should be taken in most buildings is to look for conservation opportunities, such as reducing hours of equipment operation. If equipment is being operated when the building is unoccupied, i.e. lighting, then putting programs or technology in place to ensure it is turned off, is energy conservation.

Both energy efficiency and conservation provide utility bill savings, and benefit the environment by reducing emissions from power plants. Energy efficiency measures can permanently reduce peak demand by reducing overall consumption. As noted, in buildings this is typically done by installing energy efficient equipment and/or operating buildings efficiently. Energy-efficient operations, a key objective of new building commissioning and retro-commissioning (for existing buildings), require that building systems operate in an integrated manner. Utility rebate programs are designed to drive investments in energy efficiency, such as those mentioned above, because they lower overall consumption of energy units. This allows the utility to better manage load in the short term, but it also allows them to hedge against how quickly they need to build new electricity infrastructure.

PEAK LOAD MANAGEMENT

Daily peak load management has been conducted in many buildings for decades. These strategies are designed to minimize the impact of peak demand charges and time-of-use rates. The most common types of peak load management methods include demand limiting and demand shifting. Interestingly these strategies have been forgotten, or neglected, by many building managers in recent years, but there has been a resurgence and the value they offer is significant. Understanding interval data and building operations is critical to making the best use of these strategies, while minimizing any negative impact to occupants.

Demand limiting refers to shedding loads when pre-determined peak demand limits are about to be exceeded. The manager must put equipment in place, usually with a building automation system (BAS), that monitors peak demand during the time interval dictated by the rate structure and has control capability. Demand limits can be placed on equipment (such as a chiller or fan), systems (such as cooling), or a whole building. Peak demand thresholds will be programmed into the BAS, and strategies are developed and programmed to execute an action when the peak demand limit is to be exceeded. Such actions could include turning equipment off, resetting a setpoint that causes equipment to modulate to lower operational levels and draw less electricity, etc. The system will also be programmed to restore equipment to normal operation when demand is sufficiently reduced or when the peak demand interval or period has ended. Customers implement demand limiting to save money, by flattening the load shape (kW consumption profile) when the monthly a peak demand is about to be exceeded.

Demand shifting is achieved by changing the time that electricity is used. This is more challenging for buildings because there is very little non-essential equipment operating in most facilities. It is possible though, for example thermal energy storage is a demand shifting strategy. Thermal storage can be achieved with active systems such as chilled water or ice storage, or with passive systems such as pre-cooling of building mass. In California, **time dependent valuation (TDV)*** is also in use for building energy code compliance calculations required by the state building energy code (Title 24) to take into account the time that electricity is used during the year. Time dependent valuation (TDV) is an energy cost analysis methodology that accounts for variations in cost related to time of day, seasons, geography, and fuel type. In California, under TDV the value of electricity differs depending on time-of-use (hourly, daily, seasonal) and the value of natural gas differs depending on season. TDV is based on the cost for utilities to provide the energy at different times. TDV acknowledges that some efficiency measures reduce summer peak electric demand more than others.

---

*Brook, Martha (2011) Time Dependent Valuation of Energy for Developing Building Efficiency Standards. California Energy Commission. http://www.energy.ca.gov/title24/2013standards/prerulemaking/documents/general_cec_documents/Title24_2013_TDV_Methodology_Report_23Feb2011.pdf

DISTRIBUTED GENERATION

Distributed generation (DG) presents huge potential for building owners. Investing in DG is motivated by many different factors. Some DG systems deploy micro-turbines and small-scale generation to reduce electricity cost for consumption and demand. Larger DG systems provide "combined heat and power" (CHP) to generate electricity and use the waste heat from that process to offset thermal needs in a building or on a campus. There has also been explosive growth in solar photovoltaic (PV) installations in recent years, driven by a desire for DG and by sustainability motivations to reduce carbon and improve the environment. In recent years, since Super Storm Sandy hit the coast of the northeastern United States, a new motivation is "energy (electricity) resiliency." Resiliency is about insulating facilities from the impacts of long-term power outages in the aftermath of storms and other events. The smart grid movement, for example, was instigated by a power outage in 2003 that cause the entire Eastern Seaboard to be without power for several days. Understanding interval data is critical to sizing DG installations and to operating them cost effectively.

DEMAND RESPONSE

Demand response (DR) is one of the more exciting utility programs to be deployed in recent years. DR is a great example of electricity capital, or a program that provides an ongoing revenue stream to the customer, in the form of cash payments from the utility. These cash payments are typically made monthly to customers in return for agreeing to participate in the program, and to respond a preset number of times per year. DR is a dynamic and event-driven program that can be defined as short-term modifications in customer end-use electric loads in response to dynamic price and reliability information. To clarify, first "reliability information" means an event notification that is provided to the building electronically, and typically initiates automatic execution of a pre-agreed strategy. Initially DR programs allowed customers to respond manually be physically turning off equipment when an event was called, but this approach is not always reliable. Today almost all programs require automated demand response (ADR), and these programs typically involve an electronic signal to some form of automation technology, and include a BAS which automatically executes the response by turning off equipment, changing temperature setpoints, etc. These strategies are exactly like those discussed above under demand limiting and shifting, which can be utilized for demand response.

A demand response event notice typically begins with an email notification to the customer in advance (anywhere from 10 minutes ahead to day ahead) and an electronic event signal to the BAS at the start of the event which triggers the response. There are numerous types of response strategies that may be implemented, and utility programs will dictate which ones may be executed in a particular territory. Some of these strategies might be physically shutting off non-essential equipment (i.e., a fountain pump in an atrium), reducing demand drawn by equipment (i.e., change setpoint to reduce fan speed or modulate air conditioning to lower operation mode), or operating distributed generation (DG). As noted above, another option for notification is dynamic pricing. Dynamic pricing rate structures provide customers with a "discount" on the cost per unit of electricity or demand during most days of the year, except when the local utility is having difficulty meeting demand. At those times, the customer receives an electronic notification that the cost of power per unit will be increased by some multiple (i.e. 10 times normal rates). The customer then must initiate a similar form of DR strategy to protect themselves from the price impact. DR can also be accomplished with **demand shedding**, which is a temporary reduction or curtailment of peak electric demand. Ideally a demand shedding strategy would maximize the demand reduction while minimizing any loss of building services.

Demand response (DR) programs may include dynamic pricing and tariffs, price-responsive demand bidding, contractually obligated and voluntary curtailment, and direct load control or equipment cycling. Readers who are not familiar with DR programs in their utility territories may want to research them further. In closing this topic, it is important to clarify that the customer must be intimately involved in the design of these programs. The reference to "remote initiation" in the table may be alarming, but that refers to the event notification discussed above. Before an event is ever initiated there is a detailed analysis conducted, during which the customer works with the utility, and DR is provided to develop the strategies that will be executed. The owner is fully aware of what will happen after the event notification, and is able to renegotiate the contract to change or reduce the amount of participation with a coincident reduction in the DR payment. The final point is to reinforce that the DR participation contract also sets a limit on the number of times an event can be called each year and the number of hours each event can last. All of these factors should be considered by any building manager before participating. However, energy and analytics technology that is implemented, as discussed in this chapter, can take all of the guesswork out of DR. If the customer thoroughly understands their consumption and interval data profiles and effectively deploys BAS and other technology, it is possible to accompany DR with a well-orchestrated set of higher level building operations to drive real value. For example, the building owner could pre-cool the building before an event or charge a thermal storage system, so that reducing air conditioning capacity does not impact comfort. The case study chapter, Smart Grid, Smart People, outlines just such a project that was highly successful.

ELECTRICITY MARKET PARTICIPATION

One of an owner's challenges with developing strategies for electricity is that the power business is regulated at the state level. Chapter 7 provides more background on this highly complex industry. For purposes of this discussion, the reader should research programs that exist in their utility service territory to determine if there is value. In a nutshell the idea here is that the customer sells power, which they agree not to use at a particular time, back to the utility. This may sound a bit odd, but remember that electricity is a very unusual commodity because it is created and consumed almost instantaneously, and it cannot be stored. Yes electricity can be stored using batteries and other technologies, but it cannot be stored on a scale that would allow utilities to inventory power the way that you inventory any other commodity. So this means that utilities must monitor demand instantaneously, forecast whether it is increasing or decreasing and bring on generation to meet the need. Utilities operate what they call "spinning reserves," which are power plants that are idling and ready to ramp up when demand increases. Given this highly complex environment, programs have been developed that make it possible for a customer to get paid to "not use" electricity. This reduces demand and makes it easier and less costly for utilities to keep the lights on at critical times. Again the reader is encouraged to research whether such programs exist in their utility territory and whether their properties might be candidates for participation.

The most important point for energy and analytics is still "one cannot manage what one cannot measure." Developing very detailed baseline and interval data for the building, and understanding what equipment and activities cause the consumption patterns is the price of entry for 21st century energy management. Armed with these data, the manager can evaluate every strategy that exists in the local market and develop effective optimization strategies to reduce energy use cost. Taking such action can also make the building resilient to power interruptions that negatively impact the mission, or work being done, in the facility.

Chapter 6

Analytics for Operations and Equipment Maintenance in Buildings and on Campuses

James M. Lee, CEO, Cimetrics, Inc.

IMPORTANCE OF THIS CONTENT

Thus far in this text, the stage has been set for a changing energy market, and its implications on consumption and resource management in buildings and on campuses. For purposes of this text, the term campus is used to depict an ecosystem of buildings, which could be part of a traditional corporate or higher education campus, but could extend to community energy systems for neighborhoods, districts or entire cities. Analytics bring value in all these cases by providing the opportunity to manage and operate these buildings effectively, while maximizing the value transaction associated with consuming energy to fulfill the mission being carried out in that space. This value also impacts on the larger community, as well as the planet's environment. To accomplish these goals, equipment in the building must be operated in optimum fashion, thus balancing the energy consumed by that equipment with the work being done. The work performed by that equipment could be lighting, heating, ventilation, air conditioning, vertical transport or any number of other functions. In the end this balance between energy consumption and "work" is the definition of efficiency.

The goal of analytics is to collect and analyze essential pieces of data, to understand how to achieve the same or greater levels of work with less energy, or other resources, provided as inputs. The other resources include a wide range of "inputs" such as labor and materials for maintenance or, depending on the application, any number of other commodities and resources. Jim Lee provides great insight, in this chapter, to how this is done with particular emphasis on heating, ventilating and air conditioning (HVAC) equipment. HVAC represents approximately 40% of the energy use in commercial buildings, and in more complex facilities such as labs, hospitals and industrial plants it can be an even larger percentage of consumption. HVAC is also one of the most complex systems within any building and is made up of a large number of interdependent pieces of equipment. The efficiency of each piece of equipment relies on regular maintenance and good operations, and issues at this level can create even larger problems for the building or campus as a whole. Those problems include poor comfort or disruption in the work or "mission" being carried out in the building, but of equal concern they will result in an inefficient building with higher energy cost and a poor carbon footprint. Integral to energy and analytics is a thorough understanding of the delicate balance between energy, maintenance and mission, and this is Mr. Lee's forte.

INTRODUCTION BY JAMES M. LEE

Since Cimetrics introduced automated building analytics in the year 2000, there have been many advancements in the field. Much of the discussion has focused on energy savings, but many applications of big data analytics are not specifically focused on energy. This chapter will discuss predictive maintenance in contrast to preventive maintenance, stressing the benefits of utilizing big data for predictive maintenance such as increased equipment life, improved reliability and lower labor cost. Though the specific focus here is energy, improvements in these areas will have dramatic impacts on the overall efficiency of the operation and will reduce energy use.

The goal of predictive maintenance is to save money and increase equipment reliability. Money can be saved by only making repairs or servicing equipment when necessary. The risk of equipment failure can be reduced by continuous, automated analysis of equipment performance in order to identify faults before they become critical. Whereas predictive maintenance was once limited to high-value capital assets, modern automation systems allow us to collect and store vast amounts of data, and low-cost computing power makes it possible to analyze that data.

PREVENTIVE MAINTENANCE

Definition from Wikipedia

Preventive maintenance (PM) has the following meanings:

1. The care and servicing by personnel for the purpose of maintaining equipment and facilities in satisfactory operating condition by providing for systematic inspection, <u>detection</u>, and correction of incipient failures either before they occur or before they develop into major defects.

2. <u>Maintenance</u>, including tests, measurements, adjustments, and parts replacement, performed specifically to prevent faults from occurring.

The primary goal of maintenance is to avoid or mitigate the consequences of failure of equipment. This may be by preventing the failure before it actually occurs which planned maintenance and condition based maintenance help to achieve. It is designed to preserve and restore equipment reliability by replacing worn components before they actually fail. Preventive maintenance activities include partial or complete overhauls at specified periods, oil changes, lubrication and so on. In addition, workers can record equipment deterioration so they know to replace or repair worn parts before they cause system failure. The ideal preventive maintenance program would prevent all equipment failure before it occurs.

Here are some examples of routine scheduled maintenance of equipment:

- Oil changes
- Belt changes
- Filter changes
- Linkage adjustments
- Valve seats replacement
- Steam traps replacement
- Boiler re-tubing
- Evaporator bundle cleaning
- Cooling tower water treatment chemical replenishment

Preventive maintenance has been the backbone of mechanical and industrial equipment operation for decades. When systems are constructed, the designers take note of component lifetimes, operating hours, wear parts, rated cycles and lubrication etc. Utilizing this information, manufacturers develop recommendations for maintenance to ensure effective operation and to optimize energy consumption by the equipment. Yet historically, elapsed time (run hours) has been used as the key driver for when maintenance activities should be performed. Although preventive maintenance is believed to be effective, in practice there are many shortcomings:

- The maintenance action is performed whether it is needed or not

- Labor is inefficiently deployed

- There is typically no verification of the repair action by observing system performance

- Deviation from normal operation is often limited to visual inspection

Preventive maintenance programs have frequently been auto-mated by traditional computer maintenance management software (CMMS) packages, which require a user to understand the piece of equipment in order to create regular schedules for performing main-tenance tasks. These are also coupled with spare parts inventory infor-mation, repair ticket tracking and enterprise accounting functionality. Most CMMS packages don't provide analytics capability and hence don't allow the user to gain institutional knowledge about the perfor-mance of assets over time. Furthermore, today's CMMS packages are unable to police the reliability of the repair, which is based on the skill level/training of the person performing the corrective action. In today's world of outsourced operations and repairs, how can one be certain that the repair technician knows what he is doing? By following up to analyze the data with an understanding of the models and operations of the machine or system, we can physically measure whether or not the action has been performed, and sometimes how well it has been performed.

PREDICTIVE MAINTENANCE

Definition from Wikipedia
     Predictive maintenance (PdM) techniques are designed to help deter-mine the condition of in-service equipment in order to predict when mainte-nance should be performed. This approach promises cost savings over routine or time-based <u>preventive maintenance</u>, because tasks are performed only when warranted.

The main promise of predictive maintenance is to allow convenient scheduling of corrective maintenance, and to prevent unexpected equipment failures. The key is "the right information at the right time." By knowing which equipment needs maintenance, maintenance work can be better planned (spare parts, people, etc.) and what would have been "unplanned stops" are transformed to shorter and fewer "planned stops," thus increasing plant availability. Other potential advantages include increased equipment lifetime, increased plant safety, fewer accidents with negative impact on environment, and optimized spare parts handling.

PdM also benefits equipment that operates with lower life cycle energy consumption, and that can positively impact the mission being carried out within the space this equipment serves. For example, countless studies have proven that there are improvements in productivity and learning in buildings where the environment (temperature, humidity, etc.) is optimum.

A trivial example to compare preventive versus predictive maintenance would be in the area of air filters. Preventive maintenance would attempt to calculate an average life of a filter and, perhaps enabled by a CMMS, deploy maintenance staff to replace the filter at intervals that are shorter than this average life. This implies that some filters will be replaced prematurely and some filters will be replaced too late. With predictive maintenance, technology would be measuring the differential pressure across a filter. It is possible to see it load up with dirt over time (differential pressure increasing) and hence trigger a maintenance action at the right time. When the filter is replaced, the technology will record the differential pressure drop and hence verify that the replacement was done correctly. By analyzing the pressure drop across the filters over time, it is possible to better establish when and how often to change the filter and perhaps even glean information on which filter manufacturer sells a better product. Consider the benefits of this predictive approach, when the filter in question is serving a clean room manufacturing process area and any mistakes can translate to particulate contamination, production disruptions and potential product loss.

Although it is significantly more exotic than preventive maintenance, predictive maintenance is not a new topic. Historically, thermography and oil analysis have been done, temperature and pressures have been monitored, and occasionally, vibration analysis has been applied to rotating equipment. What is new is the ability to gather and process much more physical data than in the past. By using modern analytics, or "big data" approaches, which apply algorithms to system models, the effectiveness of predictive maintenance is greatly increased. Historically, predictive maintenance has been limited to individual pieces of equipment or "islands of automation," but now with big data analytics, a systems level of predictive maintenance is possible. By having big data sets from sensors all around the process and equipment, technology can build a composite view of systems operation and even correlate maintenance data to the comfort of the building or the integrity of a manufacturing process.

In the past, predictive maintenance was limited to high-value assets. What's different today is that highly skilled professionals can deploy analytics technology to automatically collect and analyze enough data so that predictive maintenance can even be applied to small end point devices. Some of these devices might include variable air volume boxes and process utility connection points, such as water for injection and compressed air connection points. The computer does the work, so automatic fault detection and diagnostics can be scaled down to the low-cost ubiquitous devices and sensors in a system.

Driven by automatic fault detection and diagnostics, these solutions can detect even minor anomalies and failure patterns to determine the assets and operational processes that are at the greatest risk of failure. This early identification of issues helps facility managers deploy limited maintenance resources more cost-effectively, maximize equipment uptime, and enhance quality.

Predictive maintenance can include:
- Observation of equipment performance drift
- Vibration analysis
- Critical process parameter monitoring
- Verification of repair (action)—by observing the data

WHAT IS REQUIRED TO DEPLOY A PREDICTIVE MAINTENANCE PROGRAM?

There are several elements needed to deploy a predictive maintenance program. First, we need a big data, analytics, collection and analysis (condition monitoring) platform such as Cimetrics' Analytika solution, which can collect, model and perform automatic fault detection with root cause analysis. The analytics platform must comprise domain expertise so that the algorithms have a premeditated application to the system in question. The next critical element is data sufficiency—the availability of data from enough sensors, actuators and control parameters (e.g. setpoints) so that meaningful analysis can be performed. Then, equipment design information such as performance curves, rated cycles, design temperatures, and design flow rates are essential to understanding how the machine works. A system is configured by mapping the sensor data to the model and by entering static data or metadata, which describe the physical characteristics of the system. Furthermore, sensor data and equipment specifications are needed so that a model can be built defining the system we would like to maintain. This process is at the nexus of technology and technical know-how, and requires highly skilled experts who understand the equipment and the business application. Armed with the technical and business understanding, it is possible to build the system model. Unlike system simulation, this emulation of the process/equipment will take the model that is created and drive the real time data we are gathering from the real sensors and actuators through that model. After analyzing the model and real-time data with a series of algorithms, we can facilitate both equipment optimization and predictive maintenance notifications (alerts). Consider Figure 6-1 as an example of such high-level architecture, in which the Analytika predictive analytics solution is deployed.

Many equipment manufacturers have historically kept information about their design and operating characteristics proprietary. Now there is an opportunity for original equipment manufacturers (OEMs) to differentiate their products by proving a complete operating model, as well as sufficient sensors and actuators, can provide the data for predictive maintenance analytics. There has been a trend among OEMs not to include sensors on systems, because it is believed that their customers don't perceive the value. Predictive maintenance might provide the impetus to provide a new level of data sufficiency.

OEMs and consulting engineers suffer from a limited world because they do not actually operate buildings. However their system and building designs dictate to building operators what they believe adds value for long-term building operations. Given very limited direct maintenance experience among manufacturers and engineers, it is unfortunate that their roles in new building design enable them to eliminate sensors that could provide huge operational or reliability benefits. Very often these decisions are driven by "first cost" and value

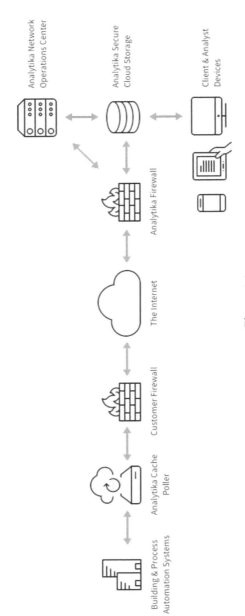

Figure 6-1

engineering efforts that fail to appreciate the importance of these elements of the system. A few years ago this author had a conversation with the manager at a chiller manufacturer, who said, "My guys know everything there is to know about chillers. Ask them anything about the machine, and they will tell you how to get 42-degree water. But they are completely ignorant of application- and systems-based issues, and of how their piece of equipment functions in a larger system." The purpose of this book is to educate the buildings industry, particularly building owners and managers, to the need for more active engagement in creating specifications for new buildings and equipment. This active engagement will ensure that overall access to energy and analytics technology can be simplified at the time of construction or in the future.

There are several ways predictive maintenance platforms can work. In their most remedial form, these systems can be used to collect data when the machine or system is working in steady state (regular operation) to create a baseline. Then statistical comparisons of current operation are made with the baseline to determine whether equipment performance is drifting. This is useful for detecting a fault in the system, but generally not as good at determining the root cause of the fault. With model-based automatic fault detection and diagnostics (FD&D), analytics systems maintain a preconceived model for the machines' ideal operating characteristics, and using real time data and sophisticated algorithms, analytics can predict where, and sometimes when, failures might occur (Figure 6-2).

Figure 6-3 is an example of a predictive maintenance finding from Analytika.

Examples of simple statistical process control techniques for predictive maintenance:
- Comparison of chiller performance curves to OEM predicitons (design curves)
- Monitoring of machine temperatures, oil viscosity, oil pressure, water pressure
- Differential pressure measurements on filters and pumps
- Pump head pressure measurements
- Vibration analysis
- Infrared thermography

Figure 6-2

Date Opened	Priority	Status	Issue #	Category	Description
5/2013	High	Updated	ABC-010	Predictive Maintenance	Equipment Rate of Travel *Tune control loop(s) to prolong equipment life and reduce the possibility of premature equipment failure.*

Figure 6-3

Table 6-1 lists the top 10 pieces of equipment with the highest actuator rate of travel during the current monitoring period. A high rate of travel may lead to premature failure of the equipment and/or the control actuator. This application is also used to identify poorly tuned control loops. Rate of travel is defined as follows:

Rate of travel: The absolute change of a signal on an hourly basis

Relative average
   rate of travel: The average of the rate of travel (per hour) over the monitoring period

Cycles during
   monitoring period: The total number of actuator cycles during the monitoring period

Cycles to date: The total number of actuator cycles since the start of monitoring

An example of a piece of equipment with a high rate of travel is shown in Figure 6-4.

BENEFITS

There are many benefits to a predictive maintenance program. Improved reliability and decreased risk of product loss and process disruptions are the most important benefits for mission critical applications such as pharmaceutical production, healthcare or manufac-

Table 6-1

EQUIPMENT	Relative Average Rate of Travel	Cycles During Monitoring Period	Cycles to Date
VAV-157 Reheat Valve	259	1,864	21,434
VAV-150 Reheat Valve	146	1,050	11,344
VAV-223A Reheat Valve	132	952	9,424
VAV-197 Damper	99	713	6,207
VAV-North Office #1 Damper	81	581	6,212
AHU-15 Reheat Valve	78	562	6,750
VAV-North Office #2 Damper	67	481	4,236
VAV-023 Damper	59	424	3,436
AHU-02 Steam Humidifier Valve	58	415	4,025
Exhaust Fan EF-12 Damper	48	342	3,524

turing. The data captured in the process of predictive maintenance analysis can be used for measurement and verification as well as providing data-historian capability for compliance reporting. Increased equipment life and an increase in mean time between failures (MTBF) can also be expected. In addition, labor savings are obtained by servicing the equipment only when necessary and dispatching repair crews with the necessary parts, thereby reducing truck rolls. Finally, in today's world, many maintenance functions are frequently outsourced to third parties. Predictive maintenance analytics allow the verification of repairs using actual operating data, allowing verification of vendor and product performance.

A predictive maintenance program aims to identify the presence of a defect in such a way as to give sufficient time for the maintenance

Figure 6-4

department to identify the root cause of the problem, efficiently order the parts, and schedule and complete the repair before a failure occurs. Consider Figure 6-4 which zone temperature and reheat value signal to determine if devices are operating properly.

Predictive maintenance program benefits:
- Police outsourced services
- Lower labor costs
- Increased reliability
- Risk mitigation
- Increased equipment life

Figure 6-5

CONCLUSION

The big data analytics revolution is beginning to enable true predictive maintenance on a large scale. Users of predictive maintenance analytics can now enjoy the benefits of cost savings, increased reliability, increased equipment life and reduced risk of process disruptions. These benefits also drive reduced energy consumption and lower energy cost. A future challenge will be the integration of predictive maintenance systems with enterprise asset management systems. Although this would seem simple at first, there is a need for a human decision maker to add business insight as to what maintenance investments should be made.

Beyond predictive maintenance, there are many other benefits to big data analytics of building systems. For example, by combining automation data with shop floor data and quality data, we can begin to gain insights that enable enterprise level risk management and process optimization. These topics and others are beyond the scope of this chapter. They highlight that we are just scratching the surface of what is possible with physical world data analytics.

Of equal importance to this book's focus on energy and analytics, is a whole new category of benefits. Any energy auditor can tell the reader that these analyses begin with a thorough evaluation of utility bills and energy consumption history. In that process it very quickly becomes evident that the explanation of consumption patterns leads to understanding how buildings and equipment are operated. During one energy audit the author conducted years ago, a fellow consultant became frustrated at how difficult it was to make the point that poor building maintenance leads to higher energy consumption and cost, and offered this analogy. The consultant expressed to the building manager that it was unlikely that anyone would maintain a $100,000 sports car as poorly as the $100,000 building chiller was being maintained, and asked why?

The power of analytics technology presents an opportunity for thorough and robust analysis of equipment and building operations to produce significant value. At the same time however, there is a diverse and complex set of functions to be carried out by these systems. This means that the reader must to be fluent in all of these functions to effectively evaluate and use analytics technology. It remains to be seen how analytics technology will be configured. Some of the initial systems on the market are one-size-fits-all, providing energy analysis, FD&D and attempting to embrace even broader feature-sets, while others offer more focused functionality. The best approach for prospective buyers is to complete a thorough needs assessment to determine both requirements and goals. With that information it will be easier to target potential solutions.

Chapter 7

Analytics for 21st Century Electricity Marketing and Energy Management

Energy and analytics are the next wave of technology evolution across industry. The term "big data" has received a huge amount of press, but these vast amounts of information are more the problem statement. Making sense of that data by summarizing and analyzing it to look for anomalies that point to problems and/or improvement opportunities, requires analytics and begins to unlock real value. Even more exciting, leveraging energy and analytics to unlock new market opportunities enhances value exponentially. That is really what 21st century energy management is all about. To be clear, the focus in this chapter will be on 21st century electricity management. As stated in earlier chapters, electricity is the highest quality fuel on the planet, while at the same time being the most capital intensive and environmentally impactful source of energy as well. Figure 7-1 is from the Galvin Electricity Initiative (www.galvinpower.org) and sheds more light on this fact. The "supply side" of the electricity system includes power production, and has inherent inefficiencies. That said, the electricity system is a marvel of technology. In 2003 the National Academy of Engineering in the United States published "A Century of Innovation: Twenty Engineering Achievements that Transformed our Lives." In that report the authors outlined what they believed to be the top 20 engineering achievements of the 20th century, and electrification was at the top of the list.

This book has already covered a good deal of content relating that the time is now for energy and analytics, particularly with electricity. The purpose of this chapter is to talk about how these analytics solutions may be applied to the new electricity marketplace. It will also

Figure 7-1

provide concrete examples of how this technology may be applied, and point out a few very strategic opportunities that could transform energy management in the 21st century. This dialog will begin with what the author calls the electricity triple threat. This triple threat came into focus with the June 2, 2014, Environment Protection Agency's ruling on coal-fired power plants, which was discussed in Chapter 5. The ruling is intended to tackle the carbon impact on climate change that is produced by electricity from the "plant to the plug."

This bold policy initiative may be controversial, but it puts a spotlight on an "electricity triple threat." EPA Administrator Gina McCarthy outlined the "Clean Power Plan" and its goal to cut carbon pollution from existing coal-fired power plants. The new rule mandates a 30 percent reduction in carbon dioxide emissions from these power plants by 2030. Each state was given customized goals, based upon local conditions, and the Obama Administration gave states until 2017 to develop local plans to meet those limits. In the original announcement,

Energy Triple Threat

Climate Change & Coal

Electricity Demand

Energy Economics

McCarthy highlighted local success stories in cities like Salt Lake City and St. Paul, Minnesota, which the agency hopes to see replicated across the country.

So how does this plan relate to an *"electricity triple threat?"* The triple threat for electricity emphasizes that it is a very high quality form of energy, but also that is a commodity with some very unique characteristics, including that it cannot be stored in bulk. The triple threat consists of three conditions that could blindside building and energy managers:

1. **Climate Change**—The U.S. Environmental Protection Agency (EPA) initiated rules to reduce up to 30% of the carbon emissions from the 600 U.S. coal-fired power plants. These rules may force closing plants that are too expensive to retrofit, but it is also exciting because it will very likely spur investment in energy efficiency and renewable energy. In New York, for example, Indian Point Nuclear Generating Station is scheduled to be shut down in 2016. This plant provides around 20% of the electricity consumed in New York City, but the state's primary plan to replace that energy is not to build another plant. Instead efficiency is a key strategy being used by New York's Con Edison to help offset this supply-side gap. In fact, Con Edison launched a $200+ million per year program to drive that strategy in mid-2014. California utilities grappling with the shutdown of San Onofre Nuclear Generating Station are engaged in a similar strategy. The EPA of course is targeting coal-fired power plants, which could add to the challenges faced in New York, California and elsewhere. McCarthy pointed out several times in her 2014 press conference announcing the new ruling, that cities and the state have already seen proven results taking the same types of action. Regardless of the readers' beliefs about climate change, this action will dramatically affect all energy users.

2. **Electricity Demand**—With the U.S. economic recovery over the years between 2009 and 2015, U.S. electric demand saw gradual

and increasing growth. Electric utilities dodged the "load growth" bullet in the early years after the downturn due to business decline, but that changed just as the major source of electric generation (40% U.S. electricity comes from coal) was proposed to see a forcible reduction under the EPA ruling. Increasing demand for electricity can stress the grid, particularly at peak times, and that combined with potential reduction in supply sources could have an affect on energy reliability or "resiliency."

3.   **Energy Economics**—All of the changes discussed above, driven by climate change and growing electric demand, and coupled with increasing amounts of natural gas generation, can be expected to impact electric cost too. The good news is that higher electricity cost will improve the ROI of efficiency, renewable energy and distributed generation projects, but there could be real challenges in the near term. Even so, higher electricity prices may be welcomed by those who believe that energy is underpriced, and the best way to manage consumption is to raise cost. BUT, the alternative position is that our "global economy" has seen a precarious recovery that could be threatened by major price increases to a commodity that is essential to economic vitality and growth.

Without question, effectively managing buildings and their interaction with a gradually smarter electric grid, is the most effective way for owners and managers to protect themselves from the energy triple threat. To restate the obvious, energy and analytics are the best way to drive that effective building management.

Based on this brief discussion, it may be clear that the grid is reliable, but relatively inefficient, and there are some major drivers in play that are could negatively impact the electricity system. One of the most significant challenges with electricity, as an energy source and a business, is that it is regulated independently in every state. In addition, ±20 states are deregulated for electricity which can add benefits, but also makes it more confusing. The result is a complex and intricate framework of regulations for the retail electricity business at the state level, and the wholesale electricity business at the federal level. So it is important, in the context of energy and analytics, to consider how this new technology can assist energy buyers in managing electricity consumption and cost. In the 21st century, building owners will buy electricity, but they will also become much more intelligent and automated in how they use energy. At the same time, more owners will generate power at their buildings, and sell power back to the grid when it is economically feasible. All of this leads to a new reality for electricity, and even more importantly to a great need for managers to deploy analytics to optimize energy use, cost, and sale back to the grid. In Chapter 2 on *4Plex Energy* these ideas were covered, including purchasing options from the local utility or a retail energy provider. It is common knowledge that the only way to effectively manage this level of energy complexity is to baseline and benchmark buildings, as discussed in Chapter 5. As discussed, it is important to pay particular attention to "interval electric demand data" and to the occupancy and use profiles in the building that impact all of these characteristics.

Electricity purchasing is also a great example of where interval data on energy consumption (kilowatt hours per interval period) can be valuable. Having the most detailed electricity consumption analysis is a great way to negotiate the best prices. Quite simply this means that buying electricity is much more complex than contacting the local utility to turn the power on and then paying the bill each month. In closing on this topic, those who have heard this author speak on grid topics, may have heard an outline of the "urban myth" to the first great round of electricity deregulation. The myth was that more sellers will lead to lower prices, but as outlined throughout this book, electricity is a unique commodity that cannot yet be stored at scale. The belief that more sellers will translate to better prices drove the first wave of electricity deregulation. This author believes that there will be a second wave of electricity deregulation, and it will be driven by a new awareness—more sellers do not lower electricity costs, but **smarter buyers will**. Leveraging energy and analytics as outlined in this book will make buyers smarter, enable them to drive better prices and to insulate themselves from market forces and fluctuations in electricity resilience.

Electricity has been an essential energy source for over 100 years, but in the 21st century the dynamics associated with this business will demand analytics. Owners will be able to keep the lights on without this technology, but they will be leaving money on the table—perhaps large amounts of money.

The growing awareness of how complex and essential electricity analytics and management technology has become, is among the reasons that the United States Green Building Council has launched a new excellence program called PEER. PEER (Performance Excellence in Electricity Renewal) was launched at the GREEN-BUILD conference in 2014. PEER takes great strides in rais-

ing awareness of the opportunities presented by managing buildings more proactively with regard to their interaction with the electric grid. Greenbuild is the annual event put on by the United States Green Building Council (USGBC). USGBC's impact on buildings worldwide has been astounding. The LEED (Leadership in Energy and Environmental Design) certification program has changed the way new buildings are designed and existing buildings are renewed.

PEER is so critical because "technology is blurring the lines between electricity demand in the building and the power industry, driving the need for a more integrated understanding of the essential interplay between buildings and energy generation, transmission and distribution systems. PEER seeks to enhance this interconnectedness and transform the power industry by forging cross-sector, outcome-driven collaboration, and leveraging emerging technologies, policies and consumer understanding." That quote is from the USGBC announcement at GREENBUILD. More information on PEER certification at www.usgbc.org/PEER.

USGBC and the Perfect Power Institute (PPI) launched PEER at a banquet in New Orleans during GREENBUILD 2014. They invited luminaries from the green buildings and smart grid world for the launch and announcement of the first entities to receive PEER certification. The Perfect Power Institute (PPI), which was created by the Galvin Electricity Initiative, developed the PEER standard, and it has now become part of USGBC. During the smart grid era, readers may remember that Bob Galvin, former chairman of Motorola Corporation and visionary who started the cell phone industry, became very interested in electricity. This author had the honor of working with Bob and Kurt Yeager, who co-founded the Galvin Electricity Initiative, for several years. True thought leaders, these two giants of business and industry shared a vision for transforming the electricity business. Kurt Yeager is the former CEO of the Electric Power Research Institute, and it was this author's sincere pleasure to attend the USGBC banquet with him. PEER embodies much of the vision that Bob Galvin and Kurt Yeager had for electricity.

Given the significant breadth of change underway in the electricity industry, it is important to highlight the diverse nature of how the electricity business works. In the discussion of triple threat, the ideas of electricity regulatory policy, and therefore how the business works, were touched on. The first thing for any reader to do in defining their "electric reality" is to research and develop an understanding of how electricity is regulated where they own property. A good place to start is the Energy Information Administration, which publishes a status update (www.eia.gov/electricity/policies/restructuring/restructure_elect.html).

Next, on a state-by-state level it is helpful to go to www.dsireusa.org, and then to research at the state level through the state energy office, the Public Utility Commission and with utilities themselves. Finally the reader should research the local utility and programs that support energy and analytics. Taking time to understand the regulatory environment, as well as the programs that exist, is the big picture. This information can help to frame the strategies that should be deployed for energy and analytics in any building or complex. It is possible to point to many strategies that hold promise for any building, but the specifics will come into focus based upon the local electric reality. In the context of large opportunities however, the balance of this chapter will discuss some exciting opportunities that exist globally, and that building owners and energy managers should evaluate for individual electricity markets.

The opportunities for electricity and analytics are unparalleled, compared to any other energy type. First and foremost, all managers should explore demand response and rebate programs that may be available in local utility territories. These programs can create significant opportunities to reduce near-term operating costs and generate capital to improve buildings. Such programs include on-bill financing, which is available in many utility territories. Explore www.dsireusa.org to learn more. Electricity and analytics will be instrumental in leveraging the greatest use from these programs, using approaches such as those discussed throughout this book. Integral to this discussion is metering and interval data monitoring. First it is ideal to capture electronic data directly from utility revenue meters. Most utilities will provide the interfaces for a fee. Second it is critical to be sure that the interface is providing usage (kWh consumption), demand (kW) and interval data (kW demand or kilowatt hour per sliding window billing period). Interval data on demand is the other critical data that must be captured. As discussed in this book, it is unquestioned that you cannot manage what you cannot measure and these are the data that must be measured.

This book emphasizes that discussions of electricity must first be categorized based on whether they refer to electric supply (traditionally the utility side of the meter) and electric demand (the customer side of the meter). However, the lines are truly blurring, and there is no better example than the resurgence of "distributed generation" (DG). DG is the term that will be used here, but this technology may also be called microgrids, micro turbines, onsite generation, cogeneration, combined heat and power (CHP) or solar photovoltaic (PV) power. This is a topic that most utilities loathe and, for more than four decades, it is a practice that they have discouraged. The Public Utility Regulatory Policies Act (PURPA) opened up the opportunity in 1978, and there have been several waves of implementation. Many large electricity users, particularly university campuses have deployed CHP successfully for decades. The main distinction with CHP is that it is almost universally applied in applications where all of the energy is consumed on the customer's side of the meter.

There is an "interconnect" required with the grid, and the power from the grid is intermingled with the DG electricity, but the number of universities that use the power on campus is much larger than those that sell back to the grid. The term microgrid has been used in recent years to refer to those systems that are capable of two-way power transactions, meaning to buy or to sell back to the grid. The term transactive power has also been used. This author is chairman emeritus of the GridWise Architecture Council, and that body has published content on this topic at www.gridwiseac.org. According to Gridwise, "the term transactive energy" is used here to refer to techniques for managing the generation, consumption or flow of electric power within an electric power system through the use of economic or market based constructs while considering grid reliability constraints. The term "transactive" comes from considering that decisions are made based on a value. The transaction itself may be based on the sale of electricity, or if the regulatory environment is prohibitive, it may be a purely financial transaction. An example of an application of a transactive energy technique is the double auction market used to control responsive demand-side assets in the GridWise Olympic Peninsula Project. More on The Olympic Peninsula Project may be found in the paper "Pacific Northwest GridWise™ Testbed Demonstration Projects: Part I. Olympic Peninsula Project," PNNL-17167, October 2007, Pacific Northwest National Laboratory, Richland, WA.

Solar photovoltaic (PV) systems may be the best example of the lines blurring between the supply and demand sides of electricity. The growth in solar PV installations over the last decade has been exponential, and it is not uncommon for cities, universities and others to be generating 25% to 50% of the electricity they use from PV panels onsite. Yet PV may also be the best example of a huge gap in "intelligence." DG systems, as described above, nearly always have a high degree of control and instrumentation, and have also been hot spots for early adoption of energy and analytics technology. PV, on the other hand, is almost always on a "communication island." This means that the only instrumentation on a PV system is usually the utility meter installed to capture data for renewable energy credits (RECs). These meters may use AMI technology for remote reading, but they do not communicate with anything else. This means that the opportunity to leverage renewable energy, in the form of PV, for value beyond the kilowatt hours that come from the system at any time, is often lost. For example, PV systems obviously reduce peak demand, but this author has never seen a system that actively managed the PV system and also included a demand (limiting) management strategy. Implementing energy and analytics to leverage the combined power of PV and demand limiting offers tremendous energy and economic value.

Most PV companies don't understand peak demand, or how to control it, so they exclude any evaluation of this opportunity from their analysis. They also exclude strategies to manage PV and demand from implementation plans. This is a huge mistake. Consider how much value could be gained if building automation system (BAS) technology were combined with energy and analytics technology to control the overall system. Such technology would balance three criteria: 1) optimal efficiency, 2) maximum value form PV generation, and 3) active control of building electric use, through demand limiting, when PV output drops. This combination of strategies would maximize cost effectiveness. This is the next frontier for buildings that deploy any form of DG, but particularly solar PV.

In summary, the electricity business is highly complex, and yet electricity itself remains the essential ingredient for every aspect of the 21st century lifestyle as well as every aspect of business and the economy. Energy and analytics for management of electric supply, demand and cost are untapped, and can be expected to see huge growth in the near future.

Part II—System Technology

Ken Sinclair AutomatedBuildings.com

I am very pleased to provide perspective on system technology, Chapters 8 through 18, of this amazing book. I have known Jack McGowan for over 30 years. When I first met him he was writing a book, and I was honored when he used some of my material for one of the chapters. He has spent much of his life as an educator of our industry so we are all pleased that he has taken on this task of sharing his insight on the big picture of our industry, and the important topic of energy and analytics is this book. Jack has the ability to capture and organize all that is around him and contextualize it into value for others.

Jack has been a personal mentor plus the greatest fan ever of mine and Jane's efforts at creating and maintaining what is AutomatedBuildings.com.

He is the rare combination of a teacher and a doer, hence his ability to prepare a book of this magnitude, volume and embodied wisdom.

It is important to understand this book is written for people—people like you. People are our only asset, technology may come and go, but at the core of the industry are the same people who have been there for years. The problem is these core people are growing older, and much of the discussion now is that we all need to plant new people, nourish them, and help them grow.

This book does an amazing job of providing a base, the actual ground where these new younger people can grow.

Your company's and the industry's technologies may come and go, but the people are the only true assets that remain and recreate new businesses to keep the industry strong. This greatly increases the importance of the induction of new blood—younger folks with IoT smarts—into our industry. If we are to build on our existing assets, the people, then we need to invest in education and transfer of the knowledge of our assets. We need to look at new talent as an investment that can greatly increase our existing assets. As you read the following chapters, stay focused on how our assets, the people, are needed to make these technologies achieve their full potential.

Buildings connected with open protocols to the powerful internet cloud and its web services are redefining the building automation industry. The result of that redefinition is that the reach and the visibility of the industry have never been greater, nor has change been so rapid. Our "clouded" future includes new virtual connections to buildings, from the communities they are part of, with both physical and social interactions. An example is digitally displayed energy/environmental dashboards to inform all of the building's impact in real-time energy use, plus the percentage generated from renewable sources. And connections to the smart grid make buildings a physical part of their supply energy infrastructure.

The ability to operate buildings efficiently via the internet cloud from anywhere allows the building automation industry to be better managed and appear greatly simplified. Web services, or software as a service (SaaS) as it is sometimes called, coupled with powerful browser presentation are changing how we appear and interact with clients.

The data cloud for our industry has become real. As we see applications and services moved "off-site," you can imagine the opportunities for managing real estate, reducing energy and providing value-added applications for buildings.

We must unhinge our minds and find new pivot points from which to build our future. We must embrace the power of the cloud while increasing our comfort level in using the solutions within.

Cloud Opportunities

New applications and infrastructure do not reside in end users premises; instead, the end user accesses the application on demand via a web browser on any device. This means he can concentrate on using the application for its purpose, without investing in capital expenditure, while avoiding the overhead of installation, networking and maintenance.

With the emergence of open system protocols, wired and wireless, and worldwide emphasis on energy management and sustainability, the rate of adoption of new technology by building automation vendors has increased dramatically, particularly in the use of web technology and open system architecture to integrate and converge with IT networks to create new features in a more cost effective and time efficient manner.

Online Commissioning

Connectivity of everything is a growing reality, and with each new connection come new opportunities and new perspectives. Just as low-cost powerful connectivity is changing and actually simplifying our personal lives with internet extensions (i.e. "apps") to our handheld devices, building automation is caught up in the same connectivity growth.

In today's complex buildings, even small problems can have big impacts on building performance. Lighting, heating, ventilating and air conditioning systems need continuous performance tracking to ensure optimal energy efficiency. Yet, a formal process for data gathering and analysis is not commonplace in the nation's building stock. Plus, there's often a disconnect between the energy modeling done in isolated, one-time re-commissioning or energy audit projects, and what happens in day-to-day operations.

What's needed is a systematic approach to tracking energy utilization that helps detect problems early, before they lead to tenant comfort complaints, high energy costs, or unexpected equipment failure. That's why new robust energy monitoring technologies and monitoring-based commissioning (MBCx) techniques are now at the forefront in building energy management.

The continuing question is how to convert data into meaningful information that is contextual and actionable. The operations center is an environment where meaningful information can be extracted and presented to produce a high level of situational awareness, align related work processes, minimize workload and errors, enhance task performance, and provide information and reporting tools required to manage the building's operations.

I am very pleased that Jack has included a chapter on Haystack Connect and the Next Generation of Energy Standards, and a Chapter on The Internet of Things. It shows how this far-reaching book has information created only a few years ago and provides connections (words to Google) to evolving online resources.

When you have read this book completely, you will grasp the scope and complexity of *Energy and Analytics—Big Data and Building Technology Integration*. Please share your new-found knowledge with your peers in discussions and on social media. Reach out to involve the people who are rising to be the new assets of our industry. Teach them what Jack taught you in this book, become their mentors, lead them to the resource of this "Theory of Everything Book" for our industry.

Chapter 8

Building Systems Technology: The Foundation of Analytics

A recurring assertion in this book is that there is significant potential for analytics. Yet there has also been emphasis on the importance of providing quality data to the analytics technology, and the fact that it is extremely costly to build entire new networks of instrumentation for this purpose. As a result it becomes very important to identify existing systems that have access to necessary data, and devise strategies to extract those data and make them available to analytics tools. Well, that is easier said than done. That is why the next several chapters in this book will provide in-depth coverage of the building systems that house important data. These systems include building automation systems (BAS), sometimes called energy management systems (EMS), and other building systems. It is the author's hope that the reader read the independent foreword that was provided for this section of the book. It was written by one of the most respected, and knowledgeable, professionals in the building technology, Ken Sinclair. Ken had a distinguished career as a consulting engineer in British Columbia, specializing in building systems, before starting the most prestigious electronic magazine in the industry, www.automatedbuildings.com. With automatedbuildings. com, Mr. Sinclair has created the "go to" resource for professionals seeking content on buildings, BAS, systems deployed throughout facilities and communications, and networking/web-based technology that is utilized by and interfaced with those systems. With Mr. Sinclair's introduction and deep technical knowledge, it is the authors' intent to expand the reader's view of energy and analytics to embrace building systems. Therefore this section of the book begins with a recognition that this may be new content for many readers, but also with the recognition that these systems are essential to implementing a robust and effective analytics program. It is of particular import that these systems will also provide implementation tools to enable recommendations that come from energy and analytics tools. It cannot be overemphasized that deployment of analytics requires an interdependence with building systems. Further this interdependence goes beyond the initial implementation, but requires ongoing diligence by management staff to ensure that the flow of quality data is uninterrupted, a topic that has been referred to as "data quality."

This series of chapters begins with an outline strategic planning and enterprise energy management from a team at the University of Louisiana in Lafayette. Though focused on energy management, this document highlights the need to inventory all building equipment including lighting, HVAC, etc., as discussed in Chapter 5. This type of rigorous inventory, energy history and planning process is essential to understanding the full breadth of the facilities involved, and to clearly understand the data points that will be needed. This will allow managers to determine whether data points may be accessed from existing systems. The section will go on to provide a detailed treatise on building automation and other facilities systems, as well as the underlying data communication systems that this technology deploys. All of this information is critical to avoid the need for implementing completely new sensor networks. The section will then delve into the topics of integration and IT/middleware technology. Accessing data from disparate systems requires specialized techniques and technologies that readers should understand well enough to evaluate proposals from solution providers.

As discussed in the author's note and in the initial chapters of this book, this is a complex topic that is impacted by wide ranging policy, business and technology trends. Energy management in the 21st century will require energy and analytics technology. Armed with this technology, building owners/managers and certified energy managers CEMs will be able to fully optimize their buildings and campuses. The goal of this series of chapters, and Section II of this book, is to assist the reader in this process of optimization, by providing detailed content regarding the fabric of underlying building and energy technology that is critical for analytics to drive maximum value. Ken Sinclair's foreword along with this chapter are here to provide insight on how these technologies are interconnected and interoperable, and what that could mean for energy and analytics. These underlying systems must exist to capture enough data for meaningful analytics. As noted, in many cases they are also required to execute the changes recommended by analytics engines.

Chapters in this section will discuss applications that are driven by the analytics but will also address new technology and practice. One such important technology evolution discussed is the Internet of Things (IoT). IoT is most appropriate because all of the technology discussed in this book has become interconnected with communication networks, and the internet. Access to the internet makes it possible for analytics to enable and automate smart decision making. This will impact energy and buildings in a profound way. It will be similar to the impact that the internet has had on consumers, enabling them to explore options, and compare and select products and services, in ways unlike at anytime in the past. Another important topic that could unleash even more profound market growth is data modeling and the exciting work of Project Haystack. Haystack represents the efforts of numerous emergent technology companies that have chosen to band together and tackle a major challenge of analytics. That challenge is devising data standards that make it possible to capture data from myriad systems quickly without the need for mapping and converting points. Finally this section will touch briefly on the topics of financing and measurement and verification for energy projects. Whether the financing discussion focuses on mechanisms that may be used to acquire systems, or on measurement and verification to ensure that these system investments perform as intended, it is an important topic for readers to consider.

Chapter 9

Six-Sigma Approach to Energy Management Planning

Jim Lee, Kirkrai Yuvamitra, Theodore A. Kozman, Kelly Guiberteau
Department of Mechanical Engineering
University of Louisiana at Lafayette, Lafayette, Louisiana 70504

INTRODUCTION

The first step for any energy and analytics program is planning. It may seem out of order therefore to provide this content as Chapter 9 of the book. This is because the first section of the book was designed to provide introductory content that outlined the full breadth of market and industry potential that exists for energy and analytics. If given that content, readers determine that it is time to implement energy and analytics, this section will be very useful in providing an understanding of what is required. This chapter from a team at the University of Louisiana at Lafayette is highly effective, and equally exciting as it incorporates the idea of Six-Sigma. At its core the idea behind energy and analytics is to create a framework that optimizes systems performance for both efficiency and operation effectiveness. Any program of this type must be able to accomplish those goals in a fashion that is repeatable. The beauty of integrating Six-Sigma is that it underscores that continuous improvement is essential, and also provides a framework that has been highly effective in analyzing processes and developing improvements. It is particularly poignant for this author, because I had the opportunity to work with Bob Galvin, in many ways the father of Six Sigma, until his death. As discussed in Chapter 7, Bob founded the Galvin Electricity Initiative with Kurt Yeager because he believed that the power industry was in dire need of an excellence program. He believed that the regulatory business model stifled creativity and innovation and was to the detriment of all electricity consumers.

There are many benefits to implementing a Six Sigma energy management program, but perhaps one of the greatest is that it is built on a framework that drives it to continuously improve. This is the ideal embodiment of a solution to the old adage "one cannot manage what one cannot measure." Building a program of this type ensures measurement, but equally important it ensures an ongoing process that continues to measure and evaluate to ensure that operations are optimized, and to identify additional steps that can be taken to further enhance the building, campus, etc. In an ideal world, the purpose of energy and analytics is to provide tools for automating analysis and evaluating performance. The next logical step is to develop an implementation program to deploy building improvements, and there again the analytics enable managers to evaluate the performance of those improvements. At each stage analytics provides timely information to make timely and effective decisions about performance and actions that are necessary. The reader should note that this planning process must also consider more than efficiency. The planning process must consider the electricity demand side, or consumption characteristics described here, as well as the electricity supply side. The electricity supply side has historically been the purview of utility companies, but as discussed in Chapter 7 the rapid advance of distributed generation (DG) at the customers premise is changing this reality. DG is increasingly important to the planning process, and could include: solar photovoltaic panels on the roof, a micro-turbine or full-scale combined heat and power (CHP). Regardless of its form, DG introduces significant change to energy management planning. The reader should incorporate that thinking into the planning process. As a final note, the content in this paper clearly refers to a manufacturing process application, and as such does not incorporate all of the systems that might be encountered in a commercial building or university campus, particularly cooling equipment. However, the focus here is more specifically on the process rather than the application, and the reader is encouraged to develop any additional information that might be appropriate for their given application.

ABSTRACT

Most companies would like to reduce costs, and at the same time the government and society are pushing for more "green" practices.

By having an energy management plan, a company can reduce energy usage and reduce operating costs because energy costs money. The main purpose for an energy management plan is to decrease energy consumption and costs. This paper will cover Six-Sigma based energy management planning procedures, to include: define, measure, analyze, improve, and control. An overview of some of the major energy consuming equipment found in most industries is discussed and different energy saving opportunities are presented in the plan. The benefits from this research will provide information and a clear understanding for establishing an energy management plan and what is to be expected when performing an energy audit to save energy and cost.

Keywords: Energy management plan, Six-Sigma approach, energy savings, energy audit, energy saving technology, ISO 50001.

INTRODUCTION

Energy management plan (EMP) is an important summary of activities that entails the information and steps that should be taken by a company to save energy and costs. The activities suggested are highly cost-effective requiring very little budget [1]. The EMP reported in this chapter was developed after an energy audit was performed by Louisiana Industrial Assessment Center for an oil service industry.

The objectives of an EMP are to improve energy efficiency, reduce cost, and conserve natural resources. The specific goals are:

- Continuously improve energy efficiency by establishing and implementing an effective energy management plan while providing a safe and comfortable work environment.

- Suggest an action plan with economic analysis to reduce energy cost.

- Encourage continuous energy conservation by employees through work and personal activities.

A Six-Sigma approach to define, measure, analyze, improve, and control is used to describe the five main steps in the energy management plan [2]. The development of EMP can be considered as the first step to achieve ISO 50001, a world-class energy management standard that integrates with ISO 9001 and ISO 14001 [3].

While an EMP is used to identify energy saving opportunities and tools, ISO 50001 is designed to help companies evaluate and prioritize the implementation of energy-efficient technology and promote efficiency throughout the supply chain. Superior Energy Performance (SEP) [4] is an ANSI/ANAB-accredited certification program that builds on ISO 50001 to provide industrial and commercial facilities with a pathway to continuously improve energy efficiency while boosting competitiveness. Demonstrations of SWEP can be found in [5].

This chapter focuses on use of the six-sigma approach in energy management planning. Figure 9-1 shows a flow chart for the Six-Sigma approach and the major steps are discussed in the following sections.

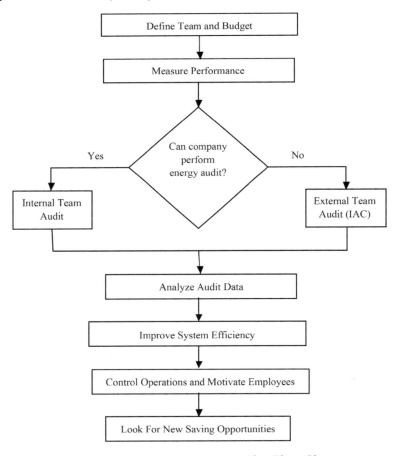

Figure 9-1. Energy Management Plan Flow Chart

DEFINE TEAM AND BUDGET

The first step in the energy management plan is to establish an energy team and to budget for implementation. They are discussed below.

Establish Energy Team

Establishing an energy team helps to integrate energy management by measuring and tracking energy performance, analyzing, planning, and implementing specific improvements. The size of the energy team will vary depending on the size of organization. In general, the energy team members are as below:

- **Energy Director**: An energy director should be a member of senior staff and have both a technical background and familiarity with the organization. Most importantly, an energy director must understand how energy management helps the organization achieve its objectives and goals. The responsibilities for energy director are:
  - Directing and coordinating the overall energy management operations.
  - Acting as the point of contact for senior management.
  - Creating the formal action plan.
  - Establishing and directing the energy team.
  - Providing budget for implementation.
  - Measuring, analyzing and monitoring progress.
  - Establishing recognition and reward program.

- **Project Engineer**: The project engineer should have a technical background and provide the team with technical specification information on production equipment. He/she is also responsible for researching new technologies, which can help improve energy savings.

- **Maintenance Supervisor**: The maintenance supervisor is responsible for providing operations scheduling information to the team to assist scheduling in the action plan.

- **Department Representative**: The department representative will cooperate with the maintenance supervisor for implementation.

Provide Budget for Implementation

Reasonable budgeting is a must for implementing an energy management plan. This should be made available under company guidelines. Budget allocation should be known to the energy team at the start of the year. According to the data provided by the Louisiana Industrial Assessment Center [6], the average implementation budget for a mid-sized manufacturer is around $40,000 to cover insulation, maintenance, and installation of energy-saving devices. The flowchart for the define step is shown in Figure 9-2.

MEASURE PERFORMANCE

Understanding how energy is used in the past and present will help the organization identify energy performance and saving opportunities. In this step, the method for measuring performance is energy audit. Energy audit can be performed either by an internal audit team(s) or by an outside service. An outside service like those provided by Industrial Assessment Centers throughout the US will look at basic energy consump-

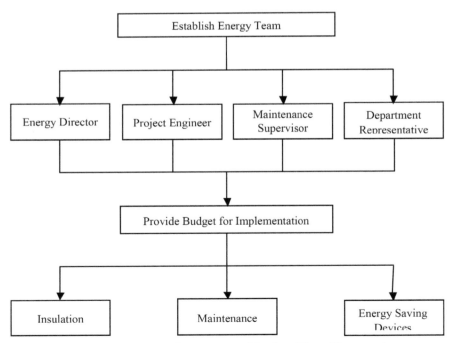

Figure 9-2. Define Team and Budget Flow Chart

tion practices and will not often get involved within specific processes key to the manufacture or maintenance of a product.

The advantage of an internal audit is that the energy team would be more familiar with the manufacturing process and more comfortable making suggestions for reductions of energy within a specific process. The main disadvantage of an internal team is being too comfortable with current practices, and the team will sometimes miss obvious opportunities for improvement. Another disadvantage of an internal audit is a lack of experience or knowledge of means of reducing energy.

The best way to perform an energy audit is to initially have an outside team come in and give an internal energy team the stepping stones of where to start reducing energy. There are two steps in an energy audit: pre-audit data collection and onsite technical audit. See the tables below.

Collect Pre-energy Audit Data

A pre-energy audit is the preparation step for a technical energy audit session, which includes collecting basic data on utilities' bills (types of energy usage, amount of energy usage, energy costs), types of equipment (size, hours of operation) involved in the processes, waste and recyclable, and production data. The data gathered during this step will allow the energy team to identify what they need to be looking for and what data they must gather while walking through the plant. A sample data collection form for pre-energy audit is shown in Table 9-1.

Perform Technical Energy Audit

During the technical energy audit, all real-time data are recorded and any missing information from the pre-energy audit is gathered. This step is a detailed audit of the entire facility. The data gathered during this part of the audit will be analyzed later for saving opportunities and implementation. The focus areas during the audit are:

- Heat loss for boilers

- Cooling equipment specifications and peration time and settings for HVAC systems

- Lighting count: including type, how it is being used and lighting intensity (lux)

- Air decay test and operating pressure for air leaks in compressed air systems

Table 9-1. Sample of Pre-energy Audit Data Collection Form

Company: ABC Manufacturing	Plant Supervisor: John Crisler

Energy Data	
Energy Usage per Year	19,152,000 kWh/yr (Electricity) and 4,227 MMBtu/yr (Natural gas)
Energy Cost ($/unit)	0.05353 $/kWh (Electricity) and 11.63 $/MMBth (Natural gas)
Energy Tax ($/unit)	0% (Electricity) and 0% (Natural gas)
Energy Cost ($/yr)	1,025,232 $/yr (Electricity) and 49,152 $/yr (Natural gas)
Comment:	

Plant Production Data

Shift	Time	Hours	Days/Week	Weeks/Year	Hours/Year
Shift 1	07.00 am – 3 pm	8	5	52	4080
Shift 2	3 pm – 11 pm	8	5	52	4080
Shift 3	-	-	-	-	-
Comment:					

Equipments

Types	Location	# Units	Size	Operating Condition	Time of Operation
Boilers (gas)	Boiler room	1	150 Hp	Steam pressure 75 psi 250 F	7 am – 11 pm
Compressed air	Outside	1	185 HP	120 psi	7 am – 11 pm
HVAC	Office	3	24,000 Btu	72 F	7 am – 4 pm
Comment: 1 HP of boiler is equal to 33,475 Btu/Hr					

As an example of data required, a sample data collection form for boilers is shown in Table 9-1. The flow chart for the measure performance step is shown in Figure 9-3, following Table 9-2. An external technical energy audit for Cameron was performed by Louisiana Industrial Assessment Center. Future work will entail performing internal energy audits to identify new saving opportunities.

ANALYZE AUDIT DATA

Analyzing data collected from the audit can help an organization gain better understanding of the current and future energy usage and

Table 9-2. Sample of Technical Energy Audit Data Collection Form for Boilers

Company: ABC Manufacturing					Plant Supervisor: John Crisler	
Boilers Data						
Type	**Location**	**Boiler Number**	**Size**	**Time of Operation**	**Operating Condition Include Operating Temp**	
Gas	Boiler room	1	150 HP	7 am – 11 pm	75 psi 250 F	
Infrared Pictures						
Picture No.	**Boiler Number**	**Hot Spot Area (ft²)**	**Hot Spot Length/Surface Area (ft)**	**Hot Spot Location**	**Hot Spot Temp (F°)**	**Ambient Temp (F°)**
1	1	25	2.36	valve	126.9	80
2	1	3	0.75	Firebox cover	333.8	80
Comment: 1 Hp is assumed to be 34.5 Lbs/Hr of saturated steam flow rate at 0 psig and 212 F° Focus on any surface temperature that is over 140 F° (Based on OSHA Safety Standards)						

Figure 9-3. Measure Performance Flow Chart

required budget for an implementing energy management plan. Saving opportunities will be identified, and energy savings, cost savings, implementation costs and payback period will be calculated. The results will later be used for developing energy saving goals and developing an action plan. Table 9-3 summarizes the results of the analyses.

Identify Saving Opportunities

The first step in analyzing audit data is to identify saving opportunities. Table 9-3 shows a list of saving opportunities based on an oil service industry audit. For example, based on OSHA safety standards and technical audit data, the saving opportunity for a boiler is to install boiler insulation.

A flow chart for analyze audit data is shown in Figure 9-4.

Table 9-3. Saving Opportunities, Resources Saving Per Year, Energy and Cost Savings, Implementation Costs and Payback Period

#	Saving opportunities	Energy savings per year	Cost savings ($/yr)	Implementation Costs ($)	Payback period (yr)
1	Insulate surface for hot processes	13 MMBtu	$145.00	$356.00	2.45
2	Preventive maintenance for group lighting replacement	3,424 labor hours	$102,711.00	$10,348.00	0.1
3	Repair leaks in compressed air system	324,606 kWh	$17,376.00	$12,200.00	0.7
4	Reduce number of lights	89,463 kWh	$4,789.00	$5,670.00	1.18
5	Install Vending Mizers	17,472 kWh	$935.00	$1,838.00	1.96
6	Insulate surface for cold processes	645 kWh	$35.00	$56.00	1.62
7	Utilization of occupancy sensor lighting controls	11,311	$606.00	$4,020.00	6.64
8	Replace lighting with more efficient lights	6,839 kWh	$366.00	$3,220.00	8.8
	Total	-	$126,963	S37,708	-

Figure 9-4. Analyze Audit Data Flow Chart

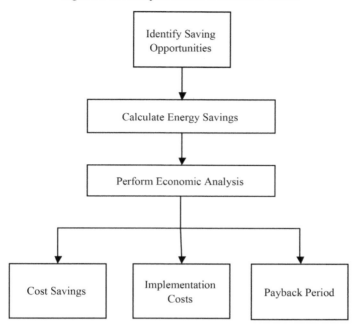

Calculate Energy Savings

Based on the saving opportunities, the next step is to calculate energy savings. For example, installing boiler insulation can be estimated using DOE tool 3E Plus with the following input parameters:

- Indoor wind speed 5 mph
- Mean surface temperature
- The ratio of length and area of hot surface
- Insulation thickness 1 inch (fiberglass foam, 450F MF BLANKET, Type II)

Perform Economic Analysis

The economic analysis includes estimating the cost savings, the implementation costs, and the payback period. The cost savings can be either energy cost savings or labor cost savings. For example, the cost saving for installing boiler insulation is calculated by energy savings multiplied by energy cost per unit.

Implementation cost is calculated based on the cost of material (capital cost) and the labor cost required for each saving opportunity.

For example, implementation cost for boiler insulation is calculated by total number of insulation needed and the labor cost. The total number of insulation needed is based on the total area of hot surface. The labor cost is calculated based on assumption that one labor hour can install insulation 3 ft^2. A simple payback period can be calculated by estimating the costs of implementation and dividing by the cost savings.

IMPROVE SYSTEM EFFICIENCY

Once the audit data have been analyzed, the next step is to develop an energy saving goal and an action plan. The improve system efficiency flow chart is shown in Figure 9-5.

Figure 9-5. Improve System Efficiency Flow Chart

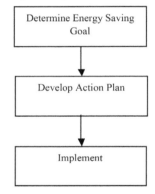

Determine Energy Saving Goal

A performance goal drives energy management activities and promotes continuous improvement. The goal must be clear and measurable. The goal for energy savings is normally between 15%-5% at the end of the first year. The following year's goal should be between 10%-3%.

Develop Action Plan

After the goal is in place, a detailed action plan must be developed for implementing recommendations. It is imperative that the energy team procures all necessary items (including budget) to achieve the implementations. The action plan must include the performance target, time line and department roles for implementations. The action plan should start with the safety issues and then move to opportunities with the highest potential cost savings. A sample action plan may include the following activities:

- Insulate surface for hot processes (approximately 10 labor hours).

- Preventive maintenance for group lighting replacement (approximately 159 labor hours).

- Repair leaks in compressed air system (approximately 305 labor hours).

- Reduce number of lights (approximately 189 labor hours).

- Install vending mizers (approximately 1.5 labor hours).

- Insulate surface for cold processes (approximately 1 labor hour).

- Utilization of occupancy sensor lighting controls (approximately 34 labor hours).

- Replace lighting with more efficient lights (approximately 15 labor hours).

Implement

After the action plan has been clearly stated, the next step is to start implementing. People can make or break an energy management plan, so it is important to gain the support and cooperation of key people at different levels within the organization.

CONTROL OPERATIONS AND MOTIVATE EMPLOYEES

In energy management, there must be a control plan to monitor the progress of the work done for implementation, make the implementation sustainable, and also monitor the savings incurred. The monitoring progress can be performed by periodic monthly reports, which can show progress on any work being done, and monitoring the electrical bills each month can also show a drop in electrical usage. The control operations and motivate employees flow chart is shown in Figure 9-6.

Perform Preventive Maintenance

After implementation, it is important to sustain the improvement and to prevent future failures by preventive maintenance. The recommended activities for various equipment are discussed below.

Figure 9-6. Control Operations and Motivate Employees

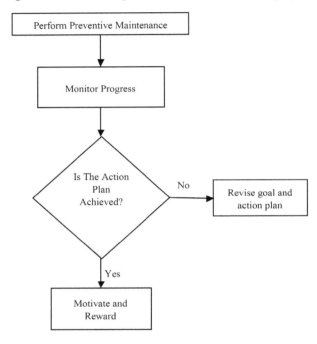

Boiler Preventive Maintenance

- Visually inspect all refractory surfaces, such as the boiler door, daily.

- Clean the surface if the fireside or waterside of boiler is dirty.

- Make sure that the air duct supply is clean, weekly.

- Check the fuel filter weekly to make sure that there will be enough fuel supplied for higher loads.

- Check wiring, monthly.

- Check weekly for leaks along the supply lines.

- Keep a daily record of fuel consumption and operating conditions.

Compressed Air Systems Preventive Maintenance

- Determine the amount of air leaks present in a system using a decay test. The test can be done by measuring the drop in air pressure in an air system over a period of time (about 120 seconds).

- Find and fix air leaks as they occur in the system. Air leaks can be found through a bubble test for small air leaks or though acoustic leaks. Once leaks are fixed the air pressure can be lowered.

- Operate system at the optimum pressure requirement, usually 100 psi.

- Turn off air system when compressed air is not in use.

Lighting Systems Preventive Maintenance

- **Cleaning of Lenses or Skylights**: Cleaning allows more light to enter the work space and reduces the need for excessive lighting fixtures. This could also be considered a safety hazard if dust collects on the lens of a light fixture and will be ignited by the heat of the fixture.

- **Group Lighting Replacement**: In most production areas high ceilings are used along with metal halide bulbs, which require the use of a man-lift to access the bulbs for changing. Group lighting is when lights are sectioned into four groups and every 6 months a maintenance team would change all of the lights in a section, regardless of whether the bulb is burnt out or not. The maintenance crew would not return to replace these bulbs until their recommended life (about 2 years) is spent. The time saved in man-hours by doing this type of light replacement is greater than the cost of throwing away some light bulbs that are not burnt out.

HVAC Systems Preventive Maintenance

- Inspect and refill refrigerant fluid to required level every 6 months
- Clean dirt and sludge from evaporator and condensate coils, annually.
- Lubricate fan motor and fan blade, annually.
- Inspect compressor and tubes for leakages, annually.
- Check all connectors, breakers, and wires for damage, annually.
- Clean or replace air filter, quarterly.

Monitor Progress

There are many ways to monitor progress of the work done for implementation as described below:

- Review weekly report for the progress of implementation.

- Review monthly report for the savings occurred.
- If the action plan is not achieved, revise the goal and action plan.
- If the action plan is achieved, go to step 5.3 and look for new saving opportunities.

Motivate and Reward

Offering incentives for energy management is one way to create interest in energy initiatives and foster a sense of ownership among employees. There are many ways to motivate employees such as [7]:

- **Internal Competition**: Use tracking sheets, scorecards, etc. to compare performance of similar facilities and foster sense of competition.

- **Recognition**: Highlight and reward accomplishments of individuals, departments, and facilities.

- **Financial Bonuses and Prizes**: Offer cash bonuses and other rewards if goals are met.

CONCLUSIONS

The purpose of having an energy management plan is to save energy and costs while a company still produces the same quality and quantity of products. Energy savings can come as a result of managing existing systems or from using new technologies. There are several areas in which most companies can save money such as lighting, HVAC, and production. These saving opportunities are identified through energy audits and implemented through preventive maintenance, replacement of old technology, and equipment workload balance.

As part of a company's initiative to lowering their costs, it is important to have an energy management plan in place along with an energy management team. For the EMP, the team must develop management commitment, energy audits, implementation, tracking of implementation, and a rewards system. Having a well-organized and devoted energy team is important in making progress on energy management.

References

[1]   Chemical Industry Digest. 2007. Effective Energy Management. http://www.energy-managertraining.com/Journal/18072007/EffectiveEnergyManagement.pdf

[2]   Summers, D. 2011. "Lean Six Sigma: Process Improvement Tools and Techniques": *Prentice Hall*. 1st ed.

[3]   US Department of Energy. 2012. ISO 50001 Energy Management Standard. http://www1.eere.energy.gov/energymanagement/.

[4]   Achieving Superior Energy Performance. 2012. Overview. http://www.superiorenergyperformance.net/index.html.

[5]   US Department of Energy. 2012. Superior Energy Performance Demonstrations. http://www1.eere.energy.gov/manufacturing/tech_deployment/sep_demonstrations.html

[6]   Kozman, T. and J. Lee, 2010. "The Results of More Than 250 Industrial Assessments for Manufacturers by the Louisiana Industrial Assessment Center for the Past Ten Years," Proceedings 2009 Industrial Energy Technology Conference (IETC). ESL-IE-10/11. New Orleans, LA.

[7]   Energy star, 2012. Guidelines for Energy Management Overview [Online] Available at http://www.energystar.gov/index.cfm?c=guidelines.guidelines_index

Chapter 10

State-of-the-art Building Automation Systems (BAS) Executing Direct Digital Control

Reviewing the breadth of building automation system technology executing direct digital control (BA^{DDC}) in one chapter, is daunting if even feasible. With that caveat therefore, the assumption here will be that the reader here will have, at least, passing familiarity with heating ventilating and air conditioning (HVAC) equipment, basic temperature and energy controls, and building automation systems (BAS). The topic of the book is energy and analytics, and the focus is on buildings and campuses, so it is hoped that this content will be useful to the reader. In the alternative, some readers might ask why this book covers building automation technology, anyway, and the answer is simple. As introduced in Chapter 8, among the most critical underlying technologies to successfully implementing energy and analytics in buildings, is the BAS. Data analytics topics are very popular in discussing all manner of complex infrastructure systems and are rapidly being deployed for public safety and a host of other applications. The single largest obstacle to wide-scale deployment of analytics across all building applications related to energy and operations, is the high cost of deploying smart sensor networks. Sensors are necessary to access the data necessary to perform the analytics and drive knowledge for management decision making. The important point for energy and buildings is that there are already extensive networks of sensors connected to BAS, meters and a host of other systems currently in place. Beyond that, the industry has also taken huge strides toward implementing "open systems" and migrating data to web based tools of all types, which means that this industry has already overcome the single greatest obstacles faced by so many others.

With that introduction, the reader should understand that the BAS is an enabling technology for energy and analytics in buildings. Therefore a brief historical perspective on BAS systems is warranted, followed by an overview of the technology. It is essential to discuss direct digital control which is executed by the BAS and to touch on critical market developments while outlining general system technology. BAS technology includes communication, networking and web services requirements for the systems which will be discussed in Chapter 11, but are clearly critical to unlocking the data from BAS sensors and energy meters to make them available for energy and analytics functionality. Finally it is critical to look at key drivers for future growth in the BAS industry, as they relate to this topic. This will be done as part of the technology discussions, yet there must be some general conclusions drawn about these trends and overall system requirements for the future.

The topic of BAS future systems is critical because ultimately these systems are, and will continue to be, restructured by technology migration from other industries and by the impact of IT based systems including middleware and web services. These IT based systems add a complex element to the BAS industry, yet as discussed, they are key to unlocking data, and the IT impact on BAS will continue pervasive and difficult to predict. Related to IT there are two critical points to make here: 1) BAS hardware components are in a dramatic state of flux and there is rapid evolution toward generic devices, and 2) HVAC and building functionality is exponentially more complex than any other IT service, such as data networking, email, etc. This means that there is no logical path to generic BAS systems with interchangeable components, and software is the key issue because of the substantial content knowledge required to develop effective BAS control strategies. As a result, the reader is cautioned to focus equal or more emphasis on finding the right company to do that work as on the technology itself. To provide a general BAS understanding, this chapter will outline the types of systems available, including the components and network infrastructure, along with a general overview of the features provided by these systems. This discussion combined with the chapters on networking/data communications and middleware should provide an excellent foundation for understanding the complexity of deploying energy and analytics functionality in a 4^{Plex} *Energy* marketplace.

HISTORICAL PERSPECTIVE

BAS have traditionally been referred to generically as control systems, and the primary focus was on heating, ventilation and air conditioning (HVAC). As early as the 1970s and 80s the topic of BAS was considered a catch-all phrase for HVAC controls, fire and life safety, as well as security, but the reference was limited. In fact, none of these systems were truly integrated for control, except in very specific examples that allow a sensed condition in one system to trigger a control sequence in another. Most important to this book is that the data in these systems were not shared; these control sequences were usually triggered by relay logic or a virtual/software point flag that caused a system to trigger the sequence. Security systems migrated to IT communication standards well before the new millennium, yet fire and life safety even at this writing are still proprietary systems that do not share data. In great part this is driven by life safety codes, but many in the industry might attribute it to a lack of willingness on the part of manufacturers in that industry to embrace change. With regard to HVAC, conventional control systems over the years have evolved from pneumatic and simplistic electro-mechanical systems to mini-computer based technologies and ultimately to the highly sophisticated microprocessor based control products and systems of today. The focus here is not to provide a discussion of older generation or non-computer based equipment, but there may be some value in researching those systems outside of this book. This is because it is sometimes easier to understand the complexity of HVAC control by breaking it down into individual elements such as temperature, pressure, equipment safety, occupant safety, etc. For overview of more recent BAS and direct digital control technology, there have been many texts published including *"Direct Digital Control, A Guide to Building Automation and Control Systems"* by John J. McGowan, CEM.

The primary intent of this chapter is provide some context for not only understanding the technology, but also the industry and marketplace drivers that have led to, and are continuing to drive, significant developments. Some examples of past technology evolutions are the move from mini computers to microprocessors and distributed direct digital control (DDC) or energy management systems (EMS); legacy systems and proprietary protocols migrating to data communications standards like BACnet™; and then middleware (i.e., Tridium), convergence, web services, the cloud and now analytics. Many of these topics will be covered in upcoming chapters, but it is worth noting that the acronyms BAS, DDC and EMS have often been used interchangeably, and for all intents and purposes they are interchangeable. In this text, the term BAS is used, but the chapter title highlights that the BAS executes direct digital control and the acronym BA^{DDC} will be used as well. The logic for using BAS as the technology descriptor is that DDC initially was a term that described where the control logic resided for a particular application. The advancement that made DDC possible was development of microprocessor-based controllers, which we now consider to be a requisite part of the BAS distributed computer architectures. These developments enabled migration of the control logic to the individual pieces of equipment, thus enhancing the granularity of control (temperature, pressure, safeties, etc.) and improving control reliability. The final point regarding system naming is that all industries are driven by markets, and when energy captures the customer's consciousness, a BAS may be called an EMS. That point provides a good segue into discussing BAS markets, prior to more discussion of technology, architecture components and features of BAS executing distributed direct digital control (DDC).

BAS MARKET

The topic of markets is important to this discussion because BAS technology has traditionally responded to "market pull." Therefore as noted, when energy efficiency is a hot topic BAS are often called EMS, but also the technology evolves to provide more solutions for that market need. At the same time when customers are concerned about stand-alone reliability and resiliency of critical applications, distributed DDC may be more important to emphasize and be the driver for new solutions. Dashboards along with energy and analytics tools are highlighted here as major market trends that may impact system naming as well, but these systems have been compartmentalized and remain independent to date. Of equal importance is that market needs, as well as technology advancements, also open up new trends that go beyond the technology itself to create new business models. These models are often the result of leveraging these technologies with "know-how" to create value by offering such services as energy savings strategies, indoor air quality, etc. All of these developments will inform and dictate how these technologies and offerings evolve in this space. Consider how the advent of distributed DDC caused a business, which was dominated by three manufacturers with vertically integrated businesses selling direct and through distribution channels, to expand into a robust market with 100 or more manufacturers selling through multiple channels. The same was true when open systems and then middleware spawned a new breed of specialty contractors called a "system integrator." Non-technology events like climate-change and the economic downturn that started in 2008, resulted in the resurgence of a retrofit market, driven by energy management and by building improvements. The savvy business people among us are trying to determine what will be the next major market driver that shakes the industry. Here is the answer: It is called *Energy and Analytics for Buildings.*

Given that introduction, it is possible to turn the clock back for a brief history of how the BAS market has evolved. The first direct digital control product was deployed at an oil refinery in Port Arthur, Texas, around 1959. Under this technology section, the book will cover architecture and device functionality in more detail with more discussion of the systems themselves and how they operate. With that project in 1959, the first of these devices providing inputs (i.e., sensors) and outputs (i.e., control relays) (I/O) were deployed at a local process. Computers were applied to process automation and heating, ventilation and air conditioning control (HVAC) for buildings in the 1960s in the form of both direct digital control (DDC), and the setpoint control market has evolved in recent years. During this time however, the primary approach was to apply minicomputers or central processing units (CPUs) for building automation. These minicomputers held all of the control algorithms and tended to execute control through conversion panels that took the digital signal through an analog interface to the pneumatic systems that were prevalent in larger more complex buildings. In spite of the limitations of this approach, significant growth occurred through the late 70s as a result of the energy shocks of 1973 and 1977. This growth further accelerated with the development of microprocessors that enabled distributed direct digital control systems. These systems were capable of complex HVAC application, as well as digital control for energy management and also applied new energy saving features for optimizing equipment operation, offsetting electrical demand, and scheduling equipment to be shut down when not necessary.

The demand for BAS has grown and continued to evolve due to a variety of market trends. The demand for technology to save energy waned in the 1980s before the green movement caused a major market resurgence later in the 1990s and beyond. During the time when interest in energy efficiency waned however, the implementation of these systems over prior decades led to an awareness of the many benefits available through automation control. Building owners saw that beyond energy cost reductions there were real benefits to better control. These benefits included longer equipment life, more satisfied tenants, and a host of new features available due to expanded building information. The communication features available through these systems allowed for managers to track their buildings more effectively and respond quickly and intelligently to problems. Intelligent response was a function of BAS communication and the ability to remotely diagnose problems, which was the precursor to development of current analytics technology. These features were extremely desirable in all types of buildings including commercial real estate. In talking with property managers, and reviewing the results of surveys by the building operators and managers associations, it is clear that tenants often begin looking for another office space when there are space comfort problems. At the same time, many tenants choose to office in "green buildings" as well. This topic has begun heating up since the early 2000s when New York, Washington DC, the State of California and others began passing laws requiring building owners to track and report on building performance. There is the belief that this "CarFax" type of reporting for buildings will make the value of energy hog buildings drop over time and create another incentive for upgrades. The BAS executing DDC market therefore continues to be driven by savings in energy but more importantly dollars, and further by enhanced control and information

Due to the market drivers listed and others in certain geographic regions, the BAS market continued to grow in the wake a limited interest in energy during the late 1980s and early 1990s. Eventually these factors fueled deployment of BAS in every new building and caused further market growth from an industry of a few hundred million in the early 1980s to a projected global market of $49.5 billion in 2018. Getting to that size was due to a continued growth trend during the years of strong construction markets in the U.S. and the Pacific Rim in the early 1990s, followed by the Middle East building booms in such areas as Dubai, Abu Dhabi in the United Emirates and elsewhere. This boom continued until the global economic crises at the end of the new millennium's first decade. The BAS became an essential component of almost all new commercial and institutional construction during those years, and that was supplemented by the growing green intelligent building movement. Emphasis on LEED and Energy Star Portfolio management scoring that could be enhance with automation, enhanced the market acceptance. Interestingly the BAS market maintained some momentum even during the downturn due to the opportunity for retrofits in existing buildings.

It should be clear at this point that the current state of BAS is made up of systems that execute direct digital control (DDC) and enable communication between components via standard data communication protocols like BACnet™. Since DDC has been highlighted, it is worthwhile to define the term. The American Society of Heating Refrigeration and Air Conditioning Engineers (ASHRAE) defines DDC as a closed loop control process implemented by a digital computer. Closed loop control, the reader may know, simply means that a condition is controlled by sensing the status of that condition, taking control actions to ensure that the condition remains in the desired range, and then monitoring that condition to evaluate whether the control action was successful. A simple example is proportional zone temperature control. The zone temperature is sensed and compared to a setpoint. If the temperature is not at setpoint, a control action is taken to add heat or cooling to the zone, and then the temperature is sensed again. A requirement to accomplish this by digital computer does not impose any particular complexity, because today even the simplest residential thermostat is likely to have electronic or digital circuitry. The author therefore expands that definition to require that the digital control be provided with a microprocessor-based device that implements a sophisticated control loop, or sequence, and is capable of communication over a standard or "open systems" network.

With the advent of web services, the market has been preoccupied with the notion of controlling devices from the internet. However this is not a likely scenario for equipment or specific building device control. The reasons quite simply go back to that first demonstration in Texas: providing control intelligence at the device level provides for the fastest and most effective processing of control algorithms. Waiting for information to be communicated over the internet for a control action will undoubtedly take longer and cause a controlled condition to float or change before the action is completed. Not all control loops require fast response, but many such as humidity or pressure control can and do require speed. As a result, web-based applications are far more appropriate for such functions as analytics, which are operating on data that include historical and current performance data to develop decision-making information. These technical progressions in this industry have been spurred by ongoing demand for energy management, but also by a variety of drivers including open systems to ease integration of legacy technologies, integration of numerous types of systems like computerized maintenance management and security, as well as standards requirements like Energy Star and LEED to name a few. The future for this market will continue to be impacted by many of the factors outlined here. Equally important is the fact that the Big Data for energy and Buildings movement will be a large driver because these systems are essential to gathering current and accurate data about building operations.

BAS TECHNOLOGY

BAS, and more specifically BA^{DDC}, technology will be discussed within the context of control architecture. Architecture in this case refers to how BA^{DDC} devices are physically wired together, but also to the notion of how they interact with one another. The BAS enterprise is the highest level of architecture and is enabled with the greatest set of capabilities. As this discussion unfolds, the reader will begin to grasp system interactions more clearly. With the advent of the internet and web-based applications the architecture can be viewed as local (in the building) or global (connected via the internet). The goal here is to ensure that the reader has a good basic understanding of BAS architecture at the local, building or campus level. Architecture, as it relates to all computer based systems, will be defined in more detail in Chapter 11, but for this discussion it may be viewed as a group of related control devices and a common communication network, such as BACnet™. Again the concept of a local area network (LAN) for building automation systems (BAS) will be discussed further in Chapter 11, but a definition of the LAN is still necessary. One comment prior to that definition however, is that this book treats the building automation system as being made up of control system components, which are referred to as controllers. The emphasis here is on energy and analytics, which again require data from the controllers within the BAS. The BAS focuses on building-wide control, and the integration of that control via many distributed devices or controllers. Distributed control devices rely by necessity on networking, within an architecture, which will be discussed in the next chapter. In addition, energy and analytics can, of course, complete equipment performance evaluations that may be used to enhance control functionality. Solutions providing such services are being introduced to the marketplace on a continuous basis.

Returning to the topic of architecture and BAS networks, a computer local area network (LAN) as defined by Thomas W. Madron "covers a limited geographic area...," where every "node on the network can communicate with every other node, and... requires no central processor."* A node is any device on the network, and for a BAS this is typically an intelligent microprocessor based controller. The control industry adds more complexity to the idea of a LAN. Unlike computer LANs, the requirement for the BAS is to provide control at an individual piece of equipment, and to also provide coordinated control for multiple pieces of equipment at multiple levels of architecture within the system. These concepts will be the focus of this chapter to set the stage for more detailed discussions of BAS protocol and networking, as a requirement for energy and analytics functionality.

The overall control architecture will be discussed in terms of the individual components. To consider the control architecture there is merit in briefly discussing a simple control application. A device within a simple BAS executing distributed DDC architecture provides control for HVAC equipment and ancillary loads such as lighting. Accomplishing this requires that distributed controllers be applied at each piece of equipment to provide application specific control. These controllers must be able to implement closed loop control via monitoring of status conditions and execution of control actions. At the same time it is also necessary to integrate overall building control provided by these devices for such functions as optimizing the building wake-up or start time. There may also be a requirement for virtual points that come from outside the control network via the internet, such as a demand response signal. These types of features for BAS systems executing DDC will be discussed in more detail throughout the book.

*Thomas W. Madron, *Local Area Networks, The Second Generation*, John Wiley & Sons, Inc., New York, N.Y., 1988, p. 3

This chapter provides the user with a basic understanding of the control architecture and technology necessary to implement a building automation system executing DDC. These systems are made possible through application of powerful microprocessor based controllers with distributed intelligence capable of equipment control, standard data communication networks such as BACnet™ and internet functionality for remote communication with energy systems, dashboards, analytics and much more.

In a typical BAS, four levels of architecture are defined: sensor/actuator, distributed controller, enterprise supervisor and dashboard. The BAS interface function is rapidly migrating from the proprietary operator interface (POI) to dashboards. All of these levels of the BAS architecture have undergone change in the last two decades and therefore each will be discussed.

The sensor and actuator technology level has traditionally been hardwired, but that is changing too. Traditionally sensors and actuators only used electrical signals rather than networking technology. Industry standard signals like 4 to 20 milliamps that are wired to a controller are most common. Controllers must then use analog to digital, or A to D, conversion technology to convert the signal to an engineering unit for use with the control sequence. For the purposes of this book, we will not delve into this technology except to note that sensor based local area networks are not far from deployment with lower cost and more compact nano-circuitry. The factors that will determine how quickly these devices achieve market acceptance will have to do with enhanced features, game changers like reliable wireless networking, cost of the technology, as well as the installation and need for the data. Interestingly, energy and analytics could be one of the factors that drives this evolution, because not all of the data are currently installed, and that will require further deployment that can be costly.

At the upper level of architecture the dashboard interface is a critical system component, yet it is ancillary to control. This level will not be discussed here, because it is covered as part of the enterprise supervisor section, an entire chapter has been devoted to the topic, and it will be treated throughout the book.

An interesting note regarding building automation systems is that there may be sublevels within the architecture. The most common implementation of distributed systems is to have both a zone level controller, tailored to simple applications like the VAV terminal unit, as well as an equipment level, or general purpose, controller for larger pieces of equipment like the VAV air handler. These two types of controllers will have different requirements and designs to accommodate the given application, yet they both fit within the level of a distributed controller. Therefore this discussion will focus on the control specific components of the system:

- The enterprise supervisor,

- BA^{DDC} equipment level controller, and

- BA^{DDC} zone level controller.

A typical building automation system executing DDC architecture will include an enterprise supervisor at the highest level and two levels of distributed controllers. The discussions of each of these levels of control will consider specific hardware and sequence of operations for that particular component. It is also important to cover the concept of building-wide or integrated control via the enterprise supervisor. Finally, this technology is extremely dynamic, so a general overview of trends will be provided for each major component of the BAS, as well as overall trends for BAS as a whole.

Enterprise Supervisor

The enterprise supervisor was selected for discussion first under this BAS technology section because it is responsible for overall building coordination. Key topics to this discussion are hardware requirements, building coordination which provides a sequence of operations for the entire system, and "analytics impact." Energy and analytics impact relates this BAS topic to the broader topic of the book, and will emphasize why BAS is so critical to accessing data and making it available to big data systems via the internet, etc. Throughout this chapter, each topic also addresses market and technology trends that can be expected to impact each level of control.

Hardware

Enterprise supervisor hardware varies greatly. In the past, approaches have been taken from custom computer based systems to dedicated personal computers (PCs), as well as to develop custom microprocessor-based equipment. It has become an increasingly common design concept to develop "platform" microprocessor-based devices.

Such devices package the microprocessor with an operating system, non-volatile (read-only memory) and volatile (random-access memory) storage, software programming and configuration capability and capabilities for data communications networking with other BA^{DDC} devices and, as appropriate, with the internet. In some cases the enterprise supervisor will include on board componentry (inputs and outputs or I/O) to sense external conditions and execute control action, but this is less common. This custom microprocessor approach is more common today in great part because of standardization, cost reduction and hardening of the technology to provide optimal performance. The custom microprocessor-based enterprise supervisor (ES) must be viewed primarily as a vehicle for managing the network, integrating building-wide control among all the distributed controllers and providing central communication functionality including the BAS device network, as well as internet access for wide-ranging capabilities. For clarification purposes, the ES is managing a device network of building automation direct digital controllers (BA^{DDCs}). By their very nature, these BA^{DDCs} execute control via distributed processing at the device, or at the individual piece of equipment, level. These concepts will be expanded significantly under sequence of operations, yet they are mentioned here to indicate the hardware complexity required at the enterprise supervisor level. In spite of the large number of variations on manufacturer approaches to development of this hardware, the author will describe a somewhat typical hardware example. A final important point is that the term "enterprise" was chosen due to the focus on a particular building or campus environment. Later in this book "middleware" and web-based systems will be discussed that interface with the enterprise and may introduce new virtual data etc., but the distinction here is that this enterprise supervisor is managing network communication and control execution for the architecture of BA^{DDCs} making up a local system.

As noted, the enterprise supervisor (ES) is typically focused on providing device networking, management of control execution and internet access functions. Therefore the ES may or may not have on-board inputs and outputs (I/O) to physically sense information and directly execute control. In some cases these devices will have a limited number of I/O, but the trend is certainly toward use of system-wide data in the form of virtual, or software, points. A virtual point is a piece of information that physically resides elsewhere in the system, or may come from an external location via the internet, but is held in a "data field" at the enterprise supervisor, for communication to other distributed controllers, or BA^{DDCs}. Perhaps the best example of this is outside air, which is needed by most BA^{DDCs}, especially HVAC. An example of an internet based virtual point might be a demand response event notification, which is shared with all BA^{DDCs} so that they may execute electrical load shed. Along with physical points, which may be connected to any particular BA^{DDC} device, both types of points can be shared via the network with all other controllers. These data-sharing functions will be discussed as part of control integration under sequence of operations. From a hardware perspective this means that the enterprise supervisor becomes the focal point for networking and communication within the system and with the outside world. Communication with the outside world is provided through an internet protocol (IP) address, and internet access, allowing access to all system data from an authorized external "dashboard" or interface. Under the networking and communication chapter the types of IP addresses, and the challenges associated with ensuring that valid addresses are maintained. Of course, there are still some older legacy systems that used modems and telephone lines, but these are rapidly vanishing. As noted, the enterprise supervisor provides overall network management functions, though in many cases these systems are self-policing. Self-policing in this context means that each network member, or BA^{DDC}, has responsibility for ensuring communication and sequences that are automatically enabled when a failure occurs. There will be much more discussion of these concepts later in this book.

The enterprise supervisor hardware described here is therefore a powerful microprocessor based system. This system is focused primarily on the two levels of system communication: networking and remote interface. The enterprise supervisor must also coordinate building-wide control functions and availability of system-wide data sharing, which will be discussed in a moment. These functions are typically implemented in one piece of hardware, however there may be other functions, or applications, required for a BAS such as life safety, fire and video surveillance/access control security systems. For purposes of this discussion, the assumption will be made that these functions are provided via separate "application-specific" enterprise supervisors. In fact there may be a system-wide requirement to integrate control between these various application areas, yet this chapter will focus on building control primarily for energy-consuming equipment. As noted previously though, it is important that some energy and analytics processing requires data from other sources to develop metrics and key performance indicators (KPIs), yet again the focus here is on buildings and energy. For the most part it will be assumed that the dashboard is only concerned with monitoring and access of these other functional systems. In summary therefore, this hardware overview defines a device with central focus on enterprise communication and networking and little or no physical I/O capability. Next it is necessary to consider building-wide coordination of control.

Building-wide Coordination

Building-wide coordination with a BA^{DDC} distributed system will be viewed in three key areas:

- control integration,

- building-wide monitoring and short-term data history, and

- remote communication with dashboards and with energy and analytics tools.

With the introduction of BAS executing DDC (BA^{DDC}) a number of new issues were raised around the accomplishment of control integration. Again these are distributed processing devices by nature, so the focus at the device level is on a specific piece of equipment or control application. The author uses the term integration because of the need to accomplish control via coordinating, or more specifically integrating, the functions of multiple microprocessors to provide control for those applications. Integrating control is important because it means the accomplishment of complex strategies that are implemented in part by more than one device. There are many functions that fit into this category and examples include morning warm-up in a VAV system, demand response or optimal start/stop for the building. On a building-wide level, the BAS must monitor functions at each device, share information about those functions via the network, and then integrate the control sequences carried out by all of the devices.

There are many design approaches taken with BA^{DDC}, due to the power of distributed processing providing by these systems. For simplicity's sake this discussion will take one of the more common approaches, enterprise supervisor integration, and discuss it further. In this approach the enterprise supervisor provides building-wide functions by monitoring building conditions or status, and based upon that data executes DDC control sequences. For example the enterprise supervisor will monitor building power consumption for the network, and based upon demand consumption and a setpoint will initiate demand shed. At the same time the enterprise supervisor will monitor the internet for a demand response (DR) event signal. The sequences executed under these two scenarios may be the same or different depending on the building and its kW electric demand profile. In either case the actual control approach focuses on control of loads that can be shed (turned off) through integrated control sequences implemented by BA^{DDCs} throughout the building. These BA^{DDCs} must physically disable loads to avoid exceeding the setpoint (or for DR the kW drop contracted with a utility) because the enterprise supervisor may not have access to actual controlled devices that can be shed. In both of these cases it also becomes critical to understand the building and use the BAS to monitor conditions, so that critical conditions do not "spin out of control" during the shed period. Many of the largest loads (most kW demand) that are easily accessible for demand limiting and DR, are HVAC. For HVAC to "spin out of control" would mean that a building exceeds the acceptable comfort conditions and becomes an unproductive environment for the work being done in that building. The real power of analytics is that operators can develop analysis routines that compare a series of variables regarding indoor comfort, outside temperature, equipment loading, etc. With that knowledge it is possible to fine-tune the building by creating sequences that can avoid unintended consequences from trial and error approaches that may result in negative outcomes.

The key to control integration is the ability of the enterprise supervisor to either "request" the implementation of local control sequences, or to override local control and force a specific sequence. In either case the enterprise supervisor must track the actions of BA^{DDCs} and be capable of taking appropriate steps if the sequence is not implemented. There are many schools of thought as to the best possible approach for accomplishing these types of functions. For this discussion however, it is only important for the reader to note that building-wide control sequences require integrated action by multiple BA^{DDCs} to be achieved.

The final topic under control integration will be system data. The term virtual point was used earlier to identify information from a sensor, etc. that is not physically connected to the ES, but the concept of system data provides even broader context. In essence the enterprise supervisor serves as the vehicle for ensuring that key information is available throughout the network. Within the BAS networks, there are two types of system data: global and shared. Global data are information needed by many or all of the controllers in the same format. There are two types of global data as well, Global^L, for data from "local" BA^{DDC}s, and Global^I, for data from "internet" sources via the ES's IP connection. Good examples of Global^L data are outside air temperature, time and enthalpy. These data are provided by one controller which has a physical point for monitoring, though for system integrity purposes backup locations may be provided. The data from that hardware point are then "broadcast" to the network and available to all BA^{DDC}s. A good example of Global^I data is a DR event signal. These data are provided by the ES from the internet and the data are then "broadcast" to the network and available to all BA^{DDC}s.

The second type of system information is shared data. This is a much more custom approach to using system data for control. A simple example that will also be discussed later is temperature reset. BA^{DDC} A is responsible for maintaining a discharge air setpoint, but that setpoint may be adjusted based upon an indication of the load. BA^{DDC} B is monitoring space temperature for local control, but this is also a good indication of the load. The shared data function provides a vehicle for controller A to get access to the space temperature with the same frequency as if it were physically connected to that device. This requires that a specific point be accessed by the enterprise supervisor with regular frequency comparable to the need for control, and that the data be transmitted to controller A. These types of functions are critical to building-wide control.

Another building-wide function of the enterprise supervisor is to serve as a vehicle for monitoring and short-term operating history data. Monitoring functions will be discussed under the dashboard portion of this section, yet the most important point is that a "window" to the network must exist. This window must allow for communication with all BA^{DDC}s via an IP address for the local building or campus network, providing internet access. Through that window a variety of monitoring and alarming features must be provided as will be discussed in a moment. Also of critical importance is short-term historical system operating information.

Historical system operating information is BAS data, and requirements for these data have been expanded dramatically. In the past these data were used primarily for alarms to identify issues that required immediate attention, and for "trend" data that could be used for trouble-shooting and diagnostics. In this new "energy and analytics era," the requirements have expanded. For purposes of this discussion, consider one application "commissioning." Commissioning requires much more data for the equipment to control or troubleshoot, and it must have those data for longer time periods, and possibly at a more granular level to achieve its purpose. Prior to the energy and analytics era, the enterprise supervisor served as a central repository for data files containing trend data on various system points. This was generally the most efficient approach to ensure that the overall cost of the system is not detrimentally impacted by the need for data storage at every BA^{DDC} device on the network. To reduce the cost burden on the overall system for storing data, the general approach was to charge one network device, the enterprise supervisor, with responsibility for history. This required the enterprise supervisor to access data from all BA^{DDCs}, and to provide data storage for later retrieval. That solution would be cost prohibitive in the energy and analytics era due to the volume of storage that would be required for commissioning alone, but add enterprise energy management (EEM) functions, plus other applications, and the system would be unsustainable. The good news is that there is now an easy solution. IP access and the evolution of server farms to provide large volumes of "cloud" storage make it possible for the ES to store data locally for a short period of time and then upload it to the cloud at specified time intervals or even stream it. From a marketing perspective, this energy and analytics era functionality points to the reason why analytics companies are typically agile technology companies rather than large BAS manufacturers. Without question many BAS manufacturers are integrating analytics into the BAS, in much the same way as an "APP" is added to the smart phone, but that may not be the only path to market. Because of the large requirement for data storage and the need for processing and analysis of the large dataset that now resides in the cloud, not at the ES, other solution providers are stepping up to perform this analytics function. The reader is encouraged to pay special attention to the technology evolution to ensure that specific requirements for any building or applications can be met by a particular architecture implementation.

The final enterprise supervisor function is to allow for remote communication "interface" via BAS software or dashboard. For simplicity purposes, all of the variations on software interface technology will be referred to generically as "dashboard." Traditionally there were three key functions required of an interface: programming, monitoring and alarming. Given the evolution of post-BACnet™ BA^{DDC}, there are currently two functions: programming and monitoring/alarming. Yet this aspect of the BAS industry is in a significant state of flux. Beginning with programming, this function requires that each BA^{DDC} network member including the enterprise supervisor may be programmed and configured using what is now called a workbench tool. Programming and integration are covered here briefly for information. Every BAS device including the ES and BA^{DDCs} must be configured with identifying information. Configuration happens only once, and it includes such information as an IP or network address and essential data to identify that device on the network, and to establish specific characteristics like whether I/O is connected. For BA^{DDCs} in particular, programming will include a sequence of operations that it is to execute and I/O devices necessary to execute that sequence. Programming will also include a variety of parameters such as control setpoints and alarm limits. It bears noting that when the building automation and control network (BACnet™) standard was promulgated, the American Society of Heating Refrigeration and Air Conditioning Engineers (ASHRAE) standards committee established that this programming function was not to be part of the standard. The reason was simple, the BAS industry is made up of companies who believe that their sustainable competitive advantage is innovation and creativity in developing and enhancing control sequences. The BACnet committee elected not to try to standardize control sequences, but rather to respond to the industry demand, which was to provide for a standardized networking and communication protocol that would allow operators and engineers to avoid being locked in to specific systems. This decision resulted in the birth of "integration" as a specialty, because companies had to develop specialized knowledge that allowed them to coordinate the operations of multiple BAS systems within a single building or campus. BACnet provided the basis for accomplishing this through the second category of interface: monitoring/alarming.

Monitoring/alarming is truly more than that for BACnet based systems, as for those that use any other network communication standard. Dashboard interfaces take their cue from BACnet by enabling monitoring, operations and alarming, and included in those categories is "data management" for analytics systems that leverage cloud computing. As will be discussed in the next chapter, BACnet enables standard-based interface to all BASs that subscribe to the standard, and equally important it enables the operator to change a number of programming parameters, such as setpoints, schedules and alarm limits. Dashboards have access to current status on all controller points, as well as access to system trend and alarm history data. Dashboard alarming is a critical feature of any BAS, and can report on critical conditions that may be defined as well as default alarms, such as sensor or controller failure. The system designer may then note whether such alarms should be logged for availability when the system is polled or should initiate notification over the IP network. IP network notification uses the internet capability to initiate communication with one or more predefined dashboards and send the alarm data. These functions will be also discussed in the networking and integration chapters.

As noted throughout this section there are a number of market trends in play at the enterprise supervisor level. This section will not repeat these trend discussions, but there is merit in a general statement about one of the trends that has not been mentioned, the growing interest in BAS from the IT industry. At the Realcomm/IBcon conference (www.realcomm.com) in 2014, the author witnessed a keynote panel with Microsoft, Google, Cisco and Intel discussing their respective positions on the future of BAS. The significant interest in green buildings, smart/connected buildings and sustainability in general, are just a few of the possible reasons for this interest, but beyond that is the obvious opportunity for these companies to create more demand for their core products. The reader is encouraged to watch these trends and see how they unfold. However, the balance of this chapter focuses on content that shows the true complexity of BAS applications. That complexity means that IT companies have a big lift to effectively match their technology expertise with building operations.

Energy and Analytics Impact

Throughout the book so far there has been a good deal of discussion about the criticality of data access and data formatting to energy and analytics tools. One of the greatest barriers to entry for analytics over time has been the cost of instrumentation to provide data for analysis. Perhaps the most important impact of BAS on energy and analytics is that these systems already have access to extensive amounts of data. Even better, in many cases it is just the equipment condition, operations, building environment and energy metering data that are essential for performance of meaningful analysis. The second critical point regarding enterprise supervisors is that these devices typically conform to data communications and networking standards. Now that does not mean the data themselves are in a standard format, but it makes accessing the data significantly easier, and through BAS IP addresses it is possible to push large amounts of data to the cloud or other server. The issue at the cloud is that metadata and tagging/naming standards do not exist, so the analytics engine can make immediate use of the data without the need to massage and convert it into a standard format. Project Haystack (see the chapter on this topic) is about making this process easier and more seamless by creating a data model. The data model create a framework to standardize data tagging, etc. Performing an extra task to convert data from many different BASs (typically called mapping) can be cumbersome and time consuming, but it is still dramatically more cost effective than installing an extensive instrumentation network. In the end, there will be many benefits to Haystack, and other data standardization efforts, but among the principle benefits will be faster technology deployment and accelerated product development of new energy and analytics tools, features and functions. As the dataset of information points from BAS, as well as all other systems that interact with the building, expands and become richer, it will be possible to drive energy and analytics functionality that we cannot conceive today.

BA^{DDC} TECHNOLOGY FOR EQUIPMENT AND GENERAL PURPOSE APPLICATIONS

The enterprise supervisor discussion focused on a top-down view of BA^{DDC} technology, yet equipment control is what actually distinguishes these systems from other types of computer-based or IT applications. This section will provide a generic overview of applications that addresses the larger and more complex equipment in a building, as well as a variety of other devices and systems such as lighting. There are many features and capabilities available with BA^{DDC}s for more complex applications. Microprocessor based control is ubiquitous with large heating, ventilating and air conditioning (HVAC) equipment, often installed at the factory by the HVAC manufacturer, but it is also common for general purpose control. The term equipment level is derived from the use of these controllers with such equipment as centrifugal chillers and air handlers. General purpose control uses the same hardware, with slightly different control sequences, for such applications as start/stop of non-HVAC loads or on/off control of lighting and other electrical equipment. BA^{DDC} control with equipment level and general purpose controllers is highly cost effective due to application complexity. In these applications there are also greater requirements for control integration due to the distributed processing nature of BA^{DDCs}. Also the equipment cost has an order of magnitude that can more easily support the cost of BA^{DDC} for multiple reasons. As HVAC manufacturers have gained market share and joined the ranks of market leaders, these companies have utilized BA^{DDC} to replace thermostats and integrated equipment controllers for static pressure, air volume etc., but also for equipment safety. It has been possible for equipment manufacturers to program a wide range of alarms, diagnostics, troubleshooting routines and protective sequences, that in the past required independent devices. The addition of such technology also makes it possible for these manufacturers to consider offering new services to the market like commissioning or energy analytics, but more on that later.

The enterprise supervisor has been discussed as a building-wide integrator of control functions. Yet the benefits of BA^{DDC} are truly realized when intelligent devices are deployed locally at a particular control application. Equipment/general purpose controllers form one of the two levels of BA^{DDC} devices noted. They provide full local control requirements, and integrate with both the enterprise supervisor and zone level controllers to provide building-wide functions. The topics which will be covered under this heading include the following and as appropriate the sections will also address relevant development trends:

- Equipment level hardware,

- Sequence of operation programming,

- Control integration,

- Networking, and

- Energy and analytics impact.

Equipment Level Control (ELC) Hardware

As with the enterprise supervisor BA^{DDC} ELCs are typically "platform" microprocessor-based devices. These devices encompass the microprocessor, as well as an operating system, non-volatile (read-only memory) and volatile (random-access memory) storage, on board componentry to sense external conditions and execute control action, software programming and configuration capability and capabilities for data communications networking with other BA^{DDC} devices and, as appropriate, with the internet. Among these characteristics, perhaps the most distinguishing feature of equipment level hardware is the number of on-board inputs and outputs (I/O), which are also referred to as "points." Devices applied at this level provide both analog and digital inputs and outputs, as well as network access to virtual points to introduce new variable information for control sequences. Input/output (I/O) requirements are generally more demanding at this level due to the expanded applications. There is generally a demand for at least eight of each point type, analog and digital inputs and outputs. Due to the fact that these controllers may be applied as general purpose devices or application specific controllers, it is not uncommon for controllers to be expanded up to as many as 64 or more total points. This may be done through add-on modules, cards, etc. It is also necessary because most equipment applications require control through digital outputs and analog or pulsed/modulating outputs, as well as monitoring of both analog and digital values. Analog values are generally used to monitor temperature or pressure, while digital points provide contact closures typically indicating an alarm. Device outputs then respond to the commands of the controller based upon the appropriate input value and the sequence of operations. These outputs will either be enabled or disabled, or may be modulated to a commanded position.

As noted, it is common for manufacturers to develop a platform device for equipment/general purpose hardware and use it with all applications. The platform will provide a base input/output capacity, and in many cases allow expansion through any of several techniques. Application of the controller is accomplished by changing software in the device. Software issues related to this approach will be discussed further under sequence of operations. Hardware design issues to be resolved also include the requirement for a full line of ancillary component products. These products include the:

•   controller,

•   sensors, transducers, other input devices and

•   electrical relays or contactors, motors, actuators, transducers and other output devices to enable control points.

A key related issue with these products is that, in the past, many manufacturers would fix the ancillary components (sensors, transducers, etc.) that could be used with a device or allow flexible application of a wide variety of industry standard equipment. This is less common today because most integrators demanded the flexibility of choosing sensors, etc. Another benefit of using generic ancillary components is that the cost of system retrofit may be greatly reduced because existing field devices can be reused. The intent of this section is not to provide a detailed discourse on ancillary devices, but it bears noting that the "Internet of Things," discussed later in the book, and the pervasive deployment of an infinite number of ancillary components has made it cost effective to begin networking these devices. This topic will not be discussed in great detail here, but the economies of scale associated with the large volume of ancillary components being applied, will lead to a new level of architecture. This level of architecture may be called instrumentation, ancillary gear or some new name, but the expectation is that networking cost declines combined with such advancements as nanotechnology will produce a great deal of advancement in this area.

There are two additional points that should also be mentioned under the category of hardware: controller size and ambient operating requirements. Controller size is typically not an issue with general purpose devices because they are often mounted in a mechanical room, above a ceiling, etc. The assumption is that these devices can be acquired with enclosures that meet standards agency approvals and local codes. With equipment controllers as noted, manufacturers generally pre-integrate BA^{DDC} devices within the control panel of HVAC equipment. This imposes a size constraint in smaller units. Another topic under hardware is the absolute requirement for equipment-level control devices to be able to operate under outdoor temperature conditions. A good example of this is a VAV rooftop air handler. It is typical for this equipment to be provided in a fully self-contained manner. A single enclosure containing the HVAC equipment and controls is provided in one package that is mounted on the roof. The package will be exposed to the full extreme of outdoor temperature and humidity, and may be shipped to any location in the world, further adding to the potential extremes. In closing, it is also important to mention "middleware" and integrated solutions. To a great degree, the proliferation of options available for BA^{DDC} systems has resulted in deployment of multiple different devices that must interoperate. The sophistication of system integrators combined with the diverse number of devices that can execute control in a "multi-vendor BACnet" environment has made this possible. Middleware and integration will be discussed further in this book, the primary reason to mention it here is that the architecture of BA^{DDC} systems has morphed over the years, and it is not possible to make simplistic statements about how equipment-level control is achieved. This is particularly true as BA^{DDC} has become standard in nearly all commercial buildings, and BACnet specifications have been developed by engineers with the idea that HVAC equipment with pre-integrated controllers will operate seamlessly with technology that is site-applied by a control contractor. These systems can be very effective, but that is by no means guaranteed. This author has said more than once that the new construction "design, bid, build" market is hopelessly broken, and without a highly qualified integrator that is goaled to be a constructive member of the design and installation team, the end result is not always positive. The reader should not imply that this is an indictment of any particular participant in this design bid supply chain, it is rather a result of the predatory nature of the model.

Sequence of Operations

Control sequences truly define BA^{DDC}, and the requirements for equipment and applications targeted at this level are significant. The author has heard this concept referred to with a simple analogy. It may be related to a civic auditorium, for example Madison Square Garden. The basic BA^{DDC} hardware platform outlined above makes it possible for that device to be applied in any number of applications, much like the functions in an auditorium. The sequence of operations is the specific program that tailors this BA^{DDC} to the application. Correspondingly the marquee and associated interior modifications in seating, etc. within the auditorium tailor it to any given event. This section will briefly touch on the techniques that are used to accomplish that programming.

For the most part, BA^{DDC} products on the market today use manufacturer-developed, "proprietary," programming tools. Generally these tools use one of two programming approaches: equation driven and library loop control parameter approach. This may come as a surprise for those readers who are not deeply immerse in the BA^{DDC}, but as has been mentioned in this text BACnet is not a standard for programming. BACnet is a communication network standard that is designed for use after the BA^{DDC} is fully programmed, configured and commissioned. Again, the term "workbench" is becoming more common as a generic way to refer to this software, and there has been significant industry effort to develop "one size fits all" tools for this purpose. However, that notion is not widely embraced by the industry. Under this heading of workbench programming, it is important to note that the "*styles*" do vary. For example, equation driven programming may be done by coding using custom software created by the manufacturer, or ever an IT language such as "C." Another very common *style* is to perform this task using a Viseo™-type of block programming. More may be learned about Viseo at www.viseo.com. There is also industry interest in using the Building Information Modeling (BIM) tool for this purpose in the future. With this Viseo graphic *style* of programming each block is actually a logic block, represented graphically, that performs a mathematical function and the programmer builds sequences in a logic driven graphical manner. For example, a logic block may compare space temperature to a setpoint and based upon a calculation determine if heating or cooling should be turned on. This section will not discuss *styles* of programming and configuration further, but the reader is encourage to ensure that they understand the *style* that is used for any BAS they procure and that this software is provided as part of the installation contract.

Regardless of programming approach, a very important point for BA^{DDC} manufacturers is that they believe their expertise in understanding the applications and creating effective control sequences is what differentiates them from competitors. Therefore they are not anxious to give up the credibility that this expertise provides them, nor are they willing to lose the intimate relationship with integrators, and building operators, that comes from selling, training and supporting the BAS. At the same time there are many other issues. Consider liability for example. If a third-party software package is used and something goes wrong with BA^{DDC} operations, who is at fault?

This author, and others, have written extensively on those topics in other books, such as the one referenced earlier. So this section will describe these approaches in limited detail as a general introduction, and tailor the discussion to equipment-level controllers (ELCs). The complexity of control sequences required for equipment, in this case HVAC, is quite sophisticated because it requires control of multiple conditions, such as temperature, pressure, possible humidity or carbon dioxide, and often much more. These types of sophisticated control sequences will expand on simple proportional control. Proportional control is the most basic sequence of operations for HVAC. Earlier in this chapter, a definition was provided for direct digital control. In that definition, the idea of a feedback loop was introduced. Proportional control is the simplest form of such feedback loops and it is also sometimes referred to as "linear control" because the response to a change in the condition, i.e. temperature being sensed, is linear. Proportional control systems are more complex than on-off control, which could be like a bi-metallic domestic thermostat that simply turns or a heating unit when the temperature drops below the setpoint, or like the special-purpose devices that will be discussed later that turn a load on or off based upon a time schedule, etc. On-off control will work where the overall system has a relatively long response time, but will result in instability if the system being controlled has a rapid response time. Proportional control overcomes this by modulating the output to the controlling device, such as a continuously variable valve. Quite simply, "feedback" means that a condition, again i.e. temperature, is sensed and compared to a setpoint, i.e. thermostat temperature setting, and an action is taken to turn an HVAC unit on or off. The feedback loop continues to sense the condition and turns the unit on when heating or cooling is needed and off when the space is at the setpoint. There are a number of issues with simple proportional control, because often the unit will run longer than necessary and overshoot the setpoint, and the temperature will drop too much before restarting the unit. These issues affect comfort in a space, but they are also inefficient. These issues were among the factors that led to development of more complex control sequences that calculate proportional control, but also perform integral and derivative computations. In this space temperature example, the function of the integral would be to calculate the distance (# of degrees) that the space temperature is from setpoint and adjust control action to avoid wide swings around the setpoint. These swings are often caused by overshot of the setpoint and delays in responding to a call for conditioning which are common with proportional control. The derivative feature is very specialized, and is used with highly dynamic applications such as pressure control. Rapid changes in a condition require that the control is adjusted to react quickly. The result of a proportional, integral and derivative (PID) control loop is a condition that is accurately maintained at desired levels with very little deviation. Combining this highly accurate control with networking standards like BACnet is an essential feature of BA^{DDC} for building control.

ELC control sequences will vary dramatically by type of equipment. These devices require complex and sophisticated control sequences tailored to the specific applications. One approach to solving this problem is to have the control designer, contractor or integrator write the sequence with an equation-driven language. This is done using "workbench" software and can address any anomalies or custom requirements, yet this task can also be time consuming. As the BAS industry has become more competitive and equipment, or integrator, selection is often made based on price alone, there has been a growing interest in development of library sequences. This is because library algorithms allow much quicker installation, startup and commissioning, but they do not allow for custom application. Another variation on this theme is to use a controller that allows flexible programming, and maintain a custom library. This allows the designer to start with a reasonably complete control sequence and edit that sequence to meet the new requirement.

The equation library approach works well for equipment level control because sequences may be maintained for chillers, boilers, air handlers, etc. Again many equipment level controllers come pre-integrated by the HVAC manufacturer and the sequences may be "locked in," meaning they cannot be modified without violating equipment warranty. So, the designer, or integrator, must determine how critical it is to modify the library, and whether these modifications will impact control reliability. If the ELC workbench software allows customer programming, it will of course be necessary to test and verify each new control sequence prior to field application. This testing can be extremely time consuming and cannot always verify every aspect of control operation. As a result the library loop control parameter approach was developed. One note is that some controllers, to a great degree zone devices to be discussed next, embed control sequences, like the pre-integrated controls mentioned above. However, it has also become common for workbench software to provide a library loop approach that allows for a variety of algorithms to be selected and downloaded to any control device.

Library loop control parameter type programming basically involves controllers that employ sequences that have been programmed, tested, verified and possibly hardcoded by the manufacturer. Hardcoded means that these sequences are held in a portion of memory that may not be accessed to review or change the sequence. As noted above, integrators often find it more convenient to access library loops on the workbench and download those into any device in the field, or during bench testing at a shop. Obviously hardcoded devices that are preprogrammed at the factory rather than allowing a workbench download are less desirable for some integrators because they must sacrifice a portion of the control flexibility available with free-form equations. Yet the engineering time and job support required to deal with writing and testing control loops is virtually eliminated. This is a strong selling point for such devices, and has led to a large number of products on the market that offer preprogrammed control sequences of various types. Another example of the library loop approach is with general purpose control. In this case general purpose is defined as simple control loops that provide either start/stop or modulating control. Examples might be time of day (TOD) scheduled sequencing of loads such as lighting and/or other electrical loads. These functions are among the first that are being completely standardized and embedded directly into BACnet. Yet these remain perfect examples of control parameter applications, because it would not be an efficient use of time to write equation programs for every TOD schedule. Another example would be a simple proportional type temperature loop. Such applications might be a three-way valve on a chilled water supply loop that is modulated to maintain a constant loop temperature. Again custom programming is not likely to be cost effective for such an application. The intent of this section is not to position one approach as desirable over the other, rather to identify the technology used.

To be more specific about the technology is difficult in this section, however there is another important concept. That concept concerns the complex nature of BA^{DDC} equipment level control. To illustrate this point, consider a variable air volume (VAV) air handler. The control for this piece of equipment must provide discharge air temperature control by sensing temperature and modulating an outside air damper for ventilation, and possibly free cooling, along with heating and cooling equipment. Often these units are cooling only, however it is not uncommon for air handlers to provide heating as well. This means that the BA^{DDC} requires one control loop to make a control decision on the mode of operation, heat or cool. Two additional control loops, one for heat and one for cool, then determine the amount of heating or cooling to provide. The control action is based on staging of independent capacity, but may also include an outdoor air economizer sequence, as noted. This fourth control sequence, the economizer, must consider another input, outside air temperature. The economizer may be required to consider enthalpy, rather than temperature alone, to make a decision about modulating the damper to provide free cooling. A fifth control loop that is common with these systems is temperature reset which will look at one of several temperature conditions, i.e. space temperature, and reset the temperature setpoint. VAV air handlers also require static pressure control to modify the amount of air delivered. Duct static pressure control is the most common approach, and makes the sixth major control loop integrated with this equipment level controller. A seventh control loop that is becoming common with VAV air handlers is to monitor space pressure and adjust supply air based upon the desire to maintain a positive or negative pressure. With the advent of demand response (DR) and related smart grid sequences, as well as a resurgence of demand limiting, an eighth control loop may be performing a reset-type control sequence on the unit to reduce electricity consumption by changing temperature setpoints. At the same time DR may address duct static pressure, fan speed or a host of other control parameter adjustments to reduce the overall energy consumption by the air handler.

One of the decided benefits to equipment-level intelligent control is the ability to monitor a variety of alarm and safety conditions. Many of these functions are now fully integrated into the BA^{DDC} equipment-level devices as previously discussed. This is particularly true for BA^{DDC}s that are developed and pre-integrated into HVAC equipment at the factory. In the past, these functions were simple control loops that monitor the condition of a contact closure or an analog value. Based on a change in state of the digital point, or an analog point exceeding a set of range limits, an alarm is initiated. As traditional HVAC manufacturers have joined the ranks of market leaders in BA^{DDC}, and leaders in HVAC, these sequences and an extensive number of troubleshooting, diagnostic and equipment-related algorithms are fully embedded into controllers. As noted before, access to such sequences would only be available to trained factory technicians using a proprietary workbench software product. Regardless of the deployment mechanism, this functionality is critical to smooth equipment operation. Though these are simple routines, when combined with the temperature and pressure loops above, it becomes clear how complex and diverse the sequences of operations must be that are provided in BA^{DDC} equipment level devices.

Sequence of operations is a complex topic, but before closing there is merit in mentioning the notion of self-learning "fuzzy logic" for BASs. This idea has been discussed for decades, but again there are articles showing up in the trade press about the benefits that could be derived from self-learning BAS. In particular, such sequences could make new smarter energy management strategies possible. For example, a demand response sequence could look at a zone infrared occupancy sensor, and add overhead light dimming to setpoint adjustment during a DR event. Of course there could be tremendous "continuous commissioning" value on a daily basis from self-learning sequences, in this case algorithms that adapt equipment operation based on a series of factors. Consider another example that has to do with telecommuting. Many buildings are lightly loaded on any day of the week because people work from home or are on travel. Enabling sequences can calculate load in the building and adjust heating, cooling and ventilation to how many people are in the building. Some large commercial building operators are already duty cycling elevators when the building occupancy is low. So the value that could be derived for comfort, energy savings, etc. is clear, but the rate at which these enhancements will hit the market is unknown. A recent article by Jim Sinopoli in www.automatedbuilding.com, discussed in the integration chapter, surfaces the idea that the Bluetooth™ signal in smart phones could be integrated into such sequences. The IT integration requirement could add a level of complexity, but this could be the optimum indicator of occupancy. Using an energy and analytics tool, Bluetooth signals could be accessed and analyzed to develop an occupancy trending rule, which could then be used to frame an algorithm that would ramp the building equipment up and down based on actual readings of occupancy based on Bluetooth signals. As with all new technology, the reader should carefully evaluate offerings, speak to references and validate the cost benefit of such offerings carefully before deployment. Given this wide ranging discussion of control sequences including the complexity of ELC control loops, and the potential for self-learning algorithms, the reader is presented with complex technology in the BAS space. This is particularly true when the reader considers that additional sequences may need to be added for control integration.

Control Integration

The concept of control integration was briefly discussed under enterprise supervisor (ES) controls and the above vignette on Bluetooth-based equipment control. The same basic definition applies to ELCs as did to ES, except that the focus shifts to appropriate integration at this level. A good example is the concept of temperature reset. One approach to reset is locating a representative sensor somewhere in the space, and making control decisions based upon that single point of information. A more integrated approach would be to monitor space temperature at any number of distributed zone controllers. The BA^{DDC} equipment-level control then might average those values or simply reset to the highest or lowest value. This function is too equipment specific to be delegated to an enterprise supervisor, yet is ideal for BA^{DDC} equipment level control. A little more complex example is morning warm-up. This sequence is used with VAV air handlers that have heating capacity. The air handler will control to the appropriate temperature sensor, and then based upon the control loop will override zone control to force the damper 100% open. This is a truly integrated sequence because control decisions are made at the ELC, but they must be integrated at zone level control.

Control integration at the equipment level is not likely to be limited to interaction with lower level devices. As noted under the enterprise supervisor, these BA^{DDC} ELCs will be integral to carrying building-wide functions such as demand limiting, optimal start/stop and more to come. It has also become much more common for new construction and retrofit specifications to require an enterprise supervisor and other BA^{DDC} devices to seamlessly integrate, at the system level, with BA^{DDC} ELCs, which come from the factory pre-integrated into building HVAC equipment. This form of integration is highly complex and requires a sophisticated integrator. Some believe that BACnet alone enables this type of integration, but is not true. System integration at such a higher level often presents requirements for a host of other software and/or hardware elements. For example, in a phase-2 construction on an existing building there may be new equipment added that has to be integrated with "legacy" equipment from the original constructions. This may require middleware devices that include "drivers" to communicate between the legacy device and a new BACnet device. These concepts will be discussed in more detail under the networking and middleware IT chapters. The primary point here is that integration of BA^{DDC} ELCs has more and more to do with IT, network communication and web services in the 21st century than it does with traditional HVAC control. Yet a thorough understanding of both content areas is necessary for success. Again a thorough understanding of HVAC is critical, but the ideal BA^{DDC} integrator must also be fully versed in IT, web services and data communication disciplines.

That is particularly true for providers' of energy and analytics, dashboards and related technology for buildings.

This is the final topic under BA^{DDC} equipment level controls, and has already been positioned as critical to building-wide control. The functions discussed under the enterprise supervisor for programming, monitoring and dashboard interface necessitate that full internet access is available with the ELC. These devices typically provide complete IP communication capability. Given that statement however, it bears noting that the devices at this level may vary in network and communication capability. These devices often require both integration and dashboard interface capability with enterprise supervisors, and yet it is also common for these devices to be integrated with legacy and other building systems via middleware components. A final topic for discussion here is that the BAS industry has undergone a merger and acquisition frenzy, resulting in major business changes in recent decades. This is relevant to BA^{DDC} ELC devices because, post-M&A, manufacturers have had to decide which BAS product families to make obsolete and which would become the next generation flagship products for that brand. Regardless of specific product decisions made by any manufacturer, companies must also determine how to support the legacy products as well. The relevance to BA^{DDC} ELC devices is that for many manufacturers these devices have become an architecture focal point for integration. It is not uncommon for these devices to incorporate "router" functionality to unify an architecture made up of multiple product families, which as a result of M&A have become one company's post-acquisition offering. The next chapter will discuss these networking concepts in much more detail, but readers should understand clearly whether products installed in their buildings have been affected by such events. If so, readers should explore how manufacturers of those products intend to provide future support and integration.

This overview of current equipment level controls is intended to provide a general view of the technology. Many of these topics will be expanded throughout the book as they relate to big data for energy and buildings. Also of critical importance to building-wide control is the provision of a BA^{DDC} zone level controller.

Energy and Analytics Impact

As previously discussed, instrumenting equipment to provide data for analysis has been one of the greatest barriers to entry for energy and analytics. BA^{DDC} ELC devices are where a large portion of the building data exist that can be made available for analytics. Equally exciting is that the enterprise supervisor and the ELCs are most often responsible for virtual points. These virtual points offer a huge source of data for analytics. Virtual point data can be trended and captured over time, so it could include kW peak demand or kWh energy consumption data (whether instantaneous or interval), kW and/or kWh cost data, temperature and humidity data from an external weather station, etc., all of which can provide insight into operating condition data and are excellent data for energy and analytics. It is particularly true that BA^{DDC} ELC devices have access to, and may be trending, extensive amounts of data on conditions, operation, etc. It is important to be aware that the memory for trending data at the ELC is very limited. However, as with the enterprise supervisor, the BA^{DDC} ELC devices should conform to data communications and networking standards, so all of that data can be uploaded to separate onsite storage or to the "cloud." Again data formatting is an issue with various propriety BAS, and other equipment. Ideally systems will migrate to data standards like Haystack. This issue will undoubtedly become more critical as adoption of energy and analytics accelerates and as data standardization efforts mature. There are also individual technology providers who are developing "drivers" and conversion tools to make use of some data. It is important not to oversimplify the idea of "data drivers"; there is a cost for all of this technology, and therefore it will not always be cost effective to access data from all sources. Because of BACnet, and other communication standards, however, it is possible to push vast amounts of data through BAS IP addresses to the cloud or other server.

BA^{DDC} TECHNOLOGY FOR ZONE LEVEL CONTROL APPLICATIONS

As noted there are two types of BA^{DDC} products: BA^{DDC} equipment-level controls which have been discussed and BA^{DDC} zone level control (BA^{DDC} ZLC). Before launching into this discussion of BA^{DDC} ZLC devices, it bears noting that there is actually a third type of product; BA^{middleware}, or simply middleware. A full chapter is devoted to middleware, and it has been discussed at some level thus far under the integration topics. As BA^{DDC} systems became more IT oriented and require networking standards and internet access, middleware devices of various types have been introduced to the market and become critical to deployment. The reader is asked to hold that topic for now, as the next two chapters cover the topics of data communications/networking and middleware in more detail. Of course it is perfectly acceptable to jump ahead to those chapters to get questions answered and then return to the BA^{DDC} ZLC discussion as well.

BA^{DDC} ZLC technology has been evolving for decades. As with the BA^{DDC} ELC, these devices may also be part of a BA^{DDC} system offering, or they may be pre-integrated by HVAC/BAS manufacturers. A great recent example of the latter is the variable refrigerant volume (VRV) and variable refrigerant flow (VRF) style heat pumps, which include controls, and have gained rapid market acceptance. That is just one example though, because BA^{DDC} ZLCs have become commonplace with such applications as variable air volume terminal units, or boxes, water source and geothermal heat pumps, and small packaged single zone units. As with the ELC level devices, these controllers are microprocessor-based distributed processing units with full capability for standard network communication.

ELC devices were discussed as both HVAC and general purpose controllers, due to the flexibility of the devices and the applications to which they may be applied. Initially BA^{DDC} ZLCs were primarily focused on unitary HVAC applications. However with the introduction of "wireless networking" and other technology evolutions that will be mentioned, ZLCs are also being used for general purpose control applications. Lighting at the zone level would be the first general purpose application to mention. Lighting controls by ZLC, particularly for dimmable florescent ballasts and LEDs, can be networked wirelessly for scheduling, but can provide space motion detector, infrared or other sensors. As many buildings seek United States Green Building Council (USGBC) Leadership in Energy and Environmental Design (LEED) points, these ZLCs can also be used to deploy control sequences like daylight harvesting to reduce light levels when ambient light is available. As with ELC integration, not all of the BA^{DDC} ZLCs deployed are part of a single manufacturer's product family. Today there's a robust ecosystem of technology companies offering stand-alone ELC and ZLC devices for many applications from demand response to pneumatic thermostat replacement. Some of these applications will be discussed in later chapters, however the focus of this book is on energy and analytics, so the emphasis here is more on the data available from such devices than on an exhaustive treatment of ZLC technology.

BA^{DDC} ZLCs provide distributed processing and BACnet, or other, standard network communication. As a result they require sophisticated control integration sequences to ensure that effective coordination is achieved through the system architecture. To provide more background, these issues will be viewed in similar categories to previous discussions along with pertinent trends that are influencing the market:

- hardware,

- sequence of operations,

- networking and control integration, and

- energy and analytics impact.

Hardware

BA^{DDC} ZLC, or more simply ZLC, technology became common due to market demand for control at this level, which ultimately provided economies of scale in production. At the same time microprocessor and associated electronic technology became cost effective, further increasing the desirability of these devices. As with ELCs, these are typically platform devices, which encompass the microprocessor, operating system, non-volatile (read-only memory) and volatile (random-access memory) storage, on-board componentry to sense external conditions and execute control action, software programming and configuration capability and capabilities for data communications networking with other BA^{DDC} devices and, as appropriate, with the internet

Further development of smaller, more powerful microprocessors for ZLC-level devices combined with pervasive deployment of the BACnet standard, resulted in robust development of these products. ZLCs are typically tailored to a specific application and fulfill the definition of direct digital control by enabling control intelligence located at each piece of controlled equipment.

The nature of ZLC products imposes requirements on these controllers that are applied to zone or unitary equipment. As with ELCs, input/output capability must be provided. BA^{DDC} ZLCs have less input and output (I/O) capability than ELCs and offer more limited expansion capability. Yet they must be well suited to a variety of applications, such as variable air volume air handlers and water source heat pumps. At the same time these devices also must be cost effective for those applications. In addition, there are several hardware related areas that are equally important. Among these are component packaging, physical dimensions, and ability to operate at outdoor ambient temperatures.

Input/output (I/O) requirements are generally less stringent than with the ELC due to the limited number of points required with zone applications. Overall there will typically be fewer points, however analog and digital inputs and outputs are still necessary. This is because most zone applications will require both monitoring and equipment control. Control is accomplished through digital and analog or pulsed modulating outputs for such equipment as dampers and valves. Again manufacturers typically develop one ZLC hardware platform and use it with all zone applications. This is accomplished by changing software in the controller. Software approaches related to this activity will be discussed further under sequence of operations.

With specific regard to inputs and outputs (I/O), an important zone hardware design issue is the available number and type of I/O channels or points. Designers must first determine the number of points that are appropriate for monitoring and control. Consideration must also be given to whether a fixed number of I/O will be available, or if expansion is to be provided. Expansion I/O may be critical if multiple applications are to be accommodated by one platform. Expansion is usually provided through boards that may be added to the base device or via a module that is applied externally to the base device. There will be trade-offs associated with any I/O expansion scheme. Two key points regarding I/O are that ZLC sequence programming capability may be limited because the device is generally intended for one relatively simple piece of equipment. As integrators consider adding more I/O they should evaluate device capacity to support code necessary for controlling those points. At the same time, with the growing application of general purpose control, programming capacity can be an issue. There is logic in using one ZLC for a particular zone and controlling HVAC, lighting and possibly other ancillary loads. There will be more discussion of these concepts under sequence of operations.

ZLC hardware design issues that are of particular importance involve the requirement for a full line of products including the controller, sensor or thermostat, static pressure measurement device, damper or valve motors and other ancillary gear depending on the application. These devices must be optional and fully compatible with each other, and the ZLC, regardless of application software. As with the ELC, the expectation is for full flexibility in selection of these components. Given the growing application of ZLC general purpose control, this is even more important. Even with target applications like VAV, the diversity in unitary equipment requires wide ranging options for electronic sensors, and as unlikely as it may seem there still may be a need in some cases for standard interface to pneumatic output devices. Across the board, ZLC devices and ancillary components are highly price sensitive. The primary recommendation here, as with BAS in general, is that the reader should be careful not to select vendors based upon price or brand name alone, but to evaluate service as well as product cost.

Component packaging is critical because zone control products tend to be self-contained in nature. Traditionally ZLCs tended to be applied by original equipment manufacturers (OEMs) in the factory, and each manufacturer offered a variety of control products. There are actually two distinct issues that are involved: packaging as it relates to easy application of zone products and packaging as it relates to physical design. As has been discussed there is a robust marketplace of third-party BAS device and component providers who offer solutions to the market. The key is for readers to educate themselves and ask the right questions during selection. VRF and VRV are a good example of this point. These heat pumps are deploying more than high efficiency solutions, they are deploying new approaches to system design. To achieve higher efficiency, direct current (DC) motors are used for fans and compressors to allow a wide range of modulation and tailor equipment loading to space comfort requirements. This makes the units very efficient but it also requires a controller that can send DC control signals to device components.

Application of ZLCs has become pervasive for all types of unitary or zone HVAC equipment including VAV boxes, air, water or ground source and VRV/F heat pumps, self-contained single zone packaged roof top units, packaged terminal air conditioners (PTACs), fan coil and most other units of this type. Using VAV as a component packaging example, it is now standard to provide one easily installed package containing the controller, sensor or thermostat, duct static pressure measurement device, and output devices for dampers and valves. Original equipment manufacturers (OEMs) of zone HVAC demand simple control interaction. More to the point, these OEMs have achieved significant market share in recent decades as leaders in the manufacturing of both the HVAC units and the controls or BAS. As will be discussed under integration, full market acceptance of BACnet coupled with significant advancement in system integration has resulted in a new BAS paradigm. There is a wide ranging belief among consultants and building owners that pre-integrated OEM ZLCs can "interoperate" with BACnet ELC and enterprise supervisor devices manufactured by other OEMs. In fact, this is possible. However, all OEM devices and all system integrators are not created equal. Achieving BAS interoperability requires a very sophisticated system integrator. Perhaps the most important point is that the ideal design process will include a system integrator, and procurement selection must evaluate the integrator as carefully as the price. Low price is not always, or even often, best.

The physical design aspect of ZLC packaging relates to the concept of ensuring that a control meets the space constraints of the application. This is actually a hardware design and selection issue. In fact, space constraints are always a concern with any control product, but are more important with the ZLC because very limited space is available. VAV boxes, for example will vary greatly in size based upon the zone CFM requirement and the type of box. A pressure dependent box with no fan or zone reheat and low CFM requirements would likely afford very little space for the ZLC. It is more common today to simply mount these devices on the outside of the box, but the designer should confirm that is an option. Also, both OEMs and building owners will require that the same ZLC be applied for all size boxes, though each for different reasons. The OEM is concerned with standardizing all facets of production including installation, manufacturing procedures and test/checkout for the ZLC. In this case the building owner is concerned with interoperability and system control integration for all of the VAV boxes and for the entire BAS. Further, as discussed above, VAV boxes are not the only application that will be controlled by a ZLC. As a result, use of any ZLC will be dictated to some degree by its ability to meet space requirements for any intended application.

Ambient temperature (where the ZLC is installed) is another important hardware consideration. Again this is a critical hardware design and selection issue, as is physical dimension. Key to the discussion of ZLC products is that the variety of applications for these devices requires that they meet a range of operating conditions. In nearly all cases, ZLCs which are mounted with VAV boxes need only operate under standard interior ambient temperature conditions; but, single zone

packaged units, which may be fitted with the same ZLC hardware platform, are likely to be exposed to exterior ambient temperature and humidity conditions. Another common ZLC general purpose application
is exterior LED lighting, which may also require outside placement.
As may be obvious, this dramatically increases the requirements, and
perhaps the cost, for these devices due to the potential for application
in Alaska or Florida. Also the control business is global, so ambient
conditions must be considered worldwide; therefore, a ZLC could con-
ceivably be applied in arctic or equatorial zones.

Sequence of Operations

As discussed under ELCs, the approach and style for programming control sequences varies dramatically by manufacturer and type
of equipment. This is true of any HVAC or load control application, yet
there are added distinctions between the ELC and ZLC. At first look, a
reasonable case could be made that ELCs must maintain more complex
and sophisticated control sequences than would be encountered in
zone applications. In many cases this may be true, yet the zone device
must be able to meet the requirements of all applicable equipment.
Throughout this chapter the VAV box has been the example; consider
again this piece of equipment. There are a number of VAV implementations, with pressure dependent being simplest and others such as pressure independent dual duct applications being more complex. As an extreme case the pressure independent system will be considered, but for
simplicity's sake we will focus on single duct. Note that the sequences
outlined are only an approximation and used for example rather than
as a direct control application.

Single duct pressure independent systems also vary in implementation. For example they may include fan-assisted systems, and
may also provide reheat. Consider one of the more common systems, a
single duct application with fan assist and one stage of electric reheat.
Assume that control is provided by a dedicated ZLC, also typical. This
system would require two primary control loops: space temperature
control and static pressure control. The space temperature control loop
modulates a damper to vary the amount of air delivered to the space
and satisfy a control setpoint. A call for heating in the space would
also sequence the electric reheat. The same algorithm would also provide occupied and unoccupied setpoints along with a sequence for the
unoccupied mode. The unoccupied mode sequence would very likely

provide at least one set of control parameters for the fan and reheat. It must also allow for starting the VAV air handler to satisfy cooling requirements. Operating concurrently with the temperature control is a static pressure loop. This loop is intended to allow for variations in cubic feet per minute (CFM) delivered to the box. Pressure control ensures that the space does not suffer from noise or discomfort due to variations in delivered CFM from the air handler. This sequence controls based upon data from a duct static pressure measuring device, and will integrate response to CFM variations with the zone damper control sequence.

The reason for this somewhat detailed discussion of one application is to raise the reader's awareness of zone control sequence complexity. Given that zone applications typically involve smaller less sophisticated equipment, and smaller numbers of I/O, it would be easy to assume that sequences are simplistic as well. Rather, sequences tend to be complex, and there are also interactive sequences to be considered. The same VAV box control requires networking communication to allow integration with the air handler (AHU) for simple functions like unoccupied override to start the AHU. Slightly more complex strategies might include reset of discharge air from zone temperature and building pressurization control with box and air handler integration. This means that it is entirely possible to use the full power of a microprocessor in the ZLC to provide sequence and communication/networking/ integration requirements, which will be discussed further below.

Networking and Control Integration

BA^{DDC} ZLCs must be networked to execute the control sequences that are carried out between modules at the zone level, as well as for integration with ELCs and the enterprise supervisor. These concepts of networking and integration are covered under the same heading for ZLCs because these devices are highly reliant on network interaction for effective building operations. At the same time, the control sequences at the ELC and building-wide rely on data from the ZLC level to provide effective operation. Networking and integration are therefore completely reliant upon one another. For example, ZLC control integration is essential because it is not possible to terminate every necessary point to this panel. At the same time, manufacturers vary on whether they choose to provide every control sequence at the ZLC. Consider scheduling for time of day on/off or setpoint functions, some ZLCs have clock functionality in the controller, while others do not. Actual time of day (TOD), or TOD and the ZLC schedule, may be maintained elsewhere, and a network broadcast from the ELC or enterprise supervisor sends this information to the controller. Typically this is done with a data point indicating to the ZLC that it is now in either occupied or unoccupied mode. These and other data points fall into the "system data" or "virtual point" category. However, it may also be necessary to implement building-wide control such as optimal start or demand limiting by issuing virtual points that initiate sequences through the ZLC.

Energy and Analytics Impact

This topic has been covered under enterprise supervisor and BA^{D-DC} ELC and is equally appropriate for the ZLC. Given the sheer volume of condition and status data available from tens, hundreds or even thousands of ZLCs in a building, it is extremely important to make this information available to energy and analytics tools. These data are crucial for continuous commissioning and enterprise energy management because data from the zone level is the best indication of how well a building is being operated. Operations in this case could focus on maintaining space environmental conditions that meet the mission of the building, but equally important could relate to operations and maintenance for equipment life as well as energy efficiency to optimize utility costs. Overall ZLC data are essential to analysis of these issues, as well as indoor air quality, measurement and verification for energy efficiency and much more.

As previously discussed, instrumenting equipment to provide data for analysis has been a major barrier to entry for energy and analytics technology, and zone equipment presented one of the greatest challenges in this area. Combine the numbers of devices mentioned above with the challenges of cabling for all of the instrumentation. These challenges were equally limiting in getting automated control to the zone level as well. This obstacle to gathering analysis data from the zone level is gradually waning, because ZLCs are being applied almost universally for HVAC. Also new ZLC features have been introduced including general purpose and lighting control. Whether these devices are networked over a hardwired or wireless network, their data can be communicated to a service, or cloud, via an enterprise supervisor, even if a middleware device is required. This is particularly important for ZLCs, because memory for trending data is extremely limited. Standard communication networks and data formatting remain a very important topic as previously discussed.

ACTIVE ENERGY AND ANALYTICS

This topic has been discussed elsewhere in this book and will not be covered in detail here except for one important point. With a more detailed understanding of BAS technology it should now be easier for the reader to understand the complexity associated with acquiring data for energy and analytics. Equally important, the reader should understand the complexity associated with using the data from the analysis performed by this technology, to optimize building operations. In many cases new sequences may be developed to further automate this optimization, but it must be an active process. The operator must:

- Actively perform analytics,

- Actively develop strategies and sequences to improve overall operations based upon the results of the analytics, and finally

- Actively perform continuous improvement to ensure that the sequences achieve the intended result.

Chapter II

Introduction to Digital Communication for Building Automation and DDC

The technology covered in this book is wide ranging by intent, because of the extensive and diverse set of "systems" that are expected to be providing data input for energy and analytics tools. These systems can range from building automation and related technology, as described in the previous chapter, to energy meters, programmable logic systems for process applications, point of sale and a multitude of other on-site computer based technologies such as Bluetooth™, but they also include the myriad data sources from the internet, cloud, etc. The diversity of these on-site systems is complicated by the fact that, in many cases, they were designed to operate independently. Therefore networking and data communications between them, and for data access from them, requires an understanding of the technology covered in this chapter. It is highly beneficial to provide a rudimentary understanding of data interchange technology as a resource for future use. Also of interest, is that the technology and many of the data communication standards discussed here are integral to the internet and data interchange between all computer systems and the cloud.

The next chapter will focus more on middleware, the internet and related web-based technology. This one addresses the underlying data communications and networking technologies and architecture. These networks are proprietary (developed by a company and kept as private intellectual property) or based upon standards (published and open for used by any company such as BACnet™). The data communication technologies that underlie energy, buildings, process, campus, plant and other systems are very important to developing strategies for accessing the data from those systems initially, as well as to ensuring the long-term reliability of those data streams.

Many readers may be unaware of how precarious system interactions can be, and how important it is to establish rigorous oversight of the data communication channels to ensure "data resilience." Cyber security is a major issue as well, and system operators must remain vigilant to avoid threats to building networks from data sharing via the internet. Developing systems that deploy cyber security strategies while data are being captured from decentralized and integrated networks is critical to managing risk. As the next two chapters unfold, it will become clear that operators must begin with a robust information architecture design. They must then develop data access systems that apply the same level of analytics to those architectures, as to the applications, to ensure that a continuing and reliable stream of data is always available. The author refers to this as data resilience.

Data resilience is a concept that becomes even more critical in light of the continuing trend for these systems to utilize web services and dashboards for all operator interface. Information interchange for many specialty systems is migrating to the internet, or web, so it is critical for customers to address cyber security and data resilience for these systems. Despite the fact that a network of businesses and independent bodies is overseeing internet security, the recommended efforts focus on specific uses of the internet and specific web applications or services. As a result, the task of maintaining the viability of data streams falls to the operator's side of the web interface. This is critical because most of the underlying technology still relies on systems that use a host of legacy and standard data communication protocols that must access the internet through some level of device that is capable of being assigned an internet protocol (IP) address, and deploying some level of web services. As has been discussed throughout this book, access to data from many of these energy and building systems requires interfaces, gateways, drivers or other mechanisms to push that data through an IP addressable device to the cloud, etc. This means that foundation-level knowledge in data communications and networking can be of great value to the reader, and that is the purpose of this chapter.

INTRODUCTION TO DIGITAL COMMUNICATIONS

This chapter will cover a wide range of topics designed to provide the reader with an understanding of data communications technology in general, including system architecture. At times these technologies are referred to as local area networks (LAN). They may also be called "sub-nets" or "sub-LANs" because the overall communications architecture in use here entails multiple levels of networking. At this sub-LAN level, the focus is on data communications for building automation and other building systems such as security, computerized maintenance management systems, energy metering or enterprise energy management systems. Multiple topics will be covered to address the protocol and networking standards related to these systems and to energy and analytics overall. Initially it is important to start with a discussion of protocol as it relates to data communication networks. For all the reasons stated thus far, this should be useful background for the reader as they consider the impact of this topic on energy and analytics. As a result the reader may need to research elsewhere for further information about data communication and related information on the local area network industry.

The basis for data communication and network is protocol. A communications protocol is a system of digital rules for data exchange within or between computers, and those rules also establish the architecture of a network. As such, protocol is a somewhat simple concept, yet the interrelationship between systems and the requirements for energy and analytics make it a large and complex topic. The focus here is on relating existing data communication and BAS technology to analytics. The author believes that an understanding of these topics will assist the reader in making better everyday decisions about operations and system design. In the end, the goal here is to exchange data in the form of computer messages, and the rules for that exchange are established by the protocol. Since the exchange of messages that contain meaningful data is the goal, it is helpful to understand the concept of messaging to gain an awareness of methods used to exchange messages within computer-based systems. The discussion will then progress through a series of protocol-related topics, each of which has a bearing on data access and data resiliency.

The term protocol will be used extensively with a focus on networks, because it is the author's contention that system networking is at the heart of energy and analytics. Networking provides the basis for BAS devices, and other computer-based systems, to communicate with one another and to communicate data to the outside world of analytics systems, etc. through the internet. Network protocol standards for BAS, energy and other building/facility systems are central to providing on-going data access necessary for operational analysis, fault diagnostics and detection (FDD) and continuous commissioning. To address these technologies, this chapter will define and discuss protocol, starting with data messaging. After a discussion of how messages are constructed, which would be necessary to request or access data, the chapter will follow with a complete review of the data communication, protocol and networking technology that exist to enable this data messaging process.

The chapter will define and describe key concepts, with expanded discussion of protocol and networking technology as it relates to energy and building data for analytics. This chapter will also cover the topic of system architecture, which was discussed with regard to BAS in Chapter 10. Perhaps of greatest import to the evolution of energy and analytics topics however, is to be aware that protocol and networking technology are mature in the IT space, as well as with buildings where standards like BACnet™ have been deployed for nearly two decades. These standards may require adaptation and evolution from time to time, but they offer a robust foundation for application to creating energy and analytics tools. Ultimately however, the informed operator will recognize that some degree of system integration will likely be required, so it is important to have a rudimentary knowledge of protocols and protocol reference models. The differences between protocols and protocol reference models will become clear as we discuss these topics further. At its most basic level however, data are the key requirement, and data must be communicated between computer-based systems and the cloud through a message.

DATA MESSAGES

The concept of messaging is essential to one of the key demands in our industry, the need to have access to the information or data that are available from many different systems. Those data are structured in the form of messages with formats that are dictated by a protocol. All the critical control and operational trend information residing in various energy and building systems are data, and at their most elemental level data are made up of binary digits.

These binary digits, often called bits, make up data consisting of two elements "0" and "1." These bits are assembled into a message with two basic types of data: control and user information (data). Control, not to be confused the BAS control application, conforms to requirements of the protocol and ensures that the information, or data, arrives at the proper end location. These control data are essential to managing individual transmissions, as well as interaction between the various computer-based devices (called "nodes") on the network. The user information, which is the primary reason for networking, may contain a space temperature, an energy consumption or demand value or any number of other types of information. The concepts associated with converting the message to an electrical signal and transmitting it over a "medium," or wire, are also the subject of published "standards" but are not germane to the focus of this book. The primary focus in this chapter is the information (data), the form they take and the process necessary to communicate them between nodes.

It may be evident at this point that the key to sharing information between two different computer-based systems, or between those systems and a cloud-based system, is ensuring that the message formats are identical. There are a number of other considerations as well, because the message format is dictated by other factors including the type of transmission that is employed. As noted, the focus here is on the data themselves and the process employed through a communication protocol to transmit them to another node on a network, another system, or to the cloud via the internet. The approach taken will be to describe message format as a concept and then to discuss the protocol that transmits that format. As an example of message formats consider the synchronous transmission process, shown below, as depicted by Uyless Black in his book *Data Communications and Distributed Networks**. The author has included Mr. Black's explanations below and incorporated, where appropriate, any issues which must be considered for messaging for analytics.

SYN Characters
    These are timing characters used to synchronize the timing of communication between two nodes residing on the network. These characters also act as start and stop bits to identify the beginning and

---

*Uyless D. Black, Data Communications and Distributed Networks, Second Edition, Prentice Hall, Inc., Englewood Cliffs, N.J., 1987, p. 252

end of a message. For analytics, such characters would serve the same purpose, yet it is important to note that microprocessor based devices on the network will likely not initiate communication. In most cases data will be "pulled" from network devices on a higher level analytics system device, therefore it is most important for that device and the analytics engine to execute the same functions.

Header or Address Field

It is critical to identify the transmitting and receiving nodes on the network. This is done through a series of characters, including numbers or letters, for each controller. In most cases there is a requirement for the node address or name to be unique for each controller on a network, and this rule holds true for energy and building networks. This address is normally for network use only, and a number of techniques are employed. Probably the most common method, however, is through a series of software or dipswitch settings that correspond to a software setting or address that is held in device memory. A corresponding address must be programmed in a device such as the enterprise supervisor discussed in the previous chapter that will be used for commissioning or monitoring the node. Allowing users to identify controller nodes by a definable name is also important for communication over the internet through an enterprise supervisor type of device.

Control Characters

Again it is important not to confuse these characters with the process of controlling equipment that is carried out by a BAS. The job of these characters is to maintain the flow of data, and ensure that it is in the correct sequence. These characters are essential to communication, and will be determined to a great degree by the protocol employed with the control network. Control characters employed and their placement will vary dependent upon the protocol and its implementation; however, in some cases the user data will be preceded and followed by control characters. Many of the efforts underway to allow connectivity must address the control aspects of messaging to allow multi-vendor networks to exist. There will be a great deal more discussion of the requirement for control of messages under the protocol section of this chapter.

User Data

In the information technology (IT) industry, these data consist of one or many fields, created by an operator or by the output of a computer program. IT industry user data are associated with the computer application. In the energy and analytics industry, user data can encompass a wide range of content, and they are also related to the application. Yet control user data may be even more critical than with IT due to the real time control decisions that are made on a second-by-second basis. At this book's writing, the intent of most energy and analytics technology is to evaluate a wide range of performance data about buildings, to analyze those data and to provide results. Those results are often reports on building performance, but they also often include recommendations to improve performance. Energy and analytics help operators to make decisions to effect a change and improve performance, but they typically do not execute any type of automatic action. In summary, data are "accessed" and analyzed by the tool to determine whether a recommendation can be made to improve a process. Consider a fault diagnostics and detection (FD&D) application with the accessed data approach, where the data accessed and the analysis conducted indicated that the mixed air function of an air handler was not operating properly. The recommendation to correct that issue might be to take any number of steps including physical activity such as replacing an actuator, programming activity such as modifying sequences, etc.

"Accessed data" from a variety of systems are critical to energy and analytic tools. However it is conceivable that systems will be developed, particularly for energy, which might also use a second type of control user data, "control integrated data." As discussed above, accessed data are generated by systems like a BAS, and may be access through the analytics systems requesting or "pulling" data, i.e. temperature information, control status, etc. for analysis. The purpose would be to ensure proper operation of the air handler by conducting FD&D on the equipment. Most often those data will be part of a larger data interchange between a site and a cloud-based analytics tool, but it is conceivable that a local operator could place the request as well. The idea behind control integrated data would be to update the information on a real-time basis, conduct the analytics and, if appropriate, to integrate a local site response. Given the fact that smart systems are installed in buildings, which can respond to an electronic message, this is achievable. As noted above, energy would be an ideal application and these types of strategies are already being used for demand response with electricity.

Error Check Data

Another essential aspect of messaging systems is to utilize schemes for error, though these will not be described here. The key issue is that data must be checked to ensure that the correct information is received. In this way, a high degree of accuracy may be verified with both accessed data and control integrated data.

Given this discussion of messages the reader should have a better understanding of the some of the concerns associated with ensuring that messages from disparate systems and other sources are accurately received by energy and analytics tools. A number of other concerns must be addressed to transmit this information between machines and allow connectivity. Another term commonly used rather than connectivity, is interoperability. Interoperability is appropriate in this case because the communication may be two-way. The goal of interoperability for energy and analytics is data access, and the definition will be that communications between the devices is successful and that data are accurately transferred between devices. When integrating BAS systems there are additional requirements, but in this case interoperability is the requirement, and it will be the focus during this chapter's discussion of protocol.

**Introduction to Data Communications
and Networking Standards**

The discussion of networks and protocols throughout this book will be limited in scope. Yet it should be evident by this point that the issues of networking and protocol are almost inseparable. It is also true that standard protocols, often simply referred to as "standards," must accommodate remote communication between the internet, a variety of BAS, metering and other hardware. Equally important, a proliferation of web-based devices are being applied for energy, buildings, etc., creating a network architecture of systems and individual devices or controllers. As a result the protocols, or standards, must accommodate both controller-to-controller communication and remote network interface via the internet. The concept of using the protocol to provide a means for integrating communications and data access between different devices, manufacturers, etc. also assumes a network of some type. There must be a means for establishing communication between multiple microprocessor based controllers, and ensuring that guidelines are established for the exchange of information or data. The means for sharing that information is a network, and the rules which define the makeup of the data are the basis for a protocol.

This chapter is intended to expose the reader to basic protocol and networking concepts. More extensive discussion of these concepts is available in texts dedicated to this discipline. The goal here however is to provide an overview of the technology with key buzzwords and acronyms, so that readers are able to analyze the requirements and complexity associated with data access via networking. Understanding networking requires an understanding of some very specialized terminology and the ability to evaluate multiple different standard implementations. Networking is also the basic building block for the internet, and is therefore a vital aspect of any modern computer or information technology (IT) system, including specialized systems like BAS. There has been a tremendous amount of effort applied to networking between and among systems, but this discussion will be confined to terms that have relevance to energy and analytics, or are relevant to its requirements.

Given that prologue, this chapter will make mention of general IT industry terminology, and will quote briefly from a *PC Magazine* article written by Frank Derfler, Jr.(1). The article may be dated, but the terms, as outlined by Derfler, are defined in exactly the same manner today as then, and are the same for the energy and buildings industry as for IT. This chapter provides definitions of communication terms as they apply to both IT and energy and analytics. In Mr. Derfler's words in that article, "before you can understand networking, you've got to speak the language." (Derfler, Frank J., "Networking Acronyms and Buzzwords," NY, NY, June 14, 1988.)

Derfler also notes that "you need a structure to hang the acronyms and buzzwords on, "therefore, you first have to know about the ISO and its OSI model. The International Standards Organization (ISO), based in Paris, develops standards for international and national data communications. The US representative to the ISO is the American National Standards Institute, or ANSI. In the early 1970s, the ISO developed a standard model of a data communications system and called it the Open System Interconnections (OSI) model. The OSI model, consisting of seven layers, describes what happens when a terminal talks to a computer or one computer talks to another. This model was designed to facilitate creating a system in which equipment from different vendors can communicate."

These data communications and IT industry notes are key to this text because the BAS industry, as a major source of analytics data, has focused a great deal of effort on the OSI model. The standardization process in buildings is led by the American Society of Heating, Refrigeration and Air Conditioning Engineers (ASHRAE) with its Communication Protocol Standard Committee 135P. That committee has elected to use the OSI model as the basis for a standard protocol.

PROTOCOLS

As discussed thus far, whether it's wired or wireless, most data communications today happens by way of packets of information travelling over one or more networks. Before these networks can work together, though, they must use a common protocol, or a set of rules for transmitting and receiving these packets of data. Many protocols have been developed. One of the most widely used is the transmission control protocol/internet protocol (TCP/IP), often associated with the internet. TCP/IP will be discussed in more detail in the next chapter. The open system interconnection (OSI) model however is a more generic protocol model that is very helpful in describing network communications, and is also useful for comparing and contrasting different protocols. Most of the buzzwords discussed here will be protocols. Frank Derfler likens protocols to "the signals that a baseball catcher and pitcher exchange for pitches, protocols represent an agreement among different parts of the network on how data are to be transferred. Though you aren't supposed to see them and only a few people understand them, their effect on system performance can be spectacular. A bad protocol can slow data transfer, but a good one can make communications possible between dissimilar systems."

A protocol consists of critical elements which define the format, structure and timing of data transmission. Format is essential to defining the organization of the data that are sent. Data structures are needed for coordination between devices and for handling data. Protocol timing involves matching transmission speeds to allow communication between devices with varying capability (for example the reader has likely experienced a time when number of users on a WiFi network slowed refresh speed). Timing is also implemented within the protocol to ensure that data are transmitted in the proper sequence to ensure that they are meaningful when they arrive at a receiving station.

The open systems interconnection (OSI) model is a means for standardizing the process of developing protocols. The reader should note that OSI is not a protocol, but a model to follow in writing new protocols. This model is intended to allow standardization by segmenting the tasks that a protocol must carry out into functional areas, called layers. The OSI model contains seven layers as noted in Figure 11-1, and has been used in the development of many protocols and protocol standards throughout the world. This model has been the choice of many organizations within the data communication and IT industries. Having been in existence since 1984, it has also been proven by experts in that industry.

The rationale above, along with a number of other factors, was taken into consideration by BAS industry experts in selecting a method for developing a standard protocol. The OSI model and associated terminology are a focus for this chapter, with the intent to provide a rudimentary understanding of networking and protocols.

Figure 11-1. OSI Reference Model Layers

Physical Layer

With the exception of this layer the OSI model consists of modular blocks of computer software. The physical layer is the only hardware element of the model and it is characterized by electrical connections, wiring and signaling, often termed "media." All of the higher layers must communicate through the physical layer. Examples of physical layer media are: Twisted-pair wiring, RS-232C cable, fiber-optic strands, and coaxial cable.

An interesting aspect of the OSI model is that each of the layers which comprise the overall protocol may be a discreet area of expertise. An example of such a standard that has been established within the physical layer is RS-232C. RS-232C is a wiring and signaling standard that is implemented via cable connections between machines or devices. These cables are connected by pins, and the standard defines which pin does what, and when a voltage level on a wire represents a 1 or a 0.

The physical layer is critical to network communication, and carries electrical signals that represent data from the higher OSI layers. Without this layer there can be no communication. Yet the upper layers are absolutely essential if there are to be meaningful communications, i.e. data access.

Data Link Layer

Given that the electrical media are in place, software must be implemented to control the information passing between network members or those members and an internet protocol (IP) connection or address. The OSI model segments this task into the data link layer which assembles characters into messages, controls the transmission of those messages over the media and then checks them before sending them on to the physical media. This layer sometimes transmits messages to notify the sending node that the data have been received. But a "receive message" is typically not sent until some type of error checking has been done to verify that the data are correct. This is a very important topic for the energy and analytics industry because critical data cannot be lost. Fortunately however, most devices have enough buffer memory to be able to resend, providing these message confirmations are timely. As with the physical layer, the data link layer also has standards or protocols that are implemented. Among these is the high-level data link control (HDLC).

Network Layer

This layer is necessary with large networks which may allow many options for transporting blocks of data from one location, typically a workstation or server in an IT local or wide area network, to another. Note that this is a good example of the interdependency that OSI incorporates between layers. These blocks of data are assembled by the data-link-layer, and the network layer allows network connection between nodes and routes the data transmission through one of a variety of paths. The actual physical pathway determined for the data will be based on network conditions such as nodes that have failed, priorities of service, and other factors. Again, this layer's function is tailored to larger IT local area networks (LANs) in IT applications.

Transport Layer

This layer performs a similar function to the network layer, except it is focused on node-to-node interaction within a smaller system, such as a LAN. The key functions of transport are to enhance data transmission reliability. This is done by ensuring that the information is passed between specified nodes, and if a failure occurs, determining another node that can pass the data. A key feature of the transport layer is that it can save data blocks if there is no appropriate transmission route on the network. This is very important in the case of a failure in the communication network, or a necessary node, to communication. The transport layer also implements data integrity features through sequence that check the data. At this layer it is possible to dissect blocks of data and confirm that information has not been corrupted.

Session Layer

This layer establishes the requirements for two network members to carry on a communication session. The session layer defines the rules for interaction between these two nodes, and perhaps the most common example of a session is between two workstations or network members on a computer network.

The primary intent of this layer is to provide a way for entities in two separate devices, potentially employing distinct protocols, to organize and synchronize their dialogue and manage the exchange of data. This is particularly important if those two entities, perhaps PCs, are operating the same application software. For example it may be necessary for the server to provide data handling for user files, while portions of the application software may reside in a workstation. Among the key functions provided at this layer, for communication over the network, are name recognition, logging, administration, and other similar functions.

Presentation Layer

This layer, as the name might imply, is oriented to the display of information. This information may be in the form of graphic- or text-based data, and still it is in the area of the presentation layer. Data passed from the lower layers must be formatted for presentation by the network software. This formatting may involve graphic representation or may require that data from another protocol be converted for presentation in a given system. A variety of related functions such as printer interface and formatting for special displays, etc. would also be done at this layer.

Application Layer

This layer is perhaps the most critical for discussion with any network, including BAS. The application layer tailors the process of data communication to specific user applications. It provides an interaction with the network software to carry out the functions necessary to achieve the network's purpose. This direct interaction with the network software is essential for interaction within any network, and for interface with the outside world via the web. The network software defines media access by the network members and provides any custom functionality that must be accomplished.

It does bear noting within this discussion that the application layer also duplicates, at a more specific level, functions that are provided at lower levels. These functions include network access, flow control and error recovery. For example, at this level, network access may be oriented toward a user password and identification code from a dashboard interface. This code will be defined in detail within the dashboard with regard to the number and type of characters. Based on an authorized code, the application layer might limit or disallow communication with the network. In much the same way, more specialized methods of flow control or error recovery might be implemented at this layer.

As Derfler states, "That's it—the top of ISO's OSI model. The concepts are pretty easy, but dozens of committees are working to define standards for little pieces of each layer, and great political fights are being waged over whose ideas should prevail." The discussion of protocols is not complete without a discussion of network software. There are two key components of this software, as noted above, media access control (MAC) and application software. The source of MAC standards is the Institute of Electrical and Electronics Engineers (IEEE).

MEDIA ACCESS CONTROL (MAC)

Derfler also states that, "the Institute of Electrical and Electronics Engineers (IEEE) developed a set of standards describing the cabling, electrical topology, physical topology, and access scheme of network products. The committee structure of the IEEE is numbered like the Dewey decimal system. The general committee working on these standards is 802. Various subcommittees, designated by decimal numbers, have different versions of the standards." Therefore the standards that have come out of this effort are often referred to as 802.X.

This chapter will provide further discussion of MAC standards under the architecture heading, but a brief overview of important topics is covered here to emphasize the significance of these standards. The reader should note that these standards directly correlate with the 1st and 2nd OSI layers. The concept of MAC is to standardize on the process of allowing a network member to gain access to the communication path. For example, there are two common approaches taken with BAS systems, and these have been defined to date by the sophistication of the control product. Media access is critical to BAS because it determines to a great degree the reliability of data communication. Control system information, particularly those data which are needed for analytics, is highly critical and losing those data would significantly diminish the value of reports and recommendations. Access control protocols that have been used in this industry are of two types: Carrier sense multiple access with collision detection (CSMA/CD) which has been used in more sophisticated systems, and token passing which has been implemented to a great degree with BAS products across the board. These MAC standards have been commonly implemented for proprietary control networks.

CSMA/CD is covered by IEEE standard 802.3. The approach to media access has been well established and proven in the computer industry. In his book on local area networks, Thomas W. Madron states that 802 standard CSMA/CD systems, particularly Ethernet have been

the most widely deployed and supported networks in the computer industry*. This approach is particularly well suited to high-speed
networking with requirements for nodes to have rapid access to the
media. As Madron and others have discussed, the CSMA/CD concept
has often been compared to a group of people talking. In such a situation each member of the group listens, and waits for an opportunity
to participate in the conversation. This is generally effective, yet there
are occasions when two members of the group will attempt to speak at
the same time. This results in the group receiving a garbled message. In
much the same way, CSMA/CD network members listen for the media
to be idle, and then transmit. This allows access to the path with a minimum of delay, yet a procedure must be establish for reinitiating communication when two nodes attempt to communicate simultaneously.
The process often called contention, requires that the network members
listen for a data collision, notify other members that a collision has occurred and then retransmit in order.

The second means of access control to be discussed, and perhaps
the most common to date in the controls industry is token passing.
Token passing is covered by two IEEE standards, however the most appropriate to BAS industry is 802.5, the Token Bus. Access control in this
case can most commonly by compared to a relay race. The token itself
is a piece of information that gives one node at a time authority to communicate. Much like the baton in a relay race, only one runner at a time
has the field for a given race team. Token passing is often referred to as
a collision avoidance technique because it disallows the possibility of
simultaneous communication. As noted, data collisions are not acceptable for BAS or any other devices that rely upon input data to analytics
systems, and this has been one of the factors in broader implementation
of this approach.

NETWORK SOFTWARE

In conjunction with the protocol and the media access control
standards, software must be implemented to provide network functionality. In IT networks it is essential to implement complex software

---

*Thomas W. Madron, *Local Area Networks, The Second Generation*, John Wiley & Sons, NY,
NY 1988

packages to interact with the application layer of the protocol, and accomplish desired user functions. These functions include accounting, database management, access and security control, as well as the network operation of a variety of application software packages. In BAS networks, a similar requirement exists, though most of these functions will be carried out at the controller or enterprise supervisor. The enterprise supervisor is a central communication master that manages communication and data interaction between panels. An enterprise supervisor may also implement data sharing and other functions to be discussed in the next section. Most important to this discussion is that this software must be transparent to the user in control applications, yet it must not be taken for granted as an integral part of the network system.

SIGNAL BOOSTING AND INTER-PROTOCOL NETWORKS

A function of communication networks that are hardwired, is that signals can travel only limited distances over the media. WiFi and wireless networks have specific limitations as well, but will not be discussed here. In most hardwired networks, including BAS, these limitations are approximately 2,000 to 4,000 feet. Another issue is that there may be a limitation to the number of nodes that can be supported by such a network. In addition, it is becoming more common to mix protocols within a given system. This limitation requires that special hardware be added to hardwired networks. There are several types of devices that have been implemented with networks to address these issues including repeaters, bridges, and gateways.

Repeaters are used to amplify and regenerate signals for the network, and this generally enables the signal to travel longer distances on the path. Boosting the signal through the repeaters is also used at times to increase the number of nodes that the network can support. This is important for nearly all networks, but particularly BAS because of the number of controllers that are being added to networks.

Two other devices that have been used extensively in the IT industry are bridges and gateways. The concept of an inter-protocol network is that more than one communication protocol is implemented within the same system. Bridges are used to provide inter-protocol functions when the two networks use the same or similar protocols. This may occur when multiple generations of the same product are installed in the same system. Another example is when the system is expanded beyond its node capacity, and the bridge is used as a way to combine two networks that employ the same protocol, but are operating independently.

Gateways are extremely important to many of the BAS, energy and other related products that will inevitably be used to provide data for energy and analytics. There have been many gateway products introduced to the energy and buildings market, and these devices have not always offered flawless operations, primarily because they typically require specialized knowledge and ongoing maintenance and management for optimum performance. Gateways are employed when communication is required between protocols that are totally incompatible. Middleware, as will be discussed in a later chapter, provides many of the functions that are discussed here, but on a larger scale and with more capability.

Gateways have been used with many conventional BAS systems from a single manufacturer. This is particularly true given the extensive number of mergers and acquisitions within this industry, and the need for a manufacturer to integrate these desperate products under the same corporate banner. Equally common is the use of gateway products to extract data from meters, computerized maintenance management systems (CMMS) and a host of other technologies. Another common application for gateways has been to integrate BAS and various distributed processing systems, which require interaction between distinct functions such as analytics for enterprise energy management (EEM) or fault diagnostics and detection (FD&D), as well as building automation for HVAC, life safety and security systems. Gateways have also been used to implement web-based dashboards and other software products. In essence, the gateway provides a data conversion process in software. It is important to note that a gateway may be an independent piece of hardware and software, but it may also be a software function that is integrated with any piece of BAS or other equipment, such as an enterprise supervisor. This may seem confusing but the optimum implementation for any market participant will vary. Ultimately the function is to handle requests for data from a dashboard, or other interface, and then to translate that request and create a message that the target system understands and transmit it. The data are then received by the gateway in the form of a message and are then converted for the dashboard, etc. and transmitted for display through a user interface. In many cases the gateway is completely transparent to the user, yet this does require that protocol be acquired by the software developer.

This discussion of the buzzwords associated with data communication, the OSI model, network hardware and software is admittedly brief. The intent is to provide a basis to better understand the role of these topics for energy and analytics. To expand on these concepts and provide the reader with a more focused view of the issues at hand, this chapter will now briefly discuss BAS industry networks and communication. BAS technology is not the only source of data for analytics technology, but it can provide significant amounts of data, and BAS networking and data communication are also representative of the approaches that are used for many metering, CMMS and other systems that are also used as sources for data. Therefore it is of interest for the reader to consider this content as a good illustration of the approach taken to access data without having to install vast networks of new sensors. Leveraging data communications and tools like gateways enables technologists to overcome the high cost of sensor networks during the implementation of technology for energy and analytics.

BAS INDUSTRY NETWORKING

This section is key to the discussion of BAS networking. Through the American Society of Heating Refrigeration and Air Conditioning Engineers (ASHRAE), and independent efforts of numerous individuals and companies within the BAS industry, there has been a tremendous amount of work done in the area of networking. The purpose of this section is to identify and define some key terms that apply to BAS network protocols. Of course many of these terms are defined the same as with IT networks. The OSI model discussion should prove to be good background, particularly given its broad acceptance within the IT and BAS industry. This section will review a BAS network example with the intent of identifying key terminology for both this specific topic and in a general context as related to IT networks.

BAS Application Example
There is a great deal of similarity between network issues for the various industries. BAS however does introduce some new concerns due to the requirement for automation and control. The application

used as an example to identify these concerns will be a medium-sized office building with packaged variable air volume (VAV) equipment. The intent here is not to fully describe the application, rather to identify key aspects of it which are network oriented.

The example application is a 50,000-square-foot office building. Primary use of this building is by commercial tenants who each occupy spaces on one of four floors. HVAC requirements for the building are met with distribution from one packaged VAV air handler. This unit is actually a self-contained VAV unit with 120 tons of cooling capacity. The air handler provides constant temperature air to pressure-independent, fan powered VAV terminal units or boxes. The VAV boxes are fitted with integral electric reheat to meet building heating needs. There are approximately 100 VAV boxes in the building with roughly 25 per floor.

Control Equipment

Control for this building is provided through a BAS with intelligent microprocessor based direct digital controllers. The BAS devices are integrated with the air handler, each VAV box, etc. Each piece of equipment is fitted with a self-contained device and includes network hardware and software components. BAS control devices of this type are capable of maintaining a control strategy, or algorithm, for any given piece of equipment. Control may include temperature, pressure, humidity and other strategies along with equipment safety monitoring for alarm or failure conditions.

The air handler (VAV-AH) is fitted with a BAS equipment level control to provide discharge air temperature and reset, along with duct static pressure, control. This BAS device may also monitor compressors for safety conditions, such as high or low pressure.

The VAV boxes are fitted with zone level BAS devices to control fans (if applicable), space temperature and pressure control in some applications. Pressure independent VAV boxes are able to integrate zone damper control with an input that monitors main supply pressure. In this way it is possible to maintain a more consistent CFM supply to the space for comfort and also to reduce noise in the building.

Many VAV-AH equipment level controllers are also capable of integrating zone data for control. The integration may be done through a higher level control or via VAV-AH communication capability on the network. An example of this would be integrating zone data with VAV-AH control functions for reset of discharge air temperature and pressure data for building pressure control. Building pressure allows a manager to operate all or part of a building at positive or negative pressure. For example, a lab could be controlled to negative pressure to avoid introducing undesirable contaminants into the rest of the building.

The final area of control is lighting for common areas which is handled by switching electrical panel circuits. Lighting may be controlled on a time-of-day basis and may be overridden along with the HVAC for after-hours tenant use. Local sensors are often integrated for occupancy or daylight harvesting, and it is possible to integrate building-wide algorithms for demand response and more extensive scheduling and sustainability routines.

Control Network Overview

Network communication, almost exclusively utilizing the BACnet™ standard for BAS, enables data communication between all devices. This would include, for example, sharing data between the equipment level device on the VAV-AH and the zone level device on VAV boxes. This network also serves to provide VAV-AH data to higher level controllers and allow commissioning as well as interrogation of controllers on the network. Of course this network may be the source of extensive amounts of data for FD&D, EEM and other analytics functionality. The most common physical layer media for such a BAS architecture was traditionally twisted pair wiring, but modern systems utilize wireless, fiber optics and any number of different media.

General Control Network Communication

It is important to discuss network communication capabilities in the context of a BAS architecture. As noted in Chapter 10, architecture refers to the rules that define the functions and capabilities of various BA^{DDC} devices, and these rules are established by the protocol in use. The goal here is to help the reader gain an understanding of the varying levels of complexity found in BAS networks. BAS network architectures allow three types of network communication: network interface, distributed network data, and integrated control. Communication types are associated with the level of controller sophistication. Network interface is a minimum requirement for any distributed network, while the other functions tend to be more powerful features. This is also the most important requirement to provide data access for energy and analytics tools. Nearly all BAS will make provisions for all three communication types, however lower end systems may be very limited in their implementation.

Network interface is critical for access to all controllers on the network. Access may be through a local terminal or web-based dashboard. In addition to access to BAS data, this interface also provides a means for commissioning a site, and all the associated controllers.

There are two types of distributed network data (DND), global and shared. These data types were discussed in Chapter 10 under the BAS. Integrated control occurs when network control commands consist of control decisions made in one BAS device and carried out by one or more other BAS devices. Integrated control is important for system-wide functions like critical alarm shutdowns, demand response (DR) or demand limit control (DLC). To implement DR, a network device must be identified to monitor the internet for a DR event notification. For DLC, one of the BAS devices will monitor the utility demand meter and determine when a pre-determined peak is imminent. When the DR event or DLC peak occurs, the BAS will execute a sequence. The intent is the same in both cases, to take action that reduces load. In the case of DR, the actions may be different and will have been agreed to between the customer and the utility. With DLC the actions may be the same or different, but rather than taking action on the event, the goal is to issue commands rapidly to the BAS devices and ensure that the demand setpoint is not exceeded. DLC commands along with other integrated control network functions must also be transmitted quickly, usually within a frequency of seconds.

This brief overview of BAS networking technology is provided to assist the reader with an understanding of one of the more common systems that provides data to analytics. Of interest is that the same approaches would be found in metering and other systems. Ultimately however, the point is that energy and analytics can be implemented in the most cost effective manner by leveraging data points from BAS and other systems, therefore it is in the reader's best interest to have a working knowledge of how such systems operate.

INTERNET AND WEB SERVICES

The previous discussion focused on BAS networks and was intended to provide a general understanding of that technology. Those systems might be referred to as "intranets," however during that discussion there were numerous references to web-enabled dashboards and the internet as a vehicle for transporting BAS data to analytics suites. It is therefore appropriate to provide a brief introduction to the internet and web services here as well. The next chapter will also provide more content on this topic. This introduction is intended to expose the reader to the next layer of architecture—worldwide architecture via the internet.

It might be helpful to begin with a discussion of web services, because these services are being used to enable data access. It may also be helpful to consider definitions for web services from IT industry powerhouses. According to **IBM Corporation** "Web services are self-contained, modular applications that can be described, published, located, and invoked over a network, generally, the World Wide Web." **Microsoft Corporation's** description is more succinct, "a web service is programmable application logic, accessible using standard internet protocols."

Others define web services as a business logic or as information made available using the XML (extensible markup language)-based SOAP (simple object access protocol). In the analytics space, however there has been a migration to other technologies such as representational state transfer (REST) and other models, as many believe these are easier to implement. REST will be discussed in Chapter 12 on middleware. In any case, web services are invoked to access data from a variety of intranet and internet data sources. To accomplish such tasks, technologies and protocols have been developed that can integrate existing business processes and resources, as well as systems data from BAS, etc., and make them available over the web. Energy and analytics tool developers looking for approaches to develop web services, have new integrated environments to choose from that offer everything from web servers to application development tools.

The BAS and analytics industries have become very aware of these trends. The site www.automatedbuildings.com has provided an incredible source of data for the BAS industry, but equally important has also become a clearinghouse for data on a wide range of emerging markets including energy and analytics. The following article is excerpted from a January, 2013 issue of AutomatedBuildings.com and is called **Information Model: The Key to Integration**, by Eric Craton, Product Development and Dave Robin, Software Development. The authors state that web services are a new breed of web application. web services are self-contained, modular applications that can be run over the internet and can be integrated into other applications. Web services perform functions that can be anything from simple requests to complicated business processes. For example, a weather bureau could offer a web service that allows a BAS to automatically retrieve temperature forecast data for use by various control algorithms. Similarly, an analytics suite can use web services to extract data from BAS and other systems to be used for analysis of critical energy and building functions. Equally important, the best analytics tools analyze that data in the context of business process, because interpretation of the data and analysis results requires a detailed understanding of the process being executed in the building. For example an analytics tool could utilize web services to extract data from a tenant's accounting system to obtain up-to-the-minute figures on energy consumption, and conduct analysis that evaluates the business process against energy consumption data to determine if changes can be made in operations. In the past, this type of data exchange would require a custom, "hard coded" data request to retrieve information that already existed in the host computer. A web service, on the other hand, is a way to allow any authorized client to actually run an application on a server in the cloud to access data and conduct analysis that previously was not possible. This provides a mechanism for building owners to not only conduct the analysis but be more timely to acting on recommendations to improve the operations. Since BACnet objects are information models, and XML is a modeling language, we could express these high level information models in XML and in so doing make them compatible with the emerging web services architecture.

Architecture

This chapter has covered data communications, networking and protocols. It also provided some background on BAS networking, with BAS being representative of many systems that are to be found in operations with energy and buildings. The term SCADA, system control and data acquisition has not be used, but SCADA is also common in this arena and is similar to BAS. This last section in the chapter will revisit the topic of architecture. As discussed there are a large number of rules or standards, which are collectively called data communications protocol. Protocol is an essential element in defining the capabilities and characteristics of a network and in defining the network's architecture. The concept of architecture is defined by both the protocol and network software, which was discussed earlier in this chapter. Architecture encompasses a broader scope because it involves both the physical and network implementation of the protocol. This section covers the physical implementation of architecture through a discussion of topology. Topology defines the structures that are possible and also the physical wire or media that may be used in connecting the network members. Topology is defined by standards that are established in layers one (physical) and two (data link) of the OSI model. Network implementation is achieved through the interaction of the protocol. The architecture allows communication between the various network members. International network standards have been developed to define architectures. These standards along with the interaction noted above, dictate the physical media and structures as well as the process for passing data between network members or nodes. Networking, the support of communication between distributed intelligent controllers, is essential to establishing a reliable flow of data for analytics. Networking is addressed here as one of two essential elements of an architecture, in terms of technology available and standards which are applicable in the controls industry. The central focus will be on understanding the interrelationships within the architecture and roles of both critical elements, protocol and network software. This will be useful because a solution to the protocol issue requires combined implementation of a standard protocol within a standard architecture. The term architecture will be used to describe the complete solution which includes the elements of protocol and topology. Network software is also of interest under the topic of architecture but this topic was covered previously with the discussion of IEEE standards for media access control.

With that introduction it becomes obvious that the concept of protocol should be transparent to the user, though all of the aspects discussed under architecture require implementation of a common protocol. So the focus here is on implementation of the complete architecture, including protocol, but discussions will be limited to topology as implemented by the protocol and network software as it interacts with the protocol.

To aid in understanding architecture, it is helpful to address the specific physical connection of network members, and the implementation of the protocol messaging through network software. This should answer these questions: What does the network look like, and how is it physically implemented? Then the discussion will view the interaction between members of the network. To clarify the residence of these components however, the reader should understand that all of the questions posed above are answered in one of the lower protocol layers. The more complex user-oriented interactions occur between the upper layers of the protocol and the network application software.

Rather than covering these topics in relationship to the specific layers in which they reside, they will be covered in conceptual terms. The intent is to cover the concepts in a way that is consistent with how system professionals view a system. The general architecture will be discussed first, followed by an overview of the physical layout or topology, and finally a review of the software applied within the architecture. The umbrella term for all of these discussions is "architecture," and it will be used in conjunction with "topology" and "network" to describe the characteristics of implementation. Again the content here is divided into two categories, architecture and topology.

It is not uncommon for these terms to be used interchangeably, so it is important here to define them very clearly. Architecture, as noted, is the overall definition of a network including protocol, topology or physical wiring connections, network implementation or rules of data link control network application software. Key aspects and capabilities of communicating controllers will be discussed within each category.

ARCHITECTURE

This section will focus on the two key elements of architecture; topology and networking software. Architecture is a much used term, and interpretations change radically based upon the context, so a definition is useful. An architecture is defined as the protocol (including electrical signaling via topology and if necessary media access standards) and networking software that allow interconnection and communication with building control system(s) and their associated components. Physical and networking standards that combine to define the architecture, as outlined by Uyless Black*,

---

*Uyless D. Black, *Data Communications and Distributed Networks*, Second Edition, Prentice Hall, Inc., Englewood Cliffs, NJ, 1987

include: hardware, software, data link controls (DLCs), standards, topologies and protocols. Communicating for IT, BAS or any other type of system began when more than one panel with intelligence was applied in an architecture. For example, the most common BAS industry architecture has been a master slave implementation in which one device is responsible for managing communication. This device more than likely contained all of the control algorithms, as well as communication responsibility. The most common approach was to implement slave panels to provide inputs and outputs, thus expanding the capability of the system.

Architecture describes the overall communication systems for any network including BAS. Within any architecture there may be a variety of devices, and among those may be specific devices that have certain capabilities for communication and interaction with other network members. A term the reader may have heard is "level of architecture." A level of architecture implies a system, or portion of a system, in which all devices communicate on a common basis. It is also possible for an architecture in this context to encompass multiple protocols. As noted above and elsewhere in this text, various styles of interconnection are possible that allow complex protocol interaction. For this chapter however, the assumption will be that the architecture shares a common protocol. This will allow the author to focus on the most important concepts of architecture to our target discussion of topology and networking software.

TOPOLOGY

Topology is defined by the 1st and 2nd OSI model layers and establishes the structures that are possible for interconnecting nodes. Topology also establishes the physical wire or media that may be used in connecting the network members. In addition to defining the rules for network interconnection, Topology also covers the associated characteristics of that connection. For that connection to occur there must be rules for attachment of each node to the local area network (LAN), and for the overall structures that are acceptable for multiple nodes. Per Uyless Black, there are four major components that define a local area network.

1.   Communication channel

2.   Interface

3.   Protocol control

4.   Intelligent device (i.e. enterprise supervisor or dashboard)

The communication channel or path is critical to a network. The path is defined by a requirement for compatibility with both the protocol and the network software, and varies significantly by the implementation. Path media ranges from the simplest twisted pairs of wire, called "twisted pair," which is low in cost and easy to install, to fiber optics with higher data transmission capacity and speed capabilities. Again the path in most cases will be defined by the lower layers of the protocol, and is the essential component of the topology. It is also relevant here to include a comparison between topology and local area network (LAN) type. LAN type is a noteworthy because it has a dramatic impact on overall network performance. Two LAN types are to be discussed: broadband and baseband. This refers, in simple terms, to the capacity of the physical media to carry data, and may also determine the physical media that is compatible. The only point here is that the amount of data that are being transmitted from any system to an analytics suite may require consideration of a LAN type that can support the desired bandwidth. The interface between the path and the protocol logic is the second key component of this discussion. Again this interface is defined by the protocol and network software or operating system. The interface is typically a software component. The orientation varies, yet in essence the interface must allow for an electrical signal from the communication path to be converted to the upper layers of the protocol. This is a good example of a data link layer function. This interface is software that interacts directly with the physical layer and its associated hardware.

Regarding topology, there are a number of options for organizing control networks including those listed below. This level of detail may be more than is necessary for readers to understand as they develop strategies to access data for analytics, so the content will be covered at a fairly general level. It may also be helpful to differentiate simple concepts from more complex topology approaches that are applied with network technology. These topics will be discussed in two categories: simple networks and network topologies.

Simple Networks
- Point-to-point
- Multipoint

Network Topologies
- Star
- Ring
- Bus
- Hierarchical

Ancillary LAN devices that directly impact the network include: repeater, gateway and bridge which were previously discussed. LANs are covered because they often define the media that is used to connect the structures noted above, and include broadband and baseband.

Simple Networks

Simple networks are oriented to IT or computer systems but provide good background for the discussion of network topologies. In this case the IT network may be enabling communication between servers or devices equivalent to an enterprise supervisor, but for simplicity this section will refer to the device as a computer. Local area computer networks are oriented to limited geographic areas and with simple networks the assumption is that only one computer is present. That computer typically supports communication to allow interface from several terminal or workstations.

The point-to-point network style is extremely simple and tends to be very much oriented to computer networks. The structure includes one computer, a communication path and a dashboard or interface of some type. This point-to-point approach barely passes for networking, yet it is considered simple networking because the terminal uses a protocol for either direct connect interaction or communication via an IP address to the internet.

The multipoint network architecture is an expansion of the point-to-point approach in which more than one interface, display or dashboard is possible. The multipoint network was developed to allow more than one interface to be connected simultaneously to a single computer or server. This is more typical with computer local area networks (LANs) that require interaction from interface terminals with the server for access to application software and a database.

Network Topologies

Network topologies are distinguished from simple networks by their more specific orientation to networks with multiple intelligent devices or servers. The star network is common with centralized computer networks. Typically these applications involve primary computing that is contained in one site, and all of the remote interfaces are connected to that site. Again interfaces in this case are more likely to be computers or dashboards. Two of the most popular local area networks (LANs) in the computer industry, ARCNET developed by Datapoint Corporation and Token-Ring by International Business Machines Inc. (IBM), allow the star network topology. The star topology enables a network which allows for a central hub and device wiring runs that can terminate at the last device. The ring topology requires that all nodes be connected to the physical media in a closed loop. With the ring concept each node is linked to the adjacent nodes on both the left and the right. Again it is common to apply ring networks in the IT industry, and in fact the IBM product noted above is a good example of a ring network. Some benefits of the ring concept are that higher data transmission speeds are possible and data collision schemes can be implemented in a simple fashion. With a ring network each station in the ring receives and retransmits a message, and as a result data collisions and errors can be minimized. There are some detriments to the concept which should be considered. First, rings have less flexibility in terms of installation, and further may add significant cost to a project due to the requirement for completion of a closed wiring circuit. Another consideration may also be the capability required of each controller node for receipt and retransmission of data.

The bus network structure is distinguished by the central "backbone" which is the physical media. The media also allows taps for arms or branches, each typically allowing one controller to be connected. The bus topology is extremely common with BAS networks because it lends itself to single wire runs without the need to loop back, as in the ring network. Generally the physical media in control bus networks is a twisted pair, which may be run throughout a building. The communication signal travels along the bus, and every controller node "listens" for the signal that carries its address. In most cases the controller both receives and transmits via the same twisted pair bus using a special signaling process. Both bus and star systems require that a "biasing resistor" or other component be used to terminate the bus. This termination is what allows the installer to establish an end point for data transmitted on the network. These topology structures have been outlined briefly for the reader's information. An interesting note is that networks are not limited to a particular topology, sometimes these approaches may coexist.

LAN type is the next topic, but it is complex, and need not be understood for analytics, so it will not be covered in detail. LAN types, broadband or baseband, also do not have a major impact on the architecture. This is a physical media issue because data are transmitted over the physical path via an electrical signal. The reader is likely aware that all computer data are, at their most basic level, zeros or ones. These zeros and ones are converted to electrical signals for transmission over the physical media. In simple terms, the greater the span of frequency that a path can support, the more information that may be transmitted at one time. The only important note for the reader regarding energy and analytics is that frequency and bandwidth are directly related. For illustration purposes, consider the analogy of an interstate freeway through a major metropolitan area. The more lanes of traffic that the freeway can accommodate, the greater the flow of automobiles in each direction, and therefore the system offers better "throughput." Throughput in data communication, as the term implies, is the measure of information traveling on the physical media for both transmission and response. In data communications networks, the concept of throughput is also impacted because greater frequency is typically accompanied by techniques for increasing transmission speed.

The concept of a computer LAN is to allow multiple devices, from small tablets and smart phones to personal computers, laptops and servers to share application software and information. A well-defined means must be established for those nodes to gain access to the media, and for recovery in the event of data corruption. This is accomplished by network software that was discussed earlier.

Data transmission media, speed and limited processing requirements at each node of a LAN are also required.

ENERGY AND ANALYTICS DATA ACCESS

This text is focused on energy and analytics as applied in a wide range of applications from buildings, plants and large-scale campus or city operations. In the end there will be a host of systems and technology already in place that can be rich sources of data for this analysis. The intent of this chapter has been to provide a limited overview of the data communications and networking that is deployed by typical systems of this type, and provide a limited understanding of the techniques that would be required to access the data in those systems. This access to system information will typically involve interface via the internet and a means of initiating data requests via an enterprise supervisor that has access. This process must be transparent to an analytics engine, allowing for a request of status on any individual point or group of points. Equally important, this process must be resilient to ensure that the flow of data is continuous, reliable and accurate.

Chapter 12

Middleware—A New Frontier for Building Systems and Analytics

This may be one of the most important chapters in this book for the long-term success of energy and analytics. With the foundation that was provided in the prior two chapters it is possible to peel a layer or two from the onion, and to begin to understand the underlying technology, or glue, that enables building systems to interoperate. Glue is a good word to describe "middleware" because these components actually provide connective tissue between systems, but a better term might be "infrastructure." The infrastructure of energy and analytics is made up of systems with hardware devices, networking and interface software and an infinite number of instrumentation devices (sensors, meters, etc.). All of these system components must be accessed by and communicate with an analytics "engine" or "tool," which conducts all of the analyses. The purpose of this chapter is to provide insight and information to the reader that will be invaluable in understanding how these systems operate, and will be useful in comparing analytics tools and system approaches between various suppliers.

Perhaps one of the most confusing things about this topic is that words like middleware are not familiar to many professionals in the energy and buildings industry. In addition, middleware, as a term, falls short of describing the full functionality of this technology. However, the industry embraces certain terms as identifiers for groups of products and services, and once a term sticks, it becomes useful to identify the technology being discussed. So the overarching term for products that will be discussed is middleware, but this simply provides a starting point, and again the goal is to provide an understanding of the underlying and interconnecting technology that makes it possible to achieve "interoperability." It may be most useful however to provide some history from the energy and buildings industry to help clarify why this functionality is needed.

In the 1980s a movement arose within the building automation systems world that demanded standardization of data communications. The term "open systems" eventually caught on as a way to describe what users wanted. Whether control technologies are referred to as building automations systems (BAS), energy management systems (EMS) or direct digital control systems (DDC), this technology performs the same work and will simply be called BAS here. Chapter 10 referred to BA^{DDC} because the emphasis was on the automation and control functionality itself. Here the reference will be BAS because the focus is on the systems themselves and the technologies that enable data sharing and interoperability between them. So BAS provides a focal point for this discussion. By the mid-1980s a number of market drivers, i.e., energy crises, development of microprocessors and demand for energy management, had resulted in hundreds of millions of dollars in BAS installations. As managers, particularly those with multiple buildings, or those who operated complex and ever changing campuses, became aware, the generation of BAS at that time presented a number of communication issues. These early-generation BAS were called "legacy systems." Recognizing the limitations and challenges presented by legacy systems led building owners and managers to drive the open systems movement for two reasons: 1) the absence of standards required independent computer interfaces for every manufacturer's BAS, and 2) expansion of systems was difficult because BAS from multiple manufacturers could not interoperate, which made owners feel locked in to a particular system. The rest is history, and by 1995 the BACnet™ had been developed, and in another decade products deploying that standard became ubiquitous. Over the period of three or more decades however, managers were still demanding solutions for those hundreds of millions in legacy systems, and that is how "middleware" came to be.

MIDDLEWARE

Middleware, as a term, was borrowed from the information technology (IT) industry, in part because of the types of devices that were used to apply the functionality. According to Wikipedia, "Middleware is computer software that provides services to software applications beyond those available from the operating system. It can be described as 'software glue.' Middleware makes it easier for software developers to enable communication between multiple systems and to access inputs/ outputs (I/O). This allows developers to focus on the specific purpose of the application being developed. Middleware is the software that connects software components or enterprise applications. Middleware is the software layer that lies between the operating system and the applications on each side of a distributed computer network."

It may be clear why the term stuck with BAS because the desire to unify systems interfaces into what we later began to call "dashboards" required software to perform communications and access input/output and other data.

The need for a type of software/hardware, which is referred to here as middleware, became even more pronounced as managers ended up with multiple generations of product from multiple manufacturers. A unifying middleware product that allowed managers to interface with all of those systems through one PC or dashboard was highly desirable. Setting aside the actual interface for a moment, one of the ways that this functionality was accomplished initially was via a gateway. In Chapter 11 gateways were described as pieces of hardware that allow the same network to have more than one protocol. The BAS task entails a bit more complex functionality, but ultimately these "BAS Gateways" were developed as pieces of hardware that could convert a legacy BAS protocol for communication over a larger network to a higher level computer, and ultimately a dashboard. Variations on this same approach are still being used today to provide interoperability that enables data to be accessed from various systems and made available to energy and analytics tools.

In 2008 Cisco Systems teamed up with Frost & Sullivan to publish a white paper called "Intelligent Middleware." Cisco had acquired Richards-Zeta, a progressive building automation company, and their platform was called the Mediator. A major focus of that paper was migration of building automation systems toward internet protocol (IP) integration. Figure 12-1 comes from that white paper, and provides a visual to emphasize Cicso's position that middleware technology was critical to allow interchange between BASs-using proprietary protocols and IT centric systems using IT protocols. The notion was that a "capability gap" existed between BAS, which were not capable of functionality beyond their intended purpose, and the internet with more sophisticated functions for a larger enterprise. Today, energy and analytics would be one of those more sophisticated, or larger enterprise, functions, but Figure 12-1 predates the emergence of analytics as it is now known. This

The Mediator – Enabling Convergence from the South to the North

North

Integrated Enterprise Application & Services, Web Services, XML-RPC, OBix

Intelligent Middleware - "The Mediator" moving data up to the network using Internet Protocol – TCP/IP

Proprietary and non proprietary Subsytems of a building such as HVAC, Lighting, Sensors, Security, Metering, etc.

Variety of systems from a variety of manufacturers including Trane, Siemens, TAC, JCI, Honeywell, Invensys, Carrier, PowerLogic, GE, Carrier and more.

Capability Gap

South

Intelligent Building Systems (IBS) infrastructure with Advanced networking enabling optimized energy management, automated demand response (ADR), remote monitoring, automated fault detection and diagnostics (AFDD), etc.

Data from the South is normalized on the Mediator

Domain layer with some level of standardization; Echelon, BacNet, Modbus, And SNMP

Limited standardization; creating closed architecture and locked down systems.
Source: Frost & Sullivan

Figure 12-1

figure assumes that the mediator provides interface to older-generation BAS-using proprietary protocols only, which have been called legacy systems in this book. However, today the concept for middleware is more expansive. In addition to legacy systems, it is not uncommon for middleware to provide interface between many systems using proprietary protocols as well as BACnet and other standards. Of equal interest, these middleware devices may also integrate an instantiation of energy and analytics functionality as well. The analysis is still occurring in the cloud, but more companies are developing their own energy and analytics tools and using middleware as a focal point for the solution. Therefore with analytics, the line sometimes blurs between *traditional middleware functionality* (providing "drivers" to execute data conversion between proprietary standards, open standards and IP), and *middleware for buildings* (providing traditional functions plus added functionality that is central to a product offering, such as enterprise energy management or analytics).

Also around 2008, Ken Sinclair, publisher of Automatedbuildings. com, authored an article on middleware. Ken began with common definitions for middleware, that it is "the 'glue' between software components, or between software and the network, or it is the slash in client/server. Middleware is used to connect applications to other applications. (See Figure 12-2.)

Middleware opens opportunities to use multiple user interfaces, such as mobile dashboards running on tablets, phones and other web-enabled mobile devices, to monitor and interact with different systems. This (middleware) brings together data from multiple systems, in multiple buildings, to give facility managers unprecedented control over their energy use, help them spot trouble with equipment early, and enable them to make adjustments in real time. In the past, it was common for this middleware to be packaged with the automation system, security and life safety systems from one vendor. While this was convenient for the purchaser, it left no room for future enhancements from other vendors—they were stuck with the vendor that installed the system. This has changed in recent years, with many vendors using open protocols, or standards, which allow customers choice. The bigger challenge today is determining what information and systems should be integrated at the building level. You can't manage what you don't measure, but careful choices have to be made regarding what sort of level you both need and want."

Figure 12-2

Another take on defining middleware came from Jim Sinopoli and Neil Gifford of Smart Buildings. In a 2008 article (www.automatedbuild-ings.com) they said that the implementation of a middleware solution would normalize and standardize the data of building automation systems. In addition, these systems can extract and digest the data and control the systems, such as set device values or set points. The word "middleware" may sound like just software, but their implementation requires software and hardware. The hardware will involve subsystem controllers likely needed for the HVAC systems and some IT hardware, such as gateways for interface to servers and dashboards. Figure 12-2 came from this article, and it identified four of the companies who dominated the industry at that time. Interestingly, all of the building-specific players mentioned were later acquired: GridLogix, acquired by Johnson Controls Inc.; Richards-Zeta acquired by Cisco; and Tridium acquired by Honeywell. Tridium is a very important participant in this industry, and will be discussed later in this chapter when more detail is provided on middleware technology solutions. Lynx Spring is a Tridium developer and BAS manufacturer and leader in this space.

Standards are a key topic that has been discussed throughout the last several chapters on data communications and protocol. Standards are key to this discussion because the more standards that are introduced to the energy and analytics industries, the easier it becomes to access data in a reliable and repeatable fashion. This has been called data resilience. Some of these standards have been discussed at length, such as BACnet™, but others are also important like MODbus™, which is used by many metering systems. Another type of standard is oBIX (Open Building Information eXchange), which is "an industry-wide initiative to define XML- and web services-based mechanisms for building control systems." oBIX is an OASIS standard. OASIS is the Organization for the Advancement of Structured Information Standards, a non-profit consortium that drives the development, convergence and adoption of open standards for the global information society. oBIX is important because its intent is to instrument control systems for the enterprise. "The purpose of oBIX is to enable the mechanical and electrical control systems in buildings to communicate with enterprise applications, and to provide a platform for developing new classes of applications that integrate control systems with other enterprise functions." The point with this standard was to overlay an IT solution that can access data in a standardized format regardless of the machine communications protocols. oBIX was ideally targeted to address the data access needs for energy and analytics, however a common theme with technology is that change is constant. Later in this chapter there will also be discussion of web services technologies that are enabling analytics developers to simplify and fast track solutions. Besides these efforts and oBIX, there are other groups working to unify data communication standards and to approach data access in different ways as well. Among these efforts are the work of the Smart Grip Interoperability Panel (SGIP) www.sgip.org, which is a spinoff of the U.S. Department of Energy Smart Grid work. This is a great example of how BAS technology has become part of much larger standards efforts and is benefiting from the work of a much larger community. This author is chairman emeritus of the DOE Gridwise Architecture Council, and represented the energy management and buildings domain with that group, but there were wide ranging other domains represented as well: industrial automation, electricity infrastructure, residential systems, IT, networking and more. An important milestone during this author's term as chairman was passage of the Energy Independence and Security Act by the United States Congress. That law directed the National Institute of Standards and Technology (NIST), which is part of the U.S. Department of Commerce) to lead a national effort to identify technology standards that could enable a Smart Grid. Interestingly, Steve Bushby was one of the managers at NIST who oversaw this work. Mr. Bushby brought strong buildings knowledge as well, because he was a founding member, and one of the leaders, of the BACnet™ standards committee with the American Society of Heating Refrigeration and Air conditioning Engineers (ASHRAE). The SGIP is actively engaged in a wide range of efforts to identify technologies and standards, which are likely to prove useful in data access for energy and analytics. Another effort that will be discussed at greater length in a future chapter is Project Haystack, an analytics industry 501.C3 organization engaged in an open source initiative to streamline working with data from the Internet of Things. Haystack is standardizing semantic data models with the goal of making it easier to unlock value from the vast quantity of data being generated by the smart devices that permeate homes, buildings, factories, and cities. Applications include automation, control, energy, HVAC, lighting, and other environmental systems.

Of particular importance to the topic of middleware is data communications and networking. The networks however are not just Ethernet or other IT networks; there are a host of network technologies in play. Therefore, the next topic is to define a number of these networks that are being managed and utilized via this middleware to make data available to analytics.

NETWORKS FOR ANALYTICS

The topic of networks was discussed at length in Chapter 11. This section may repeat some content, but the goal is to build on this topic. Again a local area network (LAN) is a system that enables data communication between multiple microprocessor-based computer devices, which must share information to perform work. Protocols and networking software were discussed as the means for enabling communications and data access between different computer devices. The network provides the means to establish communication between multiple microprocessor based devices (servers, personal computers, BAS controllers, etc.), and ensuring that guidelines are established for the exchange of messages containing information or data. The means for sharing that information is a network, and the rules which define the makeup of the data are the basis for a protocol.

With the advent of microprocessor-based systems for building applications—from BAS for HVAC, security, etc. to meter data management and enterprise energy management—data communication and networking became an integral part of the buildings world. With the advent of cloud-based systems including those providing energy and analytics services, this fabric of communication and networking has become even more complex. As discussed in Chapter 11, the local area network (LAN) is a system of computer devices that is interconnected, in a limited area, such as a building, using network media, or physical cabling. LANs for many different types of building technologies including the BAS, have been standardized by the BACnet™ standard. As noted above, there are also a number of other standards, such as Modbus for meters, that are being integrated in a meaningful way through the efforts of the American Society of Heating Refrigeration and Air Conditioning Engineers and the Smart Grid Interoperability Panel (SGIP) to name a few. That integration, particularly with legacy systems that are already installed, is typically enabled by middleware products. This is especially true for energy and analytics, because there is an expansive landscape of systems and technology that may be identified as sources to access data or as enablers to transmit data. This is why the topic of middleware is so critical to energy and analysis, and why the term "glue" seems so appropriate. Middleware technology is used to connect systems that use disparate protocols, and convert the data for presentation to energy and analytics technology. Middleware technology is also used to connect systems that utilize different network technology, and enable its presentation to energy and analytics technology. This section has focused on coverage of LANs, but will now provide some insight into the broader range of technologies that must be interoperable with for energy and analytics including:

Wide area network (WAN),

Virtual private network (VPN),

Wireless networking technologies,

Machine to machine (M2M) technologies, and

Cloud computing.

Wide area networks are applied on a very limited scale for BAS, energy and analytics, yet the concept bears noting because it provides useful context for discussion of networking via the internet, particularly virtual private networks (VPNs). A wide area network (WAN) is a network that covers a larger geographic area, rather than a building, campus, etc., (i.e., any telecommunications network that links across metropolitan, regional, national or international boundaries) using leased telecommunication lines. Business and government entities utilize WANs to relay data among employees, clients, buyers, and suppliers from various geographical locations. The key distinction between WANs and the discussions that will unfold with virtual private networks, etc. is that these networks typically utilize telecommunications systems, unlike VPNs which use the internet. Features of the internet like "always on" and the simplicity of transmitting large volumes of data using a wide range of data formats, as well as a more advantageous cost, have made internet-based solutions, such as a virtual private network, the preferred approach for analytics systems today.

A virtual private network (VPN) extends a private network across a public network, such as the internet. VPNs enable a computer, or a dashboard, to send and receive data across shared or public networks as if they were directly connected to the private network, while benefiting from the functionality, security and management policies of the private network. Quite simply for an energy and analytics application, the VPN provides all the benefits of performing these functions within a building or campus, but it also enables scale. VPNs are created by establishing virtual point-to-point connections through the use of dedicated connections, virtual tunneling protocols, or traffic encryptions. Again this is essential for multi-location building and campus owners, as well as those that have management staff in many locations. The VPN provides a vehicle for transporting the data to all of those locations, where of course the applications can be housed locally on servers. This is particularly important because energy and analytics functionality relies equally as much on human engineering knowledge and skill, as it does on technology. In many cases, the VPN is the communication enabler for the energy and analytics and other applications that are housed in the cloud, but more on that in a moment. The benefit to this is that access to data and analytics applications, from any geographic location, makes it possible to leverage human knowledge to develop a better understanding of analytics results.

The LAN, WAN and VPN as discussed thus far are complete and functional networks encompassing all of the capabilities described under the OSI model discussion in Chapter 11. An important distinction for analytics is that these LANs may incorporate multiple protocols, requiring gateways, etc., which may also requires deployment of a bridge to unify multiple communication media. Middleware is the essential technology to unify all of these differences and create seamless access to data for energy and analytics tools. In the case of VPNs, the media of interest may be a hardwired Ethernet LAN through an IP address, local area wireless technology or "WiFi" allowing an electronic device to connect to the internet. Given the challenges and first cost detriments to installing wired networks for metering and instrumentation devices, as well as the complexity of interconnecting networks where distance or construction materials such as concrete present challenges, wireless has become very popular for interoperability between these networks. Of course, one form of wireless is WiFi, which can then be used for internet access, and has become ubiquitous, enabling individual smart devices (PCs, tablets, smart phones, etc.) to access the internet.

Independent of its use with VPN technology to provide WiFi access to the internet for energy and analytics, wireless technology is also used for local area networking. This focus on wireless LANs, sometimes called WLAN, pertains to a network that has all the same characteristics as any wired LAN, except there is no physical wired connection between sender and receiver. Instead the network is connected by radio waves to maintain communications. There are many wireless networking standards that have gotten significant acceptance in the buildings space, including ZigBee™ and EnOcean™. The key point is that this is simply another form of LAN being deployed. The next major topic area here will be about building communication systems that are made up of multiple networks. Wireless networks are a good example of a "sub-LAN" or secondary network infrastructure that may be used to access data for analytics.

Machine to machine (M2M) is a term that has received more attention recently and has great implications for energy and analytics. M2M refers to multichannel networks made up a large numbers of devices, many of which are small in terms of both processing power and input/output capacity. In the context of analytics, M2M is very important because these devices can provide a significant amount of data from very granular sources. Some examples are meters, motion sensors and photovoltaic panels mounted on telephone poles. M2M is an independent topic, but in many respects it was the precursor to the Internet of Things (IoT), a topic discussed later in the book. Regarding IoT, a November 2014 report from the International Data Center estimates that there will be 30 billion autonomous things (computers, tablets, smart phones, BAS, etc.) connect to the internet by 2020. Those "things" can provide a rich and exciting source of data for analytics.

Cloud computing is the last topic that will be discussed under this heading of networking. This is also a great segue to expand beyond the infrastructure that is used to move data around, to the applications or engines of analysis that are being deployed under the heading of energy and analytics. Cloud computing is computing in which large groups of remote servers, often physically located in data centers or server farms, are networked to allow centralized data storage and online access to computer services or resources. Cloud computing is the term used to describe the use of interconnected business applications over the internet. As depicted in Figure 12-3, the applications are interconnected via web services, and the end user accesses the required service using a web browser or dashboard. Therefore, the application and the infrastructure do not reside on end users' premises. The end user accesses the application on demand, and can concentrate on using the application for its purpose, without investing capital expenditures, thereby avoiding the overhead of installation, networking and maintenance.

Cloud computing is the term used to describe the use of interconnected business applications over the internet. Nirosha Munasinghe, MBusIT BSc BE, a product development manager with Open General in Australia, published a great article on this topic called "The Future of Cloud Connectivity for BAS" (www.automatedbuilidings.com) in June 2010. An excerpt of that article defining cloud computing is provided here. Mr. Munasinghe provided Figure 12-3 to illustrate that the applications are interconnected via web services and the end user accesses the required service using a web browser.

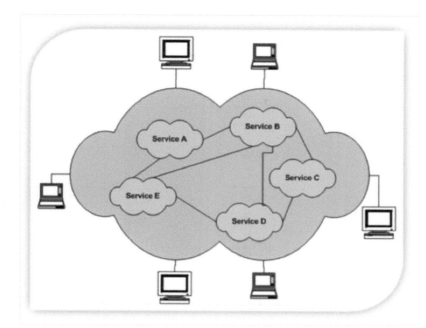

Figure 3: Set of interconnected business services/applications via web services, communicating with each other is available as a web service or via web browser over the internet for the end user.

Mr. Munasinghe goes on to explain that each service or cloud consists of detailed architecture and technology invisible to the end user. It consists of the *application/service, platform, infrastructure and storage,* shown in Figure 12-4.

Finally, Mr. Munasinghe briefly describes the functions of each element depicted in Figure 12-4.

- Application/web service: Delivers the software/application as a service (SaaS) to end user or other clouds. For example the end user in BAS can access the user interface for control networks, and it can have services for other parties to obtain data from BAS.

- Infrastructure: Computer infrastructure usually in platform virtualization environment as a service.

- Platform: Allow developers/users to extend or write new applications using the platform as a service (PaaS)

- Storage: Consists of the database to read and write data.

Figure 12-4: The detail technology behind the cloud

The early modeling of the cloud computing concept has various deployment methods in *public, private and hybrid* clouds. A public cloud service is available over the internet via direct application or web service to the end user. A private cloud is restricted to private networks that have been referred to in this book as VPNs, for data security and reliability. A hybrid cloud consists of multiple private and/or public clouds to provide enterprise solution. Which deployment model will the building automation market fit into? The vision of smart grid where the BAS communicates with other industries and the need to have a secure control network clearly indicate that BAS market will adopt a hybrid model.

Thus far, middleware has been described as a technology used to form a "glue" that merges systems composed of more than one protocol, as well as more than one network technology. The balance of the chapter will focus on providing some examples of how all of this communication and application technology comes together to be deployed as energy and analytics solutions. In that context it should be helpful to provide a limited outline of technology platforms that are used to deliver this technology. The chapter will close with a brief discussion of web services and related technologies that make up energy and analytics solutions, along with two important topics for this discipline, and building technologies as a whole—network resilience and cyber security.

ENERGY AND ANALYTICS NETWORK SYSTEMS

Professionals in the energy and buildings space have become very familiar with the idea of complex networks and topologies within building automation systems (BAS). Initial BAS technology was developed with an approach that might be called a "unified network system by design" (UNSD). To truly establish a basis for the complexity of this discussion, it is only fair to say than the notion of a UNSD is relied upon for many more systems than the BAS. It is relied upon for the entire universe of technologies, from meters to CMMS to security for access control, etc., fire systems and many more. There are some companies within the analytics space that have tried to provide comprehensive solutions to incorporate many of these systems, but the business model is extremely difficult. In the simplest terms, the reason for this has to do with the value proposition. With the exception of customers that have highly complex operational environments, such as universities, hospitals and manufacturing plants, no customer has seen value in comprehensive services. The value proposition that has been envisioned by some providers must support the cost of deploying a comprehensive system, spanning numerous independent specialty technologies, and implementing a complete new network of instrumentation along with energy and analytics software. However, there are a handful of companies which have created a compelling value proposition, using middleware solutions to create an *ad hoc* network of existing technology that may be used to provide access to comprehensive datasets from multiple existing systems, and make them available to the analytics engine or tool. The fact that this can be achieved is why the topic of middleware is so important to energy and analytics. Yet such solutions require energy and analytics providers to have sophisticated skillsets, including deep technical knowledge of networking and data communications as well as analytics, to ensure the long-term viability of the implementation.

Two terms from the previous paragraph require a bit more discussion before moving on to discuss a systems example: UNSD and *ad hoc* network. The concept of a unified network system by design (UNSD) is straightforward and should not require much discussion. It is obvious that in the case of UNSDs a company develops a complete system incorporating hardware and software. The UNSD will include an operating system and software to carry out specific functions, and will also include the data communications, networking and web services necessary to provide interface to a fully functioning system. Again this is obvious, and not unlike services that might be expected from any computer-based system manufacturer, but it is important to emphasize that with an *ad hoc* system there is no "company" with overall responsibility to make sure the system operates. More importantly, there is no company to ensure that the system continues to operate under changing conditions as well. Changing conditions, in this case, could be anything from internal network management and IP addressing schemes for any LAN to software and operating systems compatibilities, or could simply refer to general maintenance of the data communication aspects related to access the information. This is not to say that a solution provider would not attempt to provide this overarching service, but the point is that the provider does not have control over the ever-changing conditions, nor over how their technology might operate after those changes occur.

The topic of middleware really focuses on *ad hoc* networks, and this again is because it allows systems to be deployed with lower upfront cost by avoiding installation of extensive sensor and instrumentation networks. Middleware achieves this by opening up access to existing sensor and instrumentation networks through communications technology, but this requires *ad hoc* networks. So what exactly is an *ad hoc* network? *Ad hoc* networks combine multiple existing system networks for BAS, meters, etc. into a common data communications network. According to Wikipedia, *ad hoc* is a Latin term meaning "for this purpose." Wikipedia goes on to discuss the mobile internet and Wi-Fi industry for wireless *ad hoc* networks, sometimes called "WANET." The point however is that these are decentralized building networks that are *ad hoc* because they rely on a pre-existing infrastructure of building systems. These systems again include BAS, metering etc., but they also include routers in wired networks or access points in managed (infrastructure) wireless networks. All of these systems are made up of devices that are capturing data about building operations, which are "nodes" on sub-system networks.

The notion of an *ad hoc* network is that a communication infrastructure includes those nodes and systems described above, as well as middleware technology including software and hardware, like routers and gateways, which makes it possible to first communicate to an analytics tool, and second convert (or map) the data to a format that the platform can use to perform analysis. Another way to refer to these systems would be that they enable analytics solutions to access data from large numbers of disparate devices dynamically, through network interoperability. *Ad hoc* networks are predominant throughout the energy and analytics industry, and this is likely to continue to be true. That is because access to the large volumes of data needed by this industry requires access to a large set of networks, made up of large numbers of devices.

MIDDLEWARE *AD HOC* NETWORK INFRASTRUCTURE

This chapter has provided the framework for a more detailed explanation of what an *ad hoc* network looks like for energy and analytics. As mentioned, there have been numerous approaches to providing solutions by multiple companies. In Jim Sinopoli's article from 2008, mentioned above, he identified several of those companies. This discussion will provide an example based upon one of those companies, Tridium. The reader should not construe this as an endorsement, but rather should note that this company was an early leader in providing technology solutions for *ad hoc* networking. Because of that early leadership they can be used to illustrate actual examples of how many analytics providers create solutions. Again Tridium is not the only technology solution company, the space includes numerous large and small providers from the buildings industry, such as Lynx Spring, as well as from the network and IT industry. Participants in this space range from Cisco Systems and Intel to smaller entrepreneurial businesses like Sky Foundry, Cimetrics, J2 Innovations, Coppertree Analytics and more to come. The reader should recognize that there are nuances to how all of these providers have developed technology solutions, as well as how they approach the market and differentiate from their competitors. In the end however, Tridium is a good representative technology platform to use in discussing how middleware interoperability is achieved for energy and analytics tools. To provide some general background on the company, Tridium is a global software and technology company that created the Niagara Framework®, a software framework that integrates diverse systems and devices—regardless of manufacturer, or communication protocol—into a unified platform that can be easily managed and controlled in real time over the internet using a standard web browser.

This discussion on *ad hoc* networks as created using Tridium products will begin with an overview of a sample application including what data are needed for energy and analytics technology. The discussion will then go on to discuss, in general terms, how the technology might be deployed to achieve this goal. To keep things simple, the application will not be overly complex, and will entail accessing data from energy meters for analysis and from a number of HVAC units for fault detection and diagnostics. The energy data needed begin with a utility billing data history including cost, units of electricity (kWh) and kilowatt demand (kW) for electricity and billing history including cost and units (i.e. MCF) of consumption for natural gas. In addition to energy history, analytics tools will also need 15-minute interval data (typically kW demand) for energy analysis. This will be used to analyze potential benefits from participation in automated demand response and demand limiting programs, as well as the option to sell capacity into electric markets. For equipment optimization and FD&D, the application would provide predictive maintenance (PdM) for 10 large floor-by-floor variable air volume air handling units (AHUs). Repeating some of the content from Chapter 6 to elaborate on this application for these AHUs, PdM would be applied to reduce life cycle energy consumption for the equipment and to positively impact the mission being carried out within the space this equipment serves. As noted previously, countless studies have documented employee productivity improvements in buildings that maintain optimum environments (temperature, humidity, etc.). This application would use PdM for air filter maintenance, by measuring the differential pressure across the AHU filter. The technology would detect filters as they load up with dirt over time (differential pressure increasing) and trigger filter maintenance at the right time. When the filter is replaced, the technology will record the differential pressure drop and hence verify that the replacement was done correctly. By analyzing the pressure drop across the filters over time, it is possible to better establish when, and how often, to change the filter and perhaps even glean information on which filter manufacturer sells a better product. Other analytics algorithms would use the same data on space temperature and humidity, as well as perhaps CO_2 and particulates, to compare actual conditions to benchmark metrics established for environmental conditions. Many other factors could be analyzed as well, including light levels and energy metrics at a sub-meter level, etc.

To execute on this application, it is necessary to access data on all of the conditions outlined above. Accessing that data will require interface with a wide range of systems as discussed, so the balance of this section will outline review the analytics network infrastructure as well as the device nodes, and they would be configured. In other words, this is the true meat of the middleware discussion. Again, there are many manufacturers offering solutions in this space, but Tridium will be used as an example only. Interestingly, Tridium and other technology companies have not supported the use of middleware, as a term, to describe the functions that are being carried out with data communications and building systems infrastructure. It is believed that this is because use of the term in the IT industry is too narrow for the functionality that is carried out for applications such BAS, EEM, energy and analytics, etc. Devices like the Tridium JACE™ incorporate much more than self-contained software services for enterprise application. However, as previously mentioned, the energy, buildings and BAS industry have embraced the term middleware to describe the class of products that enables this network infrastructure for BAS and analytics, so it has been used here.

The analytics network infrastructure for the application discussed above could be depicted in Figure 12-5. In fact this is a generic illustration from Tridium Product literature for a product called the JACE-6. Before discussing that product, it is worthwhile to note that Tridium offers a complete portfolio of technologies that extend connectivity, integration and interoperability to millions of devices deployed in the market, but that are capable of being deployed as BAS offerings as well. The product portfolio is delivered in the form of hardware and software, but it is built around the Niagara™ software framework. This software framework is a universal, reusable software platform to develop applications, products and solutions. Software frameworks include support programs, compilers, code libraries, scripting language, an application programming interface (API) and tool sets that bring together all the different components to enable development of a project or solution. This chapter is in no way intended to be a training program for these products, rather it is providing this information to assist the reader in understanding the complexity of these network infrastructures. In the context of energy and analytics, these products are used to resolve the challenges associated with open systems integration and interoperability, by integrating diverse systems and devices, regardless of the manufacturer, or communication protocol, into a unified platform that can be managed and can access data over the internet. The hardware platform that is deployed in the building is a JACE, an acronym for Java Application Control Engine, as shown in Figure 12-5.

A JACE provides the mechanism to achieve interoperability, for access to data, from all systems in a building. By connecting common network protocols such as BACnet™, LonWorks™ and Modbus™, along with many proprietary, or legacy networks, a unified system without seams emerges. Scalability and reliability concerns are avoided with the unique distributed architecture created by a network of JACEs. This is accomplished by interfacing with standard protocols, such as those above, but the company, and members of its distribution channel, also maintain a library of "drivers" for legacy system protocols. At a simple level, the idea is that these devices can be deployed with a driver for almost any legacy protocol for BAS, meters, data loggers, etc. Figure 12-5 shows interface to all of the systems described above for this analytics application: meters with electronic interfaces for energy consumption and interval data, internet access to download billing data from utility portals and BAS systems for equipment data, etc. The reader should also note that, as with BAS, this architecture also shows a Workplace PRO as well.

Previous chapters discussed that BACnet™ and other standards are for data communication, but not for device programming, and that a "workbench" software product is used for that task. This workplace product fulfills a similar role for the architecture depicted, but the intent of this section is not to explain how the devices are programmed to accomplish these tasks. Beyond communication and gateway functionality, JACEs often have inputs and outputs, like any BAS controller, so they can actually be implemented as a direct digital control device complete with programming capability to create algorithms for equipment control. The JACE-6 for example "is part of a family of high performance embedded controllers and includes a fast (524 MHz) processor, 128 MB base memory expandable to 256, and a math coprocessor for better performance. The JACE-6 also comes with the latest NiagaraAX 3.2 software and the Web User Interface, and Niagara Connectivity built in. The product's modular design and flexibility allows for easy installation and distributing connectivity and control more widely across all types of environments." The unit is expandable and features multiple I/O modules (i.e. IO-16 below) and plug communication cards that save engineering, time and installation cost. Like many BAS devices, it comes with optional IO-16 and or IO-34 modules, internal battery backup, two 10/100Mbit Ethernet, RJ-45 ports on the CPU board, a USB port on the CPU board, and two option card slots for communication option cards (Lon, RS-232, RS-485, etc.). In closing, it is important to note that these

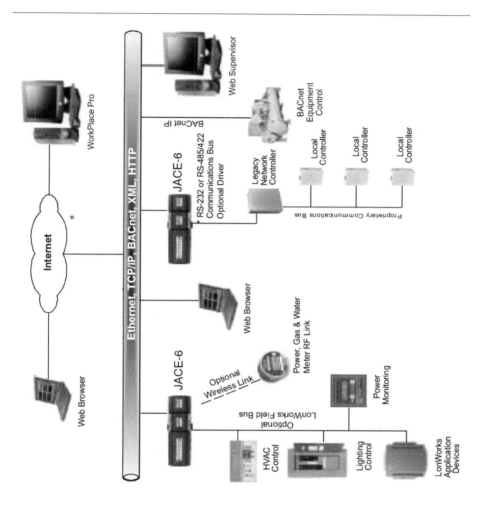

Figure 12-5

devices, and those available from a growing number of providers, are highly sophisticated and may be programmed by a capable integrator to make data available for almost any existing building system.

One last topic of particular import for energy and analytics is network resilience. This topic simply emphasizes the importance of a highly sophisticated network design, deployed by a credible integrator. As a side note, that integrator must complete a thorough commissioning which may need to be completed twice, once in heating mode and once in cooling mode, to ensure that this newly implemented system is completely functional in all seasons. Regarding network resilience, the simple challenge with energy and analytics, as with BAS, is that all of these systems typically use corporate networks, as the communication backbone, to simplify network infrastructure and reduce cabling cost. They are also often assigned an IP address so that they can use the corporate LAN to access the internet directly or through a VPN infrastructure. Again as an example, consider Cimetrics, Inc. as a best in class provider to discuss this further. This company was one of the early adopters of BACnet™, and other communications standards, used for energy and buildings solutions. They also offer a product portfolio similar to the JACE. Yet a significant distinction is that the company is also a full-service analytics provider, and has developed best practices to ensure network resilience. The ultimate goal is to achieve very high quality data access, and to enter into agreements that allow the company to perform analytics on equipment *and* the data communications interfaces put in place to access data. As discussed in Chapters 10 and 11, there are a large number of threats to a robust energy and analytics data stream. Quite simply, IT staff and network administrators are concerned solely with the computing infrastructure and business applications. The energy and analytics technology, as well as the BAS, and all of the other special systems in buildings, just do not show up on the IT radar. As a result, IT managers do not notify solution providers when network maintenance is being conducted, or when major changes are made to IT infrastructure, because they either don't think of it or don't even know these systems exist. Many new entrants to the energy and analytics space do not recognize this threat to network resilience, and therefore to their data stream, and they implement one-off middleware solutions, assuming nothing will change. Companies like Cimetrics don't make those mistakes; they leverage IT and network management systems in their design, to ensure that their systems remain viable. Equally important, they structure their design so that the network maintenance staff owns responsibility for devices that will provide data, and they communicate with IT regularly to be sure they plan for upcoming changes. They know that providers cannot tell IT one time that energy and analytics tools are in place and critical to building performance, and expect them to consider these tools every time they upgrade the IT infrastructure. The reader should become schooled in these topics so that they can ensure continuous access to data for analytics therefore protecting the integrity of their systems.

Cyber security is very much in alignment with network resilience, and its importance cannot be stressed enough. This topic was also covered in Chapter 11, but will be revisited here. As with the approach that Cimetrics takes to design resilient networks, energy and analytics staff must be aware of cyber security risks and develop strategies to mitigate those risks. In many respects this is another reason to collaborate with IT staff and ensure that risks are controlled. The intent of this book is not to provide a treatise on cyber security. Readers should know that cyber-crime costs computer users hundreds of billions of dollars annually in systems downtime, time to correct problems, etc., and should expect cyber-attacks to increase. Tools and techniques exist in the marketplace to address both the volume and complexity of cyber-attacks, so that enterprises can stay viable in the face of evolving threats. Combining energy and analytics with security technologies yields a stronger defense posture. Security analytics can provide high-speed, automated analysis to bring network activity into clear focus to detect and stop threats, and shorten the time to remediation when attacks occur. The reader is encouraged to become knowledgeable in this area and to develop strategies that protect access to data. Such strategies will also reduce down time and protect the building mission as well.

The last topic in this chapter is web services. In fact, web services have been mentioned numerous times so far in this book and this chapter. It is a term that industry professionals have become very familiar with, and it is an approach that is integral to many energy and analytics solutions. Given the importance of web services to this topic, it is worthwhile to provide some basic definitions. This is also important because coming chapters will talk about system integration and analytics tools, so may be of value to provide some content on how this technology may be architected.

So what are web services? Vangie Beal, managing editor of Webopedia.com, published this content on the term web services: "Web services describes a standardized way of integrating web-based applications using the XML (Extensible Markup Language), SOAP (Simple Object Access Protocol), WSDL (web Services Description Language) and UDDI (Universal Description, Discovery and Integration) open standards over an internet protocol backbone. It is common for web-based applications to use XML, which is designed especially for web documents to tag the data, SOAP is used to transfer the data, WSDL is used for describing the services available and UDDI is used for listing what services are available. Used primarily as a means for businesses to communicate with each other and with clients, web services allow organizations to communicate data without intimate knowledge of each other's IT systems behind the firewall. Unlike traditional client/server models, such as a web server/web page system, web services do not provide the user with a GUI. Web services instead share business logic, data and processes through a programmatic interface across a network. The applications interface, not the users. Developers can then add the web service to a GUI (such as a web page or an executable program) to offer specific functionality to users. Web services allow different applications from different sources to communicate with each other without time-consuming custom coding, and because all communication is in XML, web services are not tied to any one operating system or programming language."

Another definition for web services comes from Wikipedia, the free encyclopedia, which says that a web service is a method of communication between two electronic devices over a network. A web service is a software function provided at a network address over the web with the service *always on* as in the concept of utility computing. The World Wide Web Consortium (W3C) defines a web service generally as: a software system designed to support interoperable machine-to-machine interaction over a network. The W3C Web Services Architecture Working Group defined a web services architecture, requiring a specific implementation of a "web service." In this a web service has an interface described in a format that can be machine-processed (specifically WSDL). Other systems interact with the web service in a manner prescribed by its description using SOAP (simple object access protocol) messages, typically conveyed using HTTP with an XML serialization in conjunction with other web-related standards.

Clearly there is a great deal of content regarding web services. The author's goal however is to provide very basic information that will be useful to readers who plan to specify, buy and operate energy and analytics systems. Therefore the goal is not to understand how to develop such a system, but to understand the underlying technology that is being purchased, and how that knowledge may be used in the design/purchase process to acquire the right solution.

Given the introduction to web services, it is most important to know how this technology is used with energy and analytics. The next two chapters will consider integration and analytic tools and product configurations, so this section will not go into great detail on those topics, rather it will focus how the tools are offered. This is a marketing topic related to the product offer and how it is priced. A very popular product approach today, across multiple technology industries, is "Software as a Service" (SaaS). SaaS is exactly what is being offered with most energy and analytics tools, and it is being offered using web services. The software in this case, is the energy and analytics tool, and the SaaS approach defines how the software is structured, packaged and offered to customers. In terms of structure, SaaS can be very cost effective because the computing infrastructure made up of servers, processing power, storage (computer memory) and application software itself resides off-site. Another way to say this is that the software resides "in the cloud," and the service entails supporting all of the computing infrastructure and making it available through an internet-based web service. The energy and analytics tools provider therefore offers access to the software and computing infrastructure for a recurring fee. Of course this is a two-edged sword, these benefits are one edge of the sword, and the other edge is that these products are not "shrink wrapped" for one-time purchase and ongoing use, the SaaS model is to sell "use" of the software for that recurring fee. So the SaaS model for energy and analytics tools typically has a service, or SaaS, contract with an ongoing monthly, quarterly, etc. charge. That charge is use of the tool and computing infrastructure described above, and also includes ongoing upgrades, etc. to the tool and the infrastructure. As noted in the definitions of web services above, it is common for products to use XML and SOAP, etc.; however, for buildings applications targeting dashboard and analytics, XML and SOAP may be more sophisticated that requirements dictate. As a result, some simpler solutions have become available that are easier to develop products around and are easier to support. At this writing there are a few popular options to simplify solutions and two will be discussed: Representational State Transfer (REST) and JavaScript Object Notation (JSON).

Representational state transfer (REST) is a software architecture style consisting of guidelines and best practices for creating scalable web services. REST is a coordinated set of constraints applied to the design of components in a distributed system, which can use text, graphic and video to provide a more user-friendly and maintainable architecture. REST has gained widespread acceptance across the web as a simpler alternative to SOAP and WSDL-based web services. Systems that deploy REST typically, but not always, communicate over the hypertext transfer protocol with the same HTTP verbs (GET, POST, PUT, DELETE, etc.) used by web browsers to retrieve web pages and send data to remote servers. The REST architectural style was developed by W3C Technical Architecture Group (TAG). The World Wide Web represents the largest implementation of a system conforming to the REST architectural style. May energy and analytics systems, such as SkyFoundry are integrating "Native" REST.

The web services technologies discussed here are in some cases standards, and in others software building blocks to develop product offerings. It is also important to note that integrators are often faced with the challenge of creating "glue" to enable interface between existing systems and a web services offering. To accomplish this functionality, an API (application programming interface) is often used. One such product is the Cimetrics B6080, which is a BACnet interface to web services gateway/firewall. This product allows integration of BACnet/IP (internet protocol) devices in enterprise application systems using REST architecture. The device uses Cimetrics BACrest API (application program interface). It is a specification that allows applications to read and write data to device-centric networks using URL (uniform resource locator)-like commands. According to Cimetrics, "the meaning of the word BACrest is building automation control relational state transfer. The "REST" part of this name is a well-known IT terminology that describes the architecture used to create the internet "URL system." URL is a synonym for Web address. They have created a version of "REST" that applies to the needs of device-centric networks—the simplest yet most powerful data exchange methodology. This provides a more capable and secure interface for enterprise applications allowing access to more of the data found in building automation systems. Using this API approach, it is possible to integrate BAS with other enterprise computing applications using SOAP/XML technologies. This allows platforms such as Microsoft.Net or Java to access real time data from a building automation system. Since two isolated Ethernet ports are used, this device also acts as a firewall, meaning that no unintended communications or control is possible between the two networks. This can be a valuable feature to develop strategies that protect against cyber security threats.

Of particular interest for energy and analytics is that The Project Haystack data modeling standard has provided a documented representational state transfer, application programming interface (REST API) to define a simple mechanism to exchange "tagged" data over web services. REST servers are programmed to implement a set of ops or operations. An operation is a URI (uniform resource identifier) that receives a request and returns a response. The URI is an HTTP URI, which is used at a base address. Operations are then mapped as path names under that address. Standard operations are defined to query databases, set up subscriptions, or read/write histories of time-series data. Operations are pluggable so vendors can enhance open REST interfaces with customized, value-added functionality for their own business purposes.

JSON is another approach used by a number of technology companies in the energy and buildings space. JSON "is a lightweight data-interchange format," according to the JavaScript Object Notation Website. It is easy for humans to read and write. It is easy for machines to parse and generate. It is based on a subset of the JavaScript programming language, Standard ECMA-262 3rd Edition, December 1999. JSON is a text format that is completely language independent but uses conventions that are familiar to programmers of the C-family of languages, including C, C++, C#, Java, JavaScript, Perl, Python, and many others. These properties make JSON an ideal data-interchange language.

JSON is built on two structures:

- A collection of name/value pairs. In various languages, this is realized as an *object*, record, struct, dictionary, hash table, keyed list, or associative array.

- An ordered list of values. In most languages, this is realized as an *array*, vector, list, or sequence.

These are universal data structures. Virtually all modern programming languages support them in one form or another. It makes sense that a data format that is interchangeable with programming languages also be based on these structures."

Again, the technical details of how products might be developed and operate using JSON is beyond the scope of this book. However, it is useful for the reader to understand that tools like this exist to simplify the structure of web services offerings for energy and analytics. The result will be faster time to market for new products and faster upgrade and enhancement for existing ones, in the end this all benefits the user and operator.

In closing, this chapter has covered a diverse set of topics related to the infrastructure of energy and analytics technology. The reader should note that this "middleware" segment is in a tremendous state of flux. As discussed, these products were first introduced to the market as independent components that required separate interface, programming and installation. An analogy for consideration in coming to grips with the complexity of implementing this technology might be to local area networks (LANs). LANs are pervasive for our IT applications, as well as for internet access and web services. Yet when considering those LANs, the user/manager must understand that there are independent skills, and in many cases independent service providers, who must be hired to install and maintain separate system components. For example:

- The servers, PCs, etc. have one set of requirements for deployment,

- The LANs themselves including all of the network software, routing, switching and cabling infrastructure, while application software have another set of requirements and

- Internet service providers (ISP) have yet other requirements.

One company is typically hired to provide and implement the computer technology, a second set of companies will be hired to provide software (i.e. office suites, accounting systems, etc.) and a third company will be hired for the LAN. It is understood that companies like CISCO, 3Com, etc. have very unique skills and are certified independently from the other providers, but typiaclly cannot provide an entire end-to-end computing system complete with applications. This is true, just as an accounting software company for example would support its application, but would not be called to install a LAN. Of course companies differentiate in many ways, but the bottom line is that users understand that these products require separate content expertise.

In light of the LAN example, now consider building technologies particularly for energy and analytics. Over the years it has been common in the building space to expect one provider, often called an integrator, to combine content expertise across all applications (BAS, dashboards, energy management, analytics, etc.), as well as to be the LAN, ISP and web services provider. In many cases, each of these products and applications is manufactured by separate companies, but the building owner/manager typically uses one system integrator as the technology content expert for complete implementations. As time has progressed, the idea of bolt-on middleware components that are applied, independent of the building systems, has begun to morph, but the role of the integrator has remained constant. Many IT companies have announced plans to dominate this industry. Interestingly however, these companies usually end up coming back to the same system integrator channel to implement their solutions, because this is the only group that has the content expertise required to deploy the products properly in a building. This may or may not change over time, but one thing is changing, and that is how energy and analytics products are deploying middleware. Some companies are combining this technology into their products to simply expand the functionality, while others offer independent products for each function. The important take-away from this chapter is not how middleware is configured in particular products, or how it works today, but that middleware is, and will likely remain, a critical component for energy and analytics technology. As discussed in the beginning of this chapter, for energy and analytics middleware is essential to controlling the cost of systems implementation. For the building owner it just makes sense to utilize sensors and instrumentation, which reside in systems that have already been purchased, as sources of data for energy and analytics. This approach reduces the overall cost of acquisition for energy and analytics, while also speeding deployment. For that reason middleware will continue to be important to this topic and the reader should understand it well enough to ask informed questions about how data will be acquired and whether they can reasonably expect that data acquisition to be reliable.

Chapter 13

System Integration

The previous three chapters treated technologies related to BAS, data communications/networking and middleware in some detail. This chapter will not repeat that content, but will expand on that discussion by introducing the concept of "system integration," or simply integration. Integration implies a broader "system-wide" context, and is the practice of combining systems to achieve some level of "connectivity" or "interoperability." These terms have been used in very similar ways, almost interchangeably, in the past, but the term "interoperability" has become more universally used to describe interaction between smart systems. In the IT world there are levels of interoperability, but the focus here is on energy and analytics with systems in buildings. Therefore this chapter will focus on two levels of interoperability: data access and control integration.

Under the heading of energy and analytics, the primary concern is data access from many sources, as has been discussed. Throughout the last three chapters there have been many references to integration and system interaction. The purpose of this discussion is to address the primary issue: installing instrumentation and networks to capture data is cost prohibitive and unnecessary when exiting systems can be mined for much of the necessary data. Mining those systems is what will be referred to as "integration." Clearly there will be cases when specific data are required that cannot come from another system. In that case a decision can be made whether to add points to existing systems and access data in the same way, or to add new instrumentation. This chapter's sole purpose is to emphasize that much of the data required for energy and analytics technology can come from integration to BAS, as well as a larger ecosystem of building technologies. Other potential sources for energy and analytics suites can also include meters, CMMS, HVAC security and a host of systems that operate independently of the traditional BAS, but are essential to both, capturing data for analysis. The same systems may also be used for control integration, which is executing changes to facility operations that are recommended by the analysis.

System integration is a term that has been used extensively with BAS. It actually pre-dates the introduction of BACnet™, as a reference to this second topic "control integration."

Control integration is not the focus of this chapter, or this book, but some time must be devoted to this topic because over time energy and analytics technology can be expected to result in execution of real-time corrections, as well as report recommendations. The process today is that the analytics tool executes algorithms to analyze performance and identify anomalies; the next step is to report and ideally prioritize issues, based upon customer criteria, and make recommendations. In reality, many of the issues identified will require more detailed human interaction to identify root causes and resolve problems, however some corrections could happen automatically. For example, it could be possible to clear BAS system overrides automatically, and some control variables could be modified automatically based on learning how HVAC performs on a day-to-day, month-to-month basis. Of course the devil is in the details with all of these types of sequences. However, BAS algorithms like optimal start stop have been doing exactly the same thing for decades—learning from performance and modifying start times based upon conditions.

The new electricity market creates even more options to execute pre-approved shed sequences on kW demand status, and to fine tune those responses over time. What is really exciting about energy and analytics is that the technology can monitor many more variables than ever before. An example of such a sequence involves the way that building occupancy varies during the week. Building owners, especially those in large cities with difficult commuting, have been adapting to the growing participation of workers in telecommuting, which varies throughout the week and the year. It is very common for office buildings to be very lightly loaded on Friday afternoons, Monday mornings, etc. A great example of how applications like these are being expanded to include integration with a wider range of systems was pointed out in Jim Sinopoli's article, "Predictions for 2015" in February of that year (www.automatedbuildings.com). The article discussed Bluetooth Beaconing, a new technology for "indoor positioning, which can be used to get accurate data on building occupancy at any time based on smart phones. Beacons use Bluetooth Low Energy (BLE), which is built into most of the latest smart phones, and this could revolutionize how occupancy data are determined within a building, at a very low cost. This information opens a host of opportunities for building systems, such as HVAC, but how about cycling elevators because there is no need for four or more to be operating if the building is 50% occupied? In the past, these algorithms required occupancy data from security or lighting controls, as well as trending data on elevator operations. With BLE integration this could be done automatically without waiting for secondary analysis of the data from other systems. There are a wealth of new control integration opportunities, and these can be expected to increase exponentially as web services and integration becomes possible with many previously "siloed" systems.

BUILDING AUTOMATION SYSTEMS (BAS) AND CONTROL

In prior chapters, BAS technology was described in detail, but this chapter will begin with a simple prediction: The future of the BAS industry will not be determined by a small group of large control manufacturers. The ever expanding content knowledge of system integrators coupled with new technology will accelerate movement toward this new business reality. The BAS industry now includes companies offering many types of software and hardware, including middleware. Equally important, the role and functionality that is introduced by web services expands the power of these systems. Industry leaders agree that automation and information technology (IT) have converged, and yet neither the conventional BAS players, nor the IT companies entering this space, are obvious winners. At no time since the market explosion caused the oil embargoes of 1970s have BASs, then called energy management systems (EMS), seen such a diverse and robust marketplace. The previous hardware and software barriers to entry for BAS players have been removed due to the proliferation of microprocessor technology and system standards, while web services development tools have also made it possible to launch offerings with much lower up-front cost.

A very robust ecosystem of technology companies is participating in this market, as a result of the market changes described, and that includes energy and analytics. There are pros and cons to this market environment. Obviously it is great to have many choices, but it is also harder for the companies to differentiate and harder for the owner/manager to choose wisely. The clear outcome, however, is that new advances in building systems technology are less likely to come from the old brand name companies. In fact, advances are more likely to come from startups and small players, and this has fueled a merger and acquisition frenzy in the market as well. This is evidenced by Honeywell's acquisition of Tridium and Akuacom, Johnson Controls acquisition of Grid Logix and Energy Connect, and Schneider Electric's acquisition of TAC and Power Measurement. Therefore it is important to consider how industry participants look at the state of the BAS business. Traditionally the major industry participants were control manufacturers that developed BAS products, which have evolved from simple mechanical and electrical devices to fully networked suites of smart systems. These large companies were multinational and multidisciplinary in nature, but their vertical integration encompassed more that the BAS. Vertical integration in this case means controlling all of the raw materials, supply chains and product offerings that are necessary to offer BAS, but now these companies are also acquiring the equipment that is controlled as well. The major players are actively aligning their BAS offerings by acquiring heating, ventilation and air conditioning (HVAC) companies, just as the dominant HVAC players have acquired BAS companies since the 1980s. This may be somewhat interesting, but the reader may ask, "Why do I care?" The reason to care is that many managers and owners of buildings, particularly those that own multiple buildings in multiple locations, are faced with a dilemma. It is becoming harder and harder to rely on any one company to provide end-to-end service, and this means that managers must become more tech-savvy and better able to understand how to take control of their own BAS, energy and analytics destiny. Understanding integration is the most important first step that any manager can take in that progression. Readers who have reached this point in this book are well on their way to developing that understanding. Of course, this knowledge must be tempered with real-world experience, and requires ongoing effort for those who want to remain current.

ARCHITECTURE AND INTEGRATION

The logical place to begin understanding integration and its role with energy and analytics is to revisit the topic of architecture. From the previous three chapters the reader understands that architecture includes hardware and software, but equally important relies on an interwoven series of standards for data communications that must be compatible and interoperable. If the data communication protocols being deployed within the architecture are not interoperable, it will be necessary to abandon any data that could be accessed or to implement a solution, such as middleware technology. Therefore step one in the design of any energy and analytics solution will be to identify the business processes that require analysis, to identify the data that are needed to conduct that analysis and to determine if the data are available and resident in an existing system. If the data reside in an existing system, integration will be necessary. This is the beginning of developing the energy and analytics architecture. For each system component, web service or other data source, an element of architecture must be created and a strategy must developed to access that data. Data quality is important because access to the data must be reliable and continuous. With heightened concern about cyber security, this architecture development must also consider whether firewalls are in place, and if it is possible to work with IT and network administration staff to devise a method for interfacing to the systems that hold the data.

As stated, the term used to describe this overarching process of overcoming obstacles to interface with systems is "system integration." Definition of this term has evolved over time, and what we mean by system integration includes what we call building automation. For example, integrated systems combine HVAC control with fire/life safety and security systems. Actual integration of control sequences ranges from extremely limited, to complex approaches for smoke evacuation and after-hours access to selected areas of a building. Over the years, system integrators have evolved, and the scope of their services includes all building systems, as well as web services, energy and analytics, visualization/dashboards and a host of customer-specific services. At the simplest level these integrators develop business content expertise to help the customer identify problems that can be solved through combined system functionality. As mentioned above, that may be accomplished through data access or through a combination of data access, data analysis and integrated algorithms or "control integration." These services require that integrators be technology experts with all building systems, energy experts, and that they also be network integrators. This breadth of skill is what makes it possible to determine how an architecture must be designed and implemented to achieve optimum performance from energy and analytics.

The expanding technologies that comprise integration require industry participants to revisit training needs. Knowledge necessary to be successful in building automation starts with an understanding of BAS, web services and much more. That sentence covers a tremendous amount of ground and, in a world that demands specialization, there are two or three areas to which a person could devote an entire career. In the real world however, the industry demands more, so after mastering BAS, the system integrator must also understand data communication, networking and web services.

System integration also presents challenges for the construction procurement process on numerous levels. The industry is demanding integration throughout the enterprise—from building automation, fire alarm, access and video surveillance for security, to energy management for the enterprise, and metering and maintenance management. System integration goes beyond independent building systems such as those listed above, because it requires commonality with building application infrastructure including hardwired and wireless LANs, central databases and even network-client software, among others. The dramatic industry effort to develop standards for networking and communication has resulted in a host of BACnet™ and LON™ compatible products, but with web services and the smart grid that world is expanding dramatically. As previously discussed, the smart grid interoperability panel (SGIP) is identifying and codifying an ever-expanding number of standards that are at the integrators' disposal.

Training is, of course, needed to fully access all of the possibilities, and sources for this training are becoming available. Many technical colleges and trades associations offer seminars and short courses covering specific topics in system integration and the related data communications and web services topics that have been discussed here. Www. automatedbuildings.com launched online courses in the past, but the focus now is on up-to-date content from experts, in the form of articles and interviews. Training, however, is an important focus for trade associations such as the Association of Energy Engineers (AEE) which offers a host of face-to-face and online seminar programs. AEE face-to-face seminars are held around the country and are often co-located with their popular conferences. The online seminars are offered in both synchronous (everyone attends simultaneously through an online meeting web service) or asynchronous training environments (which allow students to learn at their own pace), while accessing real-time information from other participants via virtual seminar meetings. Training offerings should be evaluated based upon what content area the participant needs to learn about. An important consideration is that integrated systems, as discussed in relation to energy and analytics, include systems that encompass a wide range to technology elements. Again readers should look for training options that highlight their specific needs.

ENERGY MANAGEMENT, SUSTAINABILITY AND ANALYTICS

System integration that has been coupled with energy and analytics was traditionally call enterprise energy management. At its most elementary level this is primarily a technology that allows for monitoring of utility meters and energy data to develop baselines and benchmarks. Again this information can be very important for a host of functions. Ever-expanding functionality for these systems has broadened however, allowing energy and analytics to be part of full-scale integration of BAS and other building systems, as well as utility procurement, demand response, and participation in other utility programs plus effective use of onsite generation. This is clearly the future of energy management and expands the definition of system integration to its logical conclusion. At the expense of repetition, it demands that system integrators be network integrators as well. Taking this topic to its logical conclusion, one of the hottest topics today, planet-wide is sustainability. The tie between energy and climate issues is unquestioned, but the opportunity for energy and analytics to both measure and improve sustainability efforts is also significant. There is a compelling and dramatic interrelationship between the supply and demand sides of energy. This relationship has been discussed a great deal with regard to electricity in this book, but it is equally compelling as it relates to oil and natural gas. At this writing, the price of oil is just above $50 per barrel after nearly 5 years at or above $100 per barrel, and the market is highly volatile. Prices are being driven by market strategy, again on behalf of middle-eastern oil producing nations, but also by unprecedented access to low-cost oil and natural gas in the United States. For purposes of this discussion, the focus stays on the building and its owner or manager, and how energy and analytics can optimize energy performance within the building. With efficiency and operational actions achieving the best possible performance, the manager will be able to fully leverage options on the supply side more effectively. Those supply-side options may be electricity and/or natural gas procurement, participation in DR or energy markets, implementing DG or any number of other options.

Clearly an unparalleled opportunity exists to leverage BAS and integration for intelligent buildings that can fully leverage the energy opportunity. The utility industry started down this path with early smart grid strategies, but then became sidetracked building out the advanced metering infrastructure (AMI). This was a multi-billion initiative that utilities throughout North America embraced, resulting in web-enabled meters that were intended to transform the electricity business. The idea of real-time pricing, and such things as "prices to devices" to enable real-time pricing, have been deployed in the more advanced electricity markets. These markets are almost universally in states that have deregulated electricity markets, which enable energy users to make buying decisions to purchase from a variety of sellers. These buying decisions may also be extended to time-based procurement that analyzes the actual current value of the energy commodity, i.e. electricity. By the way, many of the AMI meters were deployed with very little functionality. They are like iPhones™ with only two apps, 1) the meter can be read remotely and 2) the power can be turned off if the bill is not paid. So here is the gotcha: it will take decades for expanded AMI apps, and truly price-based buying options, to become a reality for all electricity users, but in the interim, BAS integration and web services can provide the same and even greater functionality in the buildings sector. This has led to the development of system integration as a business model and to companies known as integrators to develop value propositions that sidestep the utilities and drive results. Early adopters were participating in demand response a decade ago, and this will continue to adapt and grow. Demand response is a multi-billion dollar market, and savvy system integrators have redefined themselves to deliver smart energy building solutions and to set the standard for a global solution to climate change. Energy and analytics are integral to these solutions. System integrators engaged in this higher-level thinking are considering the intersection of buildings, energy and environment to illustrate a point: buildings are at the heart of our energy and climate issues. Recent data from the Department of Energy indicate that electricity generation is responsible for 39% of greenhouse gas emissions, and the American Institute of Architects credits buildings alone with responsibility for 48% of greenhouse gas emissions. There is some overlap between these numbers since buildings are large electricity users, and the burning of fuel to produce that electricity is what causes part of the greenhouse gas emissions contributed by the building sector. There has also been solid research done to validate the fact that these emissions increase at times of peak electric demand. This is because utilities must fire their least efficient units to meet peak electric demand, and of course those higher polluting coal-fired power plants are at full capacity. This is really just another way to embrace the whole idea of green buildings, but more importantly to emphasize that HVAC, automation and energy efficiency are highly important parts of the equation. System integrators can't tell a story about how their work addresses building siting, urban redevelopment, bike racks or recycled carpet, but they can tell a story about energy and analytics, efficiency, and demand response.

The intent of this chapter has been to refocus on system integration as an enabling skill set and a set of technologies essential to deploying energy and analytics. The initial steps remain critical: 1) develop requirements, and 2) evaluate the architecture that exists, along with the system integration that is necessary to modify that architecture. System integrators are instrumental in determining how to transform systems from those that operate in independent silos of information, to those that can interoperate, and how to allow managers to access the data that are needed. The next step will be to determine whether it is also possible to develop integrated control functionality that is responsive to results from energy and analytics, as well as to push that data upstream to decision makers for prioritization and planning.

Chapter 14

Project Haystack
Data Standards

This chapter focuses on an exciting topic for energy and analytics, Project Haystack and the event it sponsors, Haystack Connect. The formation and activities of this effort are recent and in a state of rapid growth. Project Haystack was designated with 501C3 private nonprofit status less than a year before this book was published, and had held only one national Haystack Connect event. Given the emerging nature of Project Haystack, this chapter will offer on an overarching introduction to the subject including discussion of the drivers that resulted in its creation, following a brief but more specific discussion of its work. As Project Haystack continues to grow and evolve, the expectation is that its list of accomplishments will expand dramatically, and readers should follow their work. John Petze, who wrote the forward to this book and contributed the Introduction to Analytics chapter, is a partner with Skyfoundry, Inc., and is one of the founders of Project Haystack. Mr. Petze has written extensively on this topic and speaks regularly at conferences. Readers are encouraged to attend one of his presentations if possible and to read his articles on www.automatedbuildings.com and in other publications, as well as to visit www.haystackconnect.org to learn more.

CHALLENGES WITH DATA

The most important point for energy and analytics is that Project Haystack will likely transform every aspect of the work that has been described in this book, and serve to remove a significant obstacle to having this technology become pervasive. This implementation obstacle is caused by the lack of data standards to make it easy to access, understand and use data. This standards void drives higher implementation cost and slows the speed of adoption for energy and analytics technology.

This book has highlighted two important facts about energy and analytics: 1) tremendous value that can be achieved by leveraging data resident in existing systems, and 2) leveraging these data is critical, because of the high first cost to install new sensors, etc. This high cost of new sensors and instrumentation to create a data stream has been an obstacle to broader analytics deployment. Project Haystack came into being because a group of industry visionaries recognized that a problem existed with accessing data and understood how to solve the problem. Even more unusual, these visionaries were willing to develop the solution in a collaborative community, rather than to develop it as intellectual property for one company. This chapter introduces Project Haystack but it cannot provide deep technical coverage of all their work; however, this author believes it will have a transformational impact on energy and analytics.

This content may be helpful to product developers, but it is intended for system designers, implementation integrators, building operators, energy managers and consulting engineers specifying system requirements. This group may not need to be versed with the specifications and data model that has been created by Project Haystack, but they must be aware of its work and the concept of making data self-describing. A good comparison to this effort might be data communication standards, such as BACnet™, that have become pervasive. For example, most managers are not fluent with BACnet™, at the protocol level, but they understand its importance to the industry, and because they made it a purchasing requirement it has seen such widespread adoption. Another example might be the "Intel Inside™" concept, because it defines a core requirement that consumers have assigned a value to, and because it has shaped buying decisions. This author believes that Project Haystack's work is creating a standardized methodology that can be used across virtually all types of systems and data sources, which will become core requirements for a wide range of products from BAS to smart sensors to analytic tools and other building technologies. A second and equally important result of their work will be the education of an industry, perhaps multiple industries, to the importance of standards for what is known as "data semantics."

To be more specific, Project Haystack is focusing on an industry data challenge that has to do with conveying essential meaning about energy and building data. This concept is known as meta data and semantic modeling in the computer science realm—potentially daunting terms, but ones that address a very simple need, the need to include descriptive information with sensor and machine data so that external applications understand the meaning of the data. For example, is a sensor value a temperature for an occupied room or a return air duct? The Project Haystack community, which includes people from a wide range of domains has developed a flexible, extensible methodology to define and attach semantic data to all types of energy and building data.

Addressing this data modeling challenge has been difficult for a number of reasons. Most significant is that virtually none of the standard protocols that emerged in the buildings industry in the last 20 years addressed the meta data challenge. Because there has been no standard approach, implementation costs for applications that consume data from different systems have been inordinately high. This is because the data must be converted into a format that can be understood by each application such as analytics. This may sound very similar to the protocol topic that was discussed in an earlier chapter, because on the surface it looks like a formatting issue. However in this case, the focus is on data characteristics and structure that allow a system to understand the meaning of information, from its unit of measure, to the equipment system to which it is attached.

Before Project Haystack, it was necessary to convert data from building systems into a format that could be understood by analytics software, and that conversion process is a "one-off manual task" where human operators add essential descriptors to the data items. The one-off task is labor-intensive, and this is what adds more cost to implementations, but it can also create a threat to long-term data resiliency. The threat comes into play because changes to any of the systems that were part of this one-off approach can, and do, occur for any number of reasons, and that can disrupt the data flow. The Project Haystack website points out that operational data, from building systems, etc., has poor semantic modeling and requires a manual, labor-intensive process to "map" the data before value creation can begin. This mapping activity is what technologists call the "one-off" data conversion approach. Project Haystack's work focuses on pragmatic use of naming conventions and taxonomies that can make it more cost effective to analyze, visualize, and derive value from operational data. There will be further coverage of this topic in the chapter on analytics tools. Suffice it to say the data semantics challenge has been a huge issue for energy and analytics tools and Project Haystack could not have been formed at a more opportune time.

To bring the work being done by Project Haystack into focus, the project Vision is to create a standardized methodology for describing data that will make it easier and more cost effective to analyze, visualize and derive value from operational data. This of course is critical for energy and analytics. The Project Haystack website provides more detail by outlining that it "is an open source initiative to streamline working with data from the Internet of Things. The project standardizes semantic data models and web services with the goal of making it easier to unlock value from the vast quantity of data being generated by the smart devices that permeate homes, buildings, factories, and cities." These smart devices are part of applications that "include automation, control, energy, HVAC, lighting, and other environmental systems."

The Project Haystack website is very informative and provides an online forum that the community can use to collaborate and share information. Another good resource for the reader, if this topic is new to them, is an 8-minute YouTube video created by John Petze that may be viewed at: http://youtu.be/5C6GwLbYqTw. Again, the video points out that the challenge for energy and analytics is that most data contained in BAS, and other systems, suffer from poor "semantic modeling," which means that the information that describes the meaning of the data is either not easy to decipher, or in many cases is not available at all. Again as with data communication and networking, standards are essential to making data easy to interpret, and require time-consuming and costly data mapping so that it can understood by applications.

PROJECT HAYSTACK APPROACH AND ACTIVITIES

The Project Haystack community has outlined some lofty goals, and is already hard at work achieving results. Among their first steps was to up a Project Haystack website at www.project-haystack.org populated with very useful information to educate the industry, and a discussion forum that allows constituents from across the world and different industries to work together to create consensus-driven solutions. Through that effort and a lot of work behind the scenes, a first major accomplishment was for this community to conceptualize the data problem and frame the discussion to identify activities that are required to create a solution. This was done in alignment with the Project Haystack mission, which is to "...define a methodology and common vocabulary so that models of building systems and smart devices can be interpreted automatically by a variety of software and web-based applications." To state this another way, this approach provides a simple, standardized way to represent pieces of information—data. However it is more than just representing numeric values or alpha text; the software applications that use these data must be able to understand the context for the data and their characteristics. To make this possible, Project Haystack created a model, which is a method to organize data in a meaningful way.

The idea is to begin at a high level to define characteristics that explain the context for the data. The Haystack model does this by using "tags" to identify groups of data. Groups of data associated with a building or piece of equipment (i.e. air handler) use an "entity" tag, which identifies and helps to create context. There are also tags to describe the entity. Drilling down into more specific content, there are tags to identify a variety of types of information and to identify characteristics of that information (what type of number is it, is it a time of day, etc.). Simply put, tags define facts about each data item—is it a temperature sensor? Is it a room sensor or a return air sensor? Which air handler is it associated with? What is the schedule associated with that air handler and the spaces it serves? This process standardizes data so that applications can automatically interpret data, without manual intervention, allowing for the actual value add of analytics to be realized cost effectively.

The project also provided a more technical explanation of their goals for energy and building data. "The Project Haystack data modeling standard for Buildings and Equipment systems shall use a simple meta-model." As defined by Wikipedia, "meta-modeling is the analysis, construction and development of the frames, rules, constraints, models and theories applicable and useful for modeling predefined class of problems." In this case the problem is that data from building systems do not follow consistent rules and are not easily used by applications, hence the need for mapping. As noted, the Project Haystack meta-model is based on the broadly accepted concept of "tags." To provide more detail on this concept, tags are name/value pairs, associated with entities like AHUs, electric meters, etc. Tags are simple and dynamic, add structure, and provide the flexibility needed to establish standardized models of diverse systems and equipment. Tags are a modeling technique that allows easy customization of data models on a per-task, per-project or per-equipment basis, while retaining the ability to be interpreted by external applications using a standard, defined methodology and vocabulary. Using Haystack, external web-based applications are able to receive data that include essential meta data (tags) to describe the meaning of the data. This approach can be used for graphics, analytics, maintenance management and other applications, and it enables automatic interpretation of the data by software applications. This Project Haystack effort is a gift to the energy and analytics world, and it could only have been done with the expertise of this highly competent community of technologists and entrepreneurs.

The project also developed a guide specification: http://www.skyfoundry.com/file/50/Guide-Specification-for-Data-Modeling-Standard.docx. This is a highly educational document entitled "Guide Specification for Data Modeling of Building Systems and Equipment Based on Project Haystack Open Source Data Modeling Standard." In the end, to get full-scale market adoption of data modeling standards, this effort is a combination of push-pull strategies. Manufacturers and software/applications developers, such as SkyFoundry, that were early adopters of the data modeling standard are the industry leaders. The broader the adoption of the standard by others, the faster cost and implementation obstacles to analytics will be removed. At the same time, there has been a growing market pull from managers that want access applications for energy and analytics as well as maintenance management and many other applications mentioned in this book. The data model and guide specification offer significant value to all of the market participants.

Project Haystack has also been engaged in development of many technology and business enablers. These enablers take the form of protocols and tool kits to accelerate the development of new products, and the upgrade of existing ones to be compatible with the Haystack Open Source Data Model. These efforts are targeting existing *de facto* standards and widely deployed technology such as the Niagara Framework™ from Tridium, Inc., and JAVA, a high-level object-oriented programming language developed by Sun Microsystems that has been widely used for product development. Taking this approach, it is possible to reduce the cost barriers to participating in this exciting business, and to make it easier for building operators to get the full benefits of energy and analytics.

The last topic under this heading is Haystack Connect. At this writing, final preparations are underway for the 2015 event, and it has become the must-attend event for those with a passion to unlock the power of energy and building data. It is billed as "the place where the community of automation and IoT professionals come together to learn and share the latest techniques for connecting systems and using data to advance the efficiency of buildings, equipment systems and processes." To say it is a conference would be an understatement, it is the educational opportunity of the decade. After the inaugural event in 2014, Ken Sinclair wrote a review of the event saying that for data "the most significant advances are being driven not by a single company, but rather by a community of companies creating open, best-of-breed technologies that work together through a range of open protocols and software interfaces, including the rapidly growing "Haystack" standard. These new technologies reach the market through a growing group of practitioner communities, each with deep expertise in their own fields." Ken went on to say that "…for every successful event there needs to be a takeaway that changes our point of view. For me it was captured when Jason Briggs and Scott Muench of J2 Innovations took the stage and planted the seeds of change and showed us all how a connected Haystack using data modeling could alter industry dynamics as we know them." The event typically includes multiple tracks of sessions and speakers covering topics from analytics, visualization and data modeling to cyber security. An open forum filled with people who are willing to share their knowledge and experience is one of the best ways this author can think of to accelerate market change.

This has been a limited introduction to one of the most exciting and rapidly evolving movements in the industry. Again the reader is encouraged to follow developments with Project Haystack, and to make compatibility with the Open Source Data Model a requirement for every new product and system that is purchased.

Chapter 15

The Internet of Things (IoT)

Glen Allmendinger,
Harbor Research, Inc.

Glen Allmendinger of Harbor Research Inc. could almost be called the father of IoT. He founded Harbor Research Inc. more than 30 years ago and has worked with a who's who of companies internationally, helping them to develop strategies around emerging technology such as IoT. He and Harbor Research Inc. established IoT leadership more than a decade ago, so there is no better source for an overview of this extremely important topic.

We have entered an era where people, businesses and social organizations are beginning to understand the profound impacts awareness, collaboration, and intelligence that the Internet of Things will bring. In the not too distant future, hundreds of millions, then billions, of individuals and businesses, with billions, then trillions, of smart, communicating devices, will stretch the boundaries of today's business and social systems, and create the potential to change the way we work, learn, entertain and innovate.

Harbor Research, Inc.

INTRODUCTION

The Internet of Things is a global technological opportunity of unprecedented proportions. The technology behind the Internet of Things will ignite an era of smart systems that radically transforms customer service, resources allocation, and productivity in general. In this new era, manufactured objects, general infrastructure, people, and businesses will be connected and communicating constantly. As the world becomes connected, societies and governments alike will be able to respond to the needs of both citizens and assets in real time.

The internet is the profound driving force on the path to a truly connected world. First, the internet gave us e-mail and the Web, then came e-commerce and the ability of consumers and businesses to quickly purchase items, as well as the ability of retailers and businesses to build close relationships based on customer preferences. But the next phase will be much more profound. It includes shared and secure internet access for device interaction—in many cases with no human intervention at all—as well as network-based services such as status monitoring, usage tracking, consumable replenishing, and automated repair. These new services are based upon the convergence of networks, embedded computing, control, content, and sensor feedback.

Device manufacturers and service companies have important roles to play, and will be the major enablers of smart products, solutions, and systems. Virtually all markets will offer new opportunities to manufacturers, as intelligence will be embedded in categories ranging from machinery and building control systems to consumer goods.

This chapter examines the current state and evolution of the Internet of Things. It also provides a perspective on emerging opportunities enabled by intelligent device networking. More importantly, it outlines how adopters are using device networking solutions, and how device manufacturers and related service companies should leverage networking technologies to gain new operational and competitive advantages.

DEFINITIONS AND CONTEXT

Since the beginning of computing there have essentially been three waves of technology and architecture: mainframe computing, personal computing, and network computing. This next generation of IoT technology will add significant new capabilities to computing and network systems. These new capabilities will revolve around real-time situational awareness and automated analysis. As a result, technology moves beyond just proposing task solutions—such as executing a work order or a sales order—to sensing what is happening in the world around it, analyzing that new information for risks and possibilities, presenting alternatives, and taking actions.

Definition: the Internet of Things and smart systems are a new generation of systems architecture (hardware, software, network technologies and managed services) that provides real-time awareness based on inputs from machines, sensors, people, video streams, maps, newsfeeds and more that integrate people, processes, and knowledge to enable collective awareness and better decision making.

The three previous waves of technology each have had significant impacts on productivity and efficiencies: 1) Mainframes standardized transactions; 2) personal computing placed processing power into the hands of professionals; and, 3) networked systems enabled business process automation. What is important about this next wave of smart systems is the combined impact of the cycles of innovation. While there is standalone value in each of the innovations in software systems, server infrastructure, network infrastructure, and client devices, it is the combination of all these innovations that will allow computing technologies to inform smarter systems.

As networks have invaded the "physical" world, traditionally unique components and interfaces between and among electronic, as well as mechanical elements, are becoming more and more standardized. The implications of these trends are enormous. No product development organization, nor its suppliers of components and sub-systems, will be able to ignore these forces—product and service design will increasingly be influenced by common components and sub-systems. Vertically defined, stand-alone products and application markets will increasingly become a part of a larger "horizontal" set of standards for hardware, software and communications.

As it becomes easier and easier to design and develop smart systems, competitive differentiation will shift away from unique, vertically focused product features, to differentiation based on how the product is actually used, and how the product fosters interactions between and among users in a networked context. This opens nearly infinite opportunities for forward thinking product and service organizations. Businesses can begin to explore many new possibilities for system solutions unthinkable just a few years ago. The possibilities that IoT offers for energy and analytics, as discussed throughout this book, and combined with the developments in electricity and energy markets are particularly exciting.

TRENDS DRIVING THE INTERNET OF THINGS

Harbor Research Inc. expects the rate of investment in the Internet of Things and smart systems to be measurably higher than in maturing

IT systems and network infrastructure and that investment will occur in five key areas:

- Smart system platform technology to integrate systems and applications

- Purpose-built device & hardware [sensors, etc.] innovation to support new user experiences

- New generation of device data management and analytics tools

- Business process integration

- Value-added application services

Beyond mobile phones, laptops and other traditional IT devices connected to networks, the scope of what is considered an "intelligent" device is expanding, as more and different products get connected to the network: Health monitoring devices on the body, telematics in vehicles for safety, automated service scheduling, and driver convenience as well as smart grid equipment and meters that can monitor real-time electricity usage—all delivered via the internet. We are entering an age of enhanced asset awareness, where real-world assets (e.g., HVAC systems, shipping containers, shop-floor machinery, pipelines, etc.) can monitor events, execute rules, and automate business processes. Intelligent device communications is converging with IT and network infrastructure to enable vast improvements in efficiency and productivity.

The technology and market forces that are driving business and government interest in smart machine to machine (M2M) and Internet of Things solutions are many, including:

- The cost of devices will continue to plummet with advances in silicon, packaging and integration technology making them network fluent and affordable to virtually everyone;

- A ubiquitous broadband infrastructure (significantly ahead of most predictions) has been developed, which is enabling virtually everyone in the developed world to be connected both to other users, to new types of sensors and instruments and to massive processing and storing infrastructure;

- Carriers are dramatically reducing monthly fees for cellular device links—most network service providers worldwide have deployed

IP networks on a broad scale and the wider availability of 3G wireless networks is fostering market adoption;

- The storage capacity and processing power of computers will continue to grow exponentially and enable a whole new generation of infrastructure to perform an enormous variety of data management tasks—both carriers and IT infrastructure providers are working to develop software and data management platforms to support new managed services;

- The miniaturization of components and the integration of a broad range of sensing capabilities into intelligent devices will continue to provide a variety of features that support the integration of digital information and sensory inputs from the physical world, thus broadening the range of possible applications available;

- The continuing development of IT systems, the internet and next generation telecommunication network architecture will enable movement and analysis of very large amounts of information (much beyond traditional communication and messaging) which will extend the value of managed services;

- Data communication standards being developed by a wide range of bodies including professional societies/standards bodies, government sponsored organizations like the smart grid interoperability panel (SGIP) and others are making data from new and legacy (older generation) systems available to a web service and to application platforms;

- Finally, technology advances have improved and simplified system and user interfaces and interactions which, in turn, are driving adoption of new business models.

Tied to these market and technology forces are a number of regulatory and economic stimulus efforts such as smart grid and healthcare initiatives that are also fostering increased market adoption. End customers participation in the design, development and management of smart systems will rise during this next period of market development:

- End users will emerge as a force and place greater emphasis on vertical solutions that readily integrate with enterprise systems, innovative solution design and more effective service and support.

- Demand for adaptability, agility and features will grow. Innovation in product and systems design will be heavily rewarded. Customers will creatively apply and integrate technology in their work and personal lives to unimaginable levels.

- Customers will require a tailored experience from service providers. Not only do customers expect suppliers to anticipate their specific needs, they will want suppliers to project an experience for them—smart systems are driving home the importance of user experience.

- Overall, the decline in connectivity cost, coupled with declining device costs, is driving growth in virtually all device communications. This trend, plus substantial regulatory investment (e.g. smart grid) and emergence of new features from network operators and IT infrastructure suppliers, is driving the connectivity trend.

- The Internet of Things needs a universal alternative to the many existing techniques for connecting ordinary devices to the internet. The other techniques all have something to recommend them; each is optimized for a special purpose. But in return for their optimality, they sacrifice compatibility. Since most device connectivity rarely requires maximum optimality, compatibility is a much more important objective. IP is the only answer.

- The technical development in low-cost sensors and actuators combined with low-power communication technologies such as IEEE 802.15.4, low-power Wi-Fi, and power line communication has accelerated in the last few years. However, the biggest problem with the evolution of wireless sensor networks has been the large number of proprietary users.

Many IT equipment suppliers and wireless carriers have made recent pronouncements concerning the scale of the Internet of Things. Harbor Research Inc. analysis points to the many significant challenges in realizing such growth:

- Challenges in adopting new business models and making the business case to support investments.

- Complex services and solution delivery eco-systems that require businesses to relate in new and different ways.

- Anticipation of new product, service and systems innovation modes that are not widely adopted today.

- Fragmented M2M and smart systems vendor landscape that is not yet well aligned with the larger IT infrastructure and carrier players.

- Requirement for vertically focused solutions from a supply-side world that historically has been far more horizontally driven.

IoT Enables a New Generation of "Horizontal" Software to Enable Vertical Apps

Once a device becomes networked and is monitored for the primary purposes of device status, usage tracking, and consumables replenishment, it will also serve the larger business purpose of being a key driver for the vertical customization of services in general. For example, "asset management" is an important service that incorporates a number of different variables and systems (diagnostics for equipment health monitoring, location services for maintenance and spare parts planning, etc.). Application service providers need to organize the devices and system capabilities they offer configured for the environment in which they operate—factory, office, hospital, and elsewhere. A product inventory program will have a much different configuration in a factory than it will in an office building. More than ever before, the drivers, needs, and environmental conditions will determine the way technology is implemented. Ultimately, all devices and services, like asset management, will be highly configurable to match the needs of a particular arena, or even of a particular end-user. Harbor Research Inc. historically referred to these foundation/platform functions as "systems applications." This means a set of state-based application functions that are horizontal in nature and often characterized in a general sense as "middleware" that are not seen by the end user (we do not like the term middleware, as it risks generalizing capabilities that are unique to the pervasive internet and offer unique opportunities for suppliers).

In its most basic and practical form, Harbor Research Inc.'s concept of "systems applications" is based on "managed services integrated with embedded computing." But that's not as simple as it sounds. Capturing the real value of internet-connected devices goes much further than providing connectivity/interoperability, data basing, and some XML-based transport scheme. For example, real pervasive managed services will allow networked, embedded devices to execute remote applications as if those applications were part of the internal operating system. This type of enablement can bring extraordinary value to the growing population of network-embedded devices.

System applications are fairly generalized and are created by applying generic connectivity functions to a particular arena. The breakdown of system applications is as follows:

- **Status, Monitoring & Diagnostics**: Status applications capture and report on the operation, performance, and usage of a device, or the environment that the device is monitoring. Diagnostics applications allow for remote monitoring, troubleshooting, repair, and maintenance of networked devices.

- **Upgrades & Configuration Management**: Upgrade applications improve or augment the performance or features of a device. They can prevent problems with version control, technology obsolescence, and device failure. This kind of program makes site visits to upgrade products unnecessary and eliminates the need to keep track of what has been upgraded and when, thus saving time and money.

- **Control & Automation**: Control and automation applications coordinate devices into a sequenced pattern of behavior. These applications also allow for special-case discrete actions of a device under certain circumstances.

- **Location & Tracking**: Profiling and behavior-tracking applications are used to monitor variations in geography, culture, performance, usage, and sales of a device. Such applications can also be used to create a more customized or predictive response to end-users of a device.

- **Data Management & Analytics**: Business intelligence and specialized analytical software such as data mining and predictive analytics, enterprise energy management, ESCO 2.0, video image analysis, pattern recognition, and artificial intelligence algorithms.

Analytics Drives Real-time Value

"Real-time awareness" is driving renewed interest and deployment of analytic tools. Analyzing and storing the massive amounts of data that will be received is only possible with extensible and adaptable systems. Rules engines and work flow are the existing technologies for deciding which alternative courses to pursue, either automatically through the application of a rule that says, "if this happens, do this," or through human review based on work flow engines that route the anomaly and alternative courses of action to the right person to make a decision. The basic function of rules engines and work flow will stay constant—seismic leaps will be necessary in the data flow and analytical inputs in a world of vastly expanded real-time awareness.

The conversion of process applications to service-oriented architectures will allow these process apps to be adapted to business scenarios, with specific components pushed down to intelligent devices where they can execute a specified action. For example, alerting a citizen on her Smartphone to the updated arrival time of a bus that was stuck in traffic, notifying a doctor on a tablet device about the drug allergies of a patient he is about to see, or directing the thermostat in an individual home to raise the temperature by turning down the air conditioner setpoint by three degrees, perhaps for demand response.

Value-added Application [Managed] Services

An important characteristic of the smart systems opportunity will be vertically focused solutions—the bulk of which will increasingly be delivered as managed or value-added services. In conceptualizing how platforms would support managed services, system-level applications would be called upon and integrated in differing configurations to provide vertical value-added applications. For example, a combination of monitoring, diagnostic, control and tracking functions could be configured to provide basic functionality required to enable an energy management application.

Value added application services are solutions that integrate people, business processes and assets and are delivered as managed services. Examples of value-added applications services include the following:

• Asset management and optimization

• Supply chain integration & business process management

• Customer support

• Energy management

• Security management

Companies will create solutions that combine elements of industry-specialized hardware devices, vertical industry software, and industry-focused wireless/wired networks with industry-oriented analytics to optimize business processes and performance both operationally and financially. Smart systems technologies and applications will help organizations address the key challenge of optimizing the value of their balance sheets, allowing them to move beyond financial assets and liabilities to their physical assets and liabilities (like electric grids or hospitals) and then to their intangible assets and liabilities (like a skilled workforce or brand). Assets and liabilities tend to be very industry-specific, even more so than processes that may be common across industries. And the task of optimizing the value of these assets and liabilities is vertically focused because optimization requirements and goals vary dramatically from industry to industry.

Potential for New Innovations to Impact Growth

There is now substantially greater recognition of the technological capabilities and the potential benefits of connecting devices to the internet than there was even a few years ago. This represents a whole new generation of technology innovation and, if history repeats because certain conditions repeat, Harbor Research Inc. expects a significant wave of growth in smart systems across the entire economic landscape. As Moore's law takes over and the price of embedding intelligence and connectivity into devices continues to fall, networked devices will push farther and farther into the mainstream. This process is somewhat self-reinforcing as low prices are driven by high quantities, and vice versa, making these devices increasingly prevalent in human activity and businesses. Applications will spread through all areas of life. As technology, business and supplier solution challenges are met, immense growth will begin to really accelerate.

Harbor Research Inc. believes there are indications that this era is fostering new types of innovation based on new technologies that will impact the growth of IoT and smart systems. There are several phenomenon that can potentially drive significant new modes of innovation that will positively impact adoption and growth. To understand the future of networked information, it helps to remember that the Internet of Things will largely be driven by collaboration and collective intelligence. Some important forces evident in the marketplace include:

- **Collaboration and Crowd Sourcing Are Real**: It is becoming increasingly clear that "crowd sourcing," meaning that a large group of people can create a collective work whose value far exceeds that provided by any of the individual participants, including building applications that literally get better the more people use them; and, designing participatory systems that harness network effects not only to acquire users, but also to learn from them and build on their contributions. From Google and Amazon to Wikipedia, eBay, and craigslist, Harbor Research Inc. is seeing that value is facilitated by technology, but was co-created by communities of connected users. This trend towards collaborative systems continues with newer platforms like YouTube, Facebook, and Twitter, and, Harbor Research Inc. believes, will begin to spill over into new and innovative smart systems.

- **Smartphones Are Driving Innovations in User Experience and Sensory Systems**: Many people fail to understand the significant sensor innovations that are being designed into smartphones. Today's smartphones contain microphones, cameras, motion sensors, proximity sensors, and location sensors. New internet-connected GPS applications also have built-in feedback loops, reporting your speed and using it to estimate arrival time based on traffic patterns that are no longer estimated but measured and reported in real time. Sensor-based applications can be designed to get better the more people use them, collecting data that create a virtuous feedback loop that creates more usage. Sensors are dramatically improving the user experience.

- **Analytics Drive New Values**: Data analysis, visualization, and other techniques for seeing patterns in data are going to be an increasingly valuable. Sensors and monitoring programs are not acting alone, but in concert with their human partners and an increasing number of machine learning algorithms. The continuing promises of an Internet of Things will finally produce tangible value via a hodgepodge of sensor data contributing, bottom-up, to machine learning applications that gradually find more patterns and make sense of the data that are handed to them.

- **Information Signatures Drive Awareness to New Heights**: As more and more microcontrollers and sensors are embedded in everyday objects, encoded information in physical objects will also create pervasive information signatures. Seen in this way, a printed bar code, a CD or DVD disc, a house key, or even the pages of a book can have the status of an "information signature" on a network. A product on the supermarket shelf, a car on a dealer's lot, a pallet of newly produced food sitting on a loading dock— all have information signatures now. In many cases, these information signatures are linked with their real world analogs by unique identifiers: an ISBN or ASIN, or a part number. Take the smart grid as an example—neutral web services back ends for energy-related sensor data will combine smart meter and power device data from homes and businesses to discover unique energy signatures—it is possible to determine not only the wattage being drawn by the device, but the make and model of each major appliance or any electrical device plugged into any wall socket. Signatures will combine with data fusion technology to drive rapid advances in systems awareness.

- **The Internet is Becoming A Real-time Medium**: Applications driven by machines and sensors demand that data are collected, presented, and acted upon in real time. The web is no longer a collection of static pages of HTML that describe something in the world; it is becoming a real-time communication and information forum for interactions. The internet is getting faster than you might think and real time is not limited to social media. Much as Google has realized that a link is a vote, retailers like Wal-Mart realized that a customer purchasing an item is a vote and the cash register is a sensor counting that vote. Real-time feedback loops drive inventory and availability. Sensor-driven purchasing and real-time analytics is having a huge impact on the business world and customer response.

- **B2C Drives B2B and Visa Versa**: The Internet of Things and smart systems phenomenon is not limited to consumers with smartphones. Cisco's Connected Cities initiative and its "planetary skin" project with NASA, as well as IBM's Smarter Planet program demonstrate how the B2B world is being transformed by the sensors on the internet. Factories, refineries, steel mills, and supply chains are being instrumented with sensors and machine analytics that we see in mobile consumer applications. The Internet of Things and People will depend on managing, understanding, and responding to massive amounts of user and machine-generated data in real time. With more users and sensors feeding more applications and platforms, innovators and developers are able to tackle serious real-world problems. As a result, the smart systems opportunity is no longer growing arithmetically; Harbor Research Inc. believes it's growing exponentially.

BUILDINGS OPPORTUNITIES

The buildings arena includes HVAC, security and access, lighting, fire, people-moving systems and safety systems, as well as the energy they consume, that reside in facilities in commercial, institutional, industrial and residential segments. This section focuses on the applications and untapped potential enabled by Internet of Things technologies in homes, businesses, and factories. Companies can use the captive information in these products to improve customer service and marketing efforts, provide remote diagnostics and customized services, optimize their own product development, and increase arena.

Evolution of Smart Building Applications

It is clear that customers seeking building automation and control systems are beginning to demand wider integration of multiple systems within a building. Therefore customers are also demanding IP-based platform architectures for these systems, as a prerequisite for integration. IT architecture in general, and IP-based device integration specifically, combines to create a common schema towards which all building systems are converging, whether they are traditionally non-IT-based systems like HVAC, security and lighting, or native IT systems like IP telephony or a computer-to-computer data network. Key trends in the buildings arena include:

- Energy management continues to drive much of the interest in the smart buildings arena. Enterprises facing increasing pressure to cut costs and reduce environmental impact are turning to smart buildings as a means of reducing energy requirements and increasing the bottom line. In the residential market, homeowners are looking to cut costs and be more "green." Demand response systems for residential users have traditionally lagged behind commercial implementers but this trend may change with increasing investment and government support for smart grid infrastructure.

- In recent years, sales of IP-based building control systems outnumbered sales of proprietary non-IP building control systems. The move toward open IP-based building automation and away from proprietary systems continues to be an important trend as open systems permit increased interoperability and connectedness between devices made by different vendors.

- Convergence between internet-enabled IT systems and all other building automation systems (BAS), including telephone, data, video, safety, fire alarm, digital signage, energy, environmental systems, and building maintenance monitoring is clearly picking up momentum. There is pressure to be able to use open protocols to mix and match (plug and play) equipment from various vendors and generations.

- Wireless building control systems are reducing the disruptiveness that retrofits and smart building infrastructure installation entails. For continuously occupied buildings (like hospitals, apartment complexes and hotels), wireless sensor networks can be implemented without the difficulty that installing wired systems entails. Removing this barrier will continue to have a positive impact on the adoption of smart solutions in the buildings arena. Additionally, wireless technologies allow facilities managers to seamlessly add new devices and reconfigure existing systems as needs change, which is driving the growing use of many new types of sensors.

- Building automation systems are being used to monitor critical assets within facilities like server rooms, critical hospital infrastructure, and security systems. Downtime among these critical assets is unacceptable, and their health is affected by environmental factors such as temperature, ventilation and humidity. Smart monitoring solutions can mitigate these threats and ensure uptime of critical assets around the clock.

- Home automation, long predicted by futurists but slow to occur in reality, may finally begin to pick up speed as new technologies continue to penetrate homes. Smartphones and tablet computers are poised to fill a void as an inexpensive and user-friendly "universal remote." Homeowners will be able to monitor and collect data about energy usage, which lights are on, which windows are open, and whether the security system is functioning properly from anywhere in the world.

Today's Marketplace

Harbor Research Inc. estimates that as many as 40% of the new buildings could be IT-BAS convergent or intelligent over the next 8-10 years and that the retrofit rate for existing buildings may exceed 10-15%. Meanwhile, Harbor Research Inc. expects sensor demand to grow briskly over the coming decade.

The large incumbent energy system control companies such as Honeywell, Johnson Controls, Siemens and Schneider Electric and HVAC concerns such as Trane and Carrier Corporation have all developed in the past 2-3 years open protocol solutions to complement their legacy, mostly proprietary, product lines and they are now starting to offer wireless solutions as well as demand response. Some of these suppliers are expected to expand into security system applications and then propose full building intelligence systems, more comprehensive building O&M contracts and get involved in analytics technology as well. In parallel, many new players are addressing the emergent "energy intelligence," or energy and analytics, arena as it is central to the concerns of building operators. Increased building intelligence will not be restricted to new buildings (where it may be easier to sell) but it will also become increasingly applicable in existing buildings. Retrofitting an existing building is already doable with current emerging technology. Furthermore, many retrofit improvements can occur without any local utility involvement.

Increased building intelligence will mean more precise and open energy and power management in commercial premises as a result of being able to relay on demand real-time precise point-of-use data to web portals that will be openly accessible by building guests, tenants and owners alike (subject to security rules). On-demand remote metering and monitoring of any load will be possible. So, for the first time, commercial electricity management will be an open playing field where building managers, owners and tenants will all be able to truly "discover" and manage their energy needs as they want. Owners, managers, and occupants will have the ability to access precise real-time information on demand as well as the ability to retrieve information remotely via mobile phones and computers.

Open commercial energy management will not only benefit the

building engineer or manager, it will also reach the building owners' CFO, CIO, and operations executives who can now oversee large commercial real estate portfolios on a regional or national basis.

Tenants in intelligent commercial buildings will also be able to monitor and influence their demand profiles and routines to truly control their energy use, level of comfort and energy bills, all at once. This will be much better than receiving a monthly statement based on the amount of square feet they happen to rent (especially if some arcane adjustments have been made by cost accountants that do not necessarily have any idea of how the building operates and what various types of equipment different tenants use or how these tenants use their space).

This will completely change the game; more stakeholders will have a true seat at the decision table; these new constituencies will have to be recognized and catered to; new business propositions will emerge; and the marketing of energy will change. Tenants will be able to relay their site information to their headquarters which will be able to quickly aggregate for regional or national enterprises including, of course, the opportunity to shop for electricity supply. For example, building intelligence will help solve the tenant conundrum. Right now, tenants generally pay for their energy as a more or less transparent part of their rental lease payment. With building intelligence, tenants can be sub-metered (and meter any load they want) and take local, precise and cost-effective actions that affect not only the entire premises but also select parts of the rented space. This will be the end of the blind energy lease charge, the "one-size-fits-all" building management approach and the end to the tons of excuses that building owners can throw at tenants to offer them half-baked approaches.

Increased building intelligence (and the underlying IT/BAS convergence that it implies) will also enable or allow increased or better use of many new energy saving and demand-responsive technologies such as:

- Daylighting and fully programmable (luminescence-based) lighting (based on the DALI standard) will be prevalent in new buildings past 2010.

- HVAC efficiency was projected to increase 5% by 2010 over previous building stock, and around half of new buildings were expected to adopt new demand-control ventilation techniques and 20% to adopt passive cooling properly integrated in the building envelopes.

- Innovative demand-controlled ventilation designs.

- Decentralized DC (Direct Current) UPS networks in data centers.

- Packaged plug-and-play DG.

The payoff will be huge: tenants will be able to buy their energy from their own supplier in states that allow this. They will also have the freedom of participating in an individual customized or building-wide basis in local demand response schemes based on their specific supply-demand profile. Buildings will become a major source of demand response. Data show that, even though it accounts for 35% of the total US load, the commercial sector accounts for 45% on average of summer electric peak coincident demand, with a sector peak in excess of 330 GW. The ability to precisely trigger on-demand DR could help reduce the sector's peak by at least 10-15%, based on various DR experiments conducted to date. It will become possible to enroll and aggregate thousands of buildings in DR programs. The impact could be considered if we believe some estimates that show a 2.5% reduction in peak demand could reduce the costs of serving that peak by 25%.

Tenants will be able to decide whether to invest in dedicated UPS, storage or distributed generation, or rent these capabilities from the building central manager or potentially from adjacent or nearby facilities. If they do, the UPS, storage and DG systems will also be fully web-enabled and managed. There is growing use of decentralized DC-based UPS systems; smart mid-size grid-connected "active" two-way storage technologies; and the ability to deploy scalable plug and play DG (including better DG packaging and better interconnection modules). In parallel, the deployment of automation and integration technologies will usher the entry of next-generation maintenance management programs, allowing equipment condition monitoring, early fault detection, and predictive and self-healing maintenance approaches. Operating personnel will be effectively dispatched through wireless communications through their PDAs or cell phones.

Finally, one can also progressively expect a new way to design and develop new buildings, if only because the buildings of the future are likely to fulfill new functions and operate differently, especially in the office, hotel, health and education sectors. We now sense a reasonably strong momentum toward green and smart building and a better way to spec energy systems for that purpose and truly consider more long-term costing approaches. Still, many observers keep saying that the commercial real estate sector will continue to operate under an ancient and dysfunctional system where the decision maker ends up being a general contractor which is neither the end-user nor the future facility manager. As a result, the sector is served by a fragmented vendor population: architects, specialty designers (e.g., for UPS, DG), building control vendors, HVAC vendors, UPS vendors, and DG vendors.

How long the industry remains fragmented will depend on how ubiquitous new smart commercial building management systems get implemented, how quickly energy retail deregulation happens, and the speed at which DR programs get implemented.

Adoption Progress

The fundamental difficulty in achieving systems intelligence in buildings is communication, and this problem can be broken down into two types of instances. The first issue is compatibility. For example, because the company that makes light switches doesn't also manufacture water boilers, there is no reason these two devices would have been built to speak the same language. The second issue is connectivity—the fire alarm device from one manufacture is not connected to anything else. Today more than ever, there are a number of solutions that address these problems from all different angles. In fact, many experts would say that the biggest roadblock to wider adoption of intelligent systems for buildings no longer has to do with technology.

Regardless of building size, the overall goal of building managers is maintaining an environment that is responsive to the needs of those who work, shop, and live there. Managers are driven by concerns that can largely be organized into two segments of interest: comfort/convenience and safety/security. Of course, these concerns fit into a broader economic context which can best be summarized as, "Please do not add additional costs and, if possible, please reduce my costs as you add new values."

The benefits of interoperability are obvious. For example, linking life safety systems to other building systems can improve response in an emergency. The fire system could alert the HVAC system to pressurize stairwells for occupant escape; elevators could be alerted to drop off occupants at the safest, lowest floor; standby power could start up to activate emergency exit lighting. The key to attracting building managers or consumers to internet-enabled applications remains a low price point, easy installation, and simple systems management. A key challenge for technology suppliers and service providers is the fragmentation of the end markets. From a device supplier perspective, available channels are also relatively fragmented. In spite of this, interest and activity is quite high. The desire for simplicity and high uptime is largely driven by smaller staffs with less technical ability. In the case of asset management and support coordination, the objective is to fix problems remotely, or if that is impossible, to dispatch a person with the right expertise, tools, and parts.

Energy has really become the "killer app" of the buildings and home arenas. The market for energy measurement, monitoring and control devices crosses the industrial and commercial sectors and its size is difficult to assess. Each of these market sectors will benefit from the ability to control power and even reduce consumption permanently, thereby reducing carbon emissions. Demand response solutions today are doing this on a contracted basis in order to alleviate load during peak periods of the summer months, however they strive to implement more automated energy management solutions and/or those that can permanently reduce load. Remote management is an additional benefit which could further reduce operating costs in the commercial/industrial sectors and some high-end property and property management solutions. Today's solutions for building energy management are rapidly converging with IoT technologies and include:

- AMR/AMI (automated meter reading/advanced meter infrastructure),

- Demand response, and

- Utility sponsored/consumer energy efficiency products.

Unfortunately, some of these solutions are limited by a lack of cost-effective, space-efficient sensors to measure, monitor and manage energy demand and consumption. For instance, demand response solutions must rely on expensive, external control mechanisms to cycle-down large equipment and disconnect loads, so limiting their reach and their cost-effectiveness. AMR/AMI solutions are beginning to grant a much better view from utility to meter, but they still offer virtually no insight beyond the meter, offering little to no control to the occupant to monitor and manage electricity consumption. Moreover, none of these solutions addresses the huge, untapped opportunity to provide information and control of the commercial building to consumers. Clearly, energy efficiency efforts have begun, but they have a long way to go, and it is the last few yards (beyond the meter) that really matter in managing and reducing the world's energy consumption.

Combining the pervasiveness of networking with embedded energy intelligence enables for the first time new real-time capabilities for demand-side management even down to socket and appliance level. As concern grows around power quality, availability and uptime, these technologies provide a unique unobtrusive means to provide customers with detailed load profiles and usage information that will empower end users to take control of their energy use. By setting building policies, end users will be able to safely forget about their energy consumption while their buildings look after their interests—actively connecting and disconnecting unused and unnecessary loads automatically as they go about their daily lives. Areas like sub-billing/metering, easier servicing of equipment and the ability to upgrade "in-site" and set sensitivity parameters are attractive benefits. Ultimately, organizing load management without disrupting customer life styles will be key to attaining important "green" goals in society. Smart energy intelligence can enable industrial, commercial and home smart energy networks, which can be used to monitor energy quality, switch and control energy sources, reduce energy consumption, and save costs.

Future Opportunities

Harbor Research Inc. believes that the following market forces deserve the acute attention, as they will have great impact on the requirements and direction of the market for building automation systems:

- Energy efficiency—rising energy prices and government regulations are encouraging building owners to operate more efficiently;

- IT integration occurring throughout the consumer environment is driving the desire and assumption for it to occur everywhere;

- Rising cost pressures from increased outsourcing and contractor buying;

- Proliferation of IT-based service delivery platforms like XML and SOAP; and,

- Wireless technology is gaining momentum by addressing its two key drawbacks—reliability and cost.

The advent of "green" building design will also have a growing effect on the market. Most green building technologies are mature enough today that investments should not be considered high risk. The most efficient green buildings take a complete system perspective of requirements and capacities, incorporating real-time heating and cooling adjustments to reduce costs and improve effectiveness. Significant cost reduction opportunities for green projects are available for qualified investments. There is a growing interest among both traditional building equipment suppliers and IT vendors in entering the green building industry with new products and services.

Chapter 16

Energy and Analytics Tools

The topic of energy and analytics tools is really a culmination for this book and yet it is a daunting topic. After years of evaluating this technological development and surveying offers in the marketplace, it has become evident to this author that a comprehensive review of all the tools available in the marketplace is unrealistic. Therefore, this chapter will take the same approach espoused throughout the text; it will encourage the user to carefully evaluate system requirements before exploring technology or "tool" options. A thorough review of requirements should result in a framework/specification that can be used to consider solutions. Many building owners and operators have completed such an analysis only to realize that there is no offering currently available that fulfills all of their needs. In some cases, these operators have teamed with a company that they felt had a "best in class" offering, with the understanding that ongoing advancement would be necessary to retain the business and evolve the solution to meet all of that customer's needs. In other cases, some building owners have elected to create their own solution, and become a solution provider for their own properties as well as actively sell the solution to others. There are many ways to approach this issue, but every approach must start with a clearly delineated set of requirements and expectations. Of course the owner must also recognize that requirements change over time, and an assessment of the solution provider's willingness to respond with enhancements, upgrades and expanded capabilities should also be considered. This last requirement is very difficult to assess, but it is important for the customer to consider the corporate culture and ownership of the provider to make the best estimation possible of where there is alignment with the customer's business philosophy and a drive for excellence that will spur continuous offering improvement.

Once requirements are outlined, the next consideration is "best practices for analytics." This chapter will begin with an overarching review of energy and analytics Best Practices to frame the dialog for a secondary set of customer requirements. These requirements should consider the scalability, resilience and long-term viability of solutions. As part of that discussion, the chapter will review pilot implementation steps that have been drafted by SkyFoundry. The final topic of this chapter is analytics architecture. In this architecture section, the makeup and infrastructure of analytics offerings will be reviewed. This is important because much of the coverage readers will find in the media focuses on the analytics tool/engine, rules, algorithms and visualization, but not on the actual infrastructure. Previous chapters have covered topics related to what analytics are capable of and how rules, algorithms and visualization can be deployed for energy management. The focus here will be on the actual technology implementation, so that the manager can truly understand the context of implementation, how invasive it will be, and what might happen if a break-up decision is made downstream. A manager who has assimilated this knowledge will be in the best possible position to evaluate energy and analytics tools and make an informed decision about the best solution to procure. This section will close with a brief discussion of training. Training will be covered under two headings: 1) training for all customer staff on the selected solution and 2) industry training to maintain a continuously improving energy and analytics program that results in the highest level of performance for buildings and campuses.

ENERGY AND ANALYTICS BEST PRACTICES: SETTING THE BAR

Applying the science of analytics to energy management, particularly in the 21st century, transforms the work that must be done by building operators and Certified Energy Managers (CEMs). As has been discussed throughout this book, this is especially true for electricity which has seen a business transformation and redefinition of the supply and demand sides of the meter. Equally important to managing energy is also reliability (or "resiliency"), especially for electricity, and there are a host of other topics in the spotlight globally, besides resiliency, in this era of challenges including climate change. At the building and campus level, the task of managing energy use and cost remains as critical and difficult as ever. That is why it is exciting to see CEMs being presented with a new set of tools to help carry out these tasks. Energy and analytics have been covered from every perspective in the book thus far; yet there are other instances of this technology to consider, particularly the Internet of Things, which was discussed in the last chapter. In that chapter Harbor Research Inc. pointed out that CEMs who deploy IoT may be able to achieve more data and potentially higher levels of energy optimization than ever before. The Internet of Things is exciting and will be discussed here in the context of analytics tool configuration and data access. There may be unlimited applications for the Internet of Things (IoT), but analytics is one that is driving energy optimization results today. This shouldn't be surprising because building operations, with high energy cost, demand new approaches—in this case, Internet of Things-driven Analytics IoT. Before talking about the role of IoT within energy and analytics however, it is again critical to emphasize the importance of delineating requirements and expectations in any building.

So what is Analytics IoT? As this book has covered in detail, analytics is a term for discovering meaningful patterns in data. Incorporated into the definition as it has been discussed here is visualization via dashboards and other tools, but to drill down a bit deeper there are three "essential elements" that must be covered:

1.   Human expertise,
2.   High quality data, and
3.   Sophisticated analytics software.

In this section these topics will be discussed in more detail because they are essential to evaluating analytics tools. Treatment of BAS, data communication, middleware and Internet of Things (IoT) in previous chapters was provided because understanding these topics is essential to evaluating tools. The manager can apply this technology understanding to an evaluation of how these elements are packaged and addressed in any analytics tool. Tools are being offered to the industry that leverage the advanced interoperability of devices, systems, and services. Yet the tools referred to here as Analytics IoT apply the essential elements along with the energy and analytics technology/software to produce exciting results for energy management and equipment optimization in buildings and large campuses. Universities facing huge energy challenges are among the early adopters of Analytics IoT. About once a month the author receives an email from Jim Lee at Cimetrics, Inc., with stories about such early adopters. A recent story was about one Ivy League university that is achieving $315,000 in annual energy savings. This campus began with 3 buildings, two labs and an administrative building, comprising over 400,000 square feet. In this case the IoT component, includes "interoperability" with an energy management system (EMS) to connect to, and from which to collect over 5,200 physical points of sensor and actuator data. These data were collected from air handlers, terminal units, pumps and other equipment every 15 minutes, 24 hours a day, 365 days a year, for a total of approximately 500,000 data samples per day. The analytics component function performed over 1,000 software algorithms continuously analyze the data and identify opportunities to reduce energy use, improve environmental conditions and drive down operations and maintenance costs. The result was an Analytics IoT system that paid for itself in 0.23 years... yes that is 4 months! It also reduced the university's CO_2 emissions by 820+ tons for impressive sustainability performance too. This could not have been achieved without technology that is built on the essential elements of energy and analytics.

Certified Energy Managers, and the facilities industry as a whole, are demanding this type of technology, and a growing number of companies are offering options, or tools. The challenge for managers, and the focus here, is how to choose an energy and analytics tool that will deliver results. Analytics IoT solutions combine interoperability, data, software, analysis and an understanding of best practices in building operations. The key to that previous sentence is that it describes the "offering" as a service or "solution" rather than a "tool," and yet, so often in the energy and analytics world, providers only want to talk about the technology. As the manager considers an energy and analytics tool, it is important to evaluate the technology and the interoperability, but also to evaluate how the technology carries out the analytics and how a tool is interfaced with human expertise to touch all of the bases outlined as "essential elements."

The first essential element is human expertise. In fact the basis for this discussion is that Analytics IoT is a combination of data, technology and know-how. The data discussed in this book are specific to energy and buildings, and they can be accessed from a host of installed systems. Many might confuse Analytics IoT with "Big Data" and the term is valid but there are some distinctions. Big data is used for a wide variety of applications, like on-line retailing, and Wikipedia defines it as "an all-encompassing term for any collection of data set so large and complex that it becomes difficult to process using traditional data processing applications." Unlike those generic big data applications, the focus of Analytics IoT is to leverage big building data for a much more specific focus on energy management, buildings and systems which demand custom analytics software and technology. In this case it is more about understanding what the data tell CEMs about building operations and how that information can be used to develop strategies for better, more efficient, buildings. This aspect of Analytics IoT merges technology with know-how or "human expertise." Human expertise is the "essential element" of analytics that enables an understanding of what the data mean, and how to develop meaningful recommendations about what issues should be addressed. Consider a medical analogy. What if a patient is sick and told that a magnetic resonance imaging (MRI) scan must be done. What type of doctor is the patient most likely to want—an expert on MRI technology, or a doctor that understands both the technology and the patients' body, in order to understand how to use the information from the MRI to treat him or her successfully? The obvious answer is the same reason the ideal solutions for building analytics require experts, in many cases CEMs, who understand the technology and the building.

The question for managers is what should they look for in an energy and analytics tool? This section answers that question by providing a context for evaluating tools through the lens of these essential elements. The premise here is that the ideal tool combines human expertise with technology that effectively delivers the other two essential elements: high quality data and sophisticated analytics software. The right energy and analytics solution provider must deploy sophisticated technology, combining the elements above, along with world class analysts (human expertise) to adapt the technology to customer needs and provide continuous support. Analysts must be content experts, ideally engineers or CEMs, experienced with energy and buildings, as well as the equipment and environment that customers are striving to optimize. Analysts can then apply this understanding of unique customer applications, and deploy energy and analytics technology to turn data into knowledge about how to improve building efficiency and operations. The analyst plays an essential role to ensure data quality and deploy effective Analytics IoT technology.

The second essential element is high quality data, and managers begin by evaluating tools based upon two aspects of data quality: data sufficiency and data resiliency. Data sufficiency is the first step and the goal is to ensure that there are enough data available to conduct meaningful analysis. Having sufficient data is critical, but in most cases the installation cost to add hundreds of new data points to a building is prohibitive. So tool analysts and designers rely on data from existing sources including BAS or energy management systems (EMS), computerized maintenance management systems (CMMS) and meters, plus some external web-based sources such as utility databases for bill data. The energy and analytics tool must be able to build a sufficient and effective data architecture, which requires creating a wide range of expertise with technology, data communications, IT and computer systems. In many respects, this is more a question of how the tool deployment is designed than of the tool itself, but again energy and analytics is as much about the human expertise as the tool itself. However it is important for tools to be flexible in the data that can be accessed and, as will be discussed later, in the rules against which those data are evaluated. Tool providers must leverage business process experience with the type of building or campus in question, and conduct ongoing communication and coordination with client teams.

It may be helpful to illustrate the importance of data sufficiency, by discussing it in the context of one specific building type—universities. Focusing on universities and, in particular energy analysis, shows how important it is to have sufficient data. Energy metering for universities can be an issue for two reasons. First, many universities have traditionally been master metered by the electric and natural gas utilities, without building level meters, a fact that is changing. Second, universities often utilize central plants for hot and chilled water loops, so energy consumption at the building level is not easily compared with energy benchmarks for buildings that include consumption by prime movers such as boilers and chillers. Analysts must consider and identify all of the data that will be needed to conduct analysis and produce recommendations for improvement. In this case, energy may not be consumed by prime movers, but it is possible to meter the hot and chilled water loop and measure the energy content of that water entering a building as Btus. One slight issue is that this approach ignores the energy conversion losses, such as natural gas burned by a boiler to produce heat, which reflects efficiency or how well the boiler converts energy into heat. This makes it hard to compare a building with a boiler to a building served by a central plant. Yet comparing buildings on the campus to one another is very effective. This is another good reason why the Energy Star™ program provides benchmarking comparison data by building type, allowing universities to compare performance against other universities. To bring this discussion back to data quality, the point is that managers must evaluate tools based upon how data sufficiency is addressed. Tools must provide the maximum number mechanisms for accessing data needed to perform meaningful analysis from any source, underscoring the importance of leveraging interoperability with all building systems, web-sources etc. Equally important to data sufficiency is how the tool ensures that data flow or that resiliency is not interrupted.

Data resiliency is the second aspect of high quality data, and it is critical to ensuring that analytics solutions remain viable. A common threat for analytics applications involves networking and data communication. Almost any type of building today will have IT and network administrator groups that must be interfaced with, and which must give permission to implementation of energy and analytics. If middleware, such as gateways or third-party communications devices, must be installed as part of the solution, extra diligence is required, especially if that network administrator is asked to provide an internet protocol (IP) address. The manager, or analytics solution provider, will need to pay ongoing attention to the data being provided to be sure that communication, and therefore data flow, is not disrupted. IT departments and network administrators, some of whom are outsourced service providers themselves, implement "changes," almost continuously. These "changes" can disrupt data resiliency and may include building renovations that cause re-cabling or upgrades to networking routers and switches and changes to information technology (IT) and internet protocol (IP) addressing. When this happens, data flow is disrupted, and the value of energy and analytics tools is diminished. This is because the analytics tool is analyzing old data or analysis is suspended for a period of time.

There are two critical data resiliency take-aways: 1) it is important to forge robust ties between IT and plant departments, and 2) it is critical to conduct data assessments that are both technology and human driven, to ensure data resiliency. The topic points out a very important evaluation criteria that will be discussed below under sophisticated analytics software. That criteria is to evaluate how the tool operates when the data flow is interrupted; for example, does the tool keep conducting analysis with old data, does it estimate data, etc.? A final note under data resiliency is that energy and analytics tool providers, or the manager's organization itself, must have connectivity and interoperability expertise, to ensure continuous flow of reliable data. This is the single most important reason for the organization of this book. The technology section of the book has covered the full range of topics from BAS to data communications and middleware technology to emphasize how important this technology is, as a foundation for the essential elements of energy and analytics. Data resiliency is part of that foundation, and it requires a method, human or technology-oriented, to continuously monitor data integrity. This process must evaluate data access and integrity, and must also be able to create electronic alerts to notify appropriate personnel of the issue and corrective action needed.

Armed with high quality data, the next essential element for energy and analytics is sophisticated analytics software. The reader should note that there are myriad analytics technology start-ups that are promoting new offerings. So a first technology requirement should be that the offering is field proven and provides hundreds (even thousands) of sophisticated algorithms, which constantly analyze data, to identify energy savings, as well as comfort, code, regulatory, safety and equipment efficiency improvement opportunities. These algorithms must evaluate energy intensity of the building and equipment, while also providing predictive maintenance capability that has been tested and field proven. These algorithms access data, as discussed above, to determine current operating conditions and then the algorithms compare those data to rules that define either optimal operation or optimal energy performance for a piece of equipment or process. The rules used may be based on design specifications for a piece of equipment, benchmarks from high performance buildings, past performance in the building being evaluated, etc. Hence, the desire for proven technology. This is because the more robust the database of performance data in the analytics tools, the more sophisticated the analytics software. Ideally algorithms may be tailored to various building types so that facility specific characteristics can be evaluated against rules. For example, indoor air quality and ventilation requirements are very different in a laboratory, hospital intensive care unit and office buildings, so it should be possible to adapt the rules, which algorithms are compared to, for a variety of facility needs. Energy and analytics software must also provide the capability for customers to add new rules that identify recommended actions to improve the customer processes on campuses. This is particularly important because managers, particularly CEMs, tend to be highly skilled and capable of sophisticated system interactions. Strategies should be offered to use technology to react to data quality or resiliency issues, and to incorporate corrective actions to compensate for missing data, in real time. If data points are missing, alternative algorithms and calculated values are utilized to perform analytics. This ensures that results can be achieved under varying levels of data availability while data resiliency issues are addressed.

Another sophisticated analytics software feature is incorporating effective software planning tools to track and prioritize recommendations for correction and improvement. Correction, or corrective action, may be a repair, etc., while improvement could be an optimization to reprogram a BAS control sequence or a retrofit that could include an equipment upgrade—i.e. adding a VFD to a fan. This is an important analytics differentiator; some systems simply list a number of issues or anomalies. More sophisticated systems combine that technology with direct interaction by an analyst who evaluates all building systems and then meets with managers to review analysis of the energy/cost savings from each recommendation and prioritize which ones to address first. The best case is for the software to track all of the corrective action/improvement recommendations, report on them, identify prioritization for addressing those items, and to reprioritize recommendations based upon new information. Even more valuable is tracking how long it has been since the recommendation was originally made and to provide a means to review and evaluate all of the recommendations. These reports can also summarize the value of savings or avoided cost associated with each recommendation, and potentially information such as how much "avoided cost" has been incurred as a result of not addressing the issue immediately. This could be called a "do nothing" evaluation. Considering the cost of doing nothing, and its impact on the potential savings, makes it easy to decide which recommendations to address first.

Applying the energy and analytics essential elements to selecting and deploying this technology cannot be understated. Analysts provide human expertise for engineering technical support and ongoing communication with management to ensure proper and timely implementation of recommendations. Customers, or managers, benefit because they become an analytics team with the analyst. The analytics team is continuously working together to fine-tune buildings and to incorporate what the analyst/manager team has learned about how specific types of facilities operate. Addressing the essential elements also improves the value of benefits that are quantified, including but limited to energy & O&M savings calculations. Only proven sophisticated analytics software coupled with human expertise can ensure a design that maintains high quality data, and can be customized to the unique characteristics of any building type. There is one additional topic that must be addressed regarding the evaluation of analytics tools, and that is analytics architecture.

Analytics Implementation Options

To reset the context for this discussion of analytics tools, it may be helpful to frame this dialog based upon the technical content provided throughout the second half of this book. Yet the scope of the content can be daunting, so another approach might be to view analytics tools through the lens of requirements to execute an analytics pilot project. A valuable resource for accomplishing this is provided by John Petze, partner at SkyFoundry and co-founder of Project Haystack. Mr. Petze provides a resource to frame the dialog using the *SkySpark Pilot Process Overview* published on August 11, 2013. The reader may also find a more detailed overview of getting started with deployment of SkySpark software in the deployment chapter of the SkySpark documentation, http://www.skyfoundry.com/doc/docSkySpark/Deployment. These documents point out that some of the "most successful projects start with a pilot implementation." In the context of analytics tool evaluation, that is a useful point because the complexity of an implementation can be overwhelming, as can be the cost. Therefore it may be helpful to think about this in the context of a pilot project. It may also be helpful for the owner to take that approach in evaluating tool options.

This pilot project document goes on to state that "pilot projects may focus on a little bit of data from a large number of sites or a more thorough application of analytics to all major equipment in a few facilities. In either case a pilot involves using real data and an implementation effort is required." The key facets of an implementation effort include:

1. **Data Access**. Identify the source(s) of the data to be analyzed and answer the following questions:
    a. Where is the data located?
    b. How will you connect to the data?
    Typically the data include historical data from a BAS and/or metering system. It is also important to have basic facility data such as address, size (square foot or meters), equipment listing. The goal is to identify the available data, where it is, how you will connect and what format it is in.

2.   **Data Modeling**—also known as tagging or semantic modeling. Data must have meaning in order to be interpreted by analytics. The data on-boarding process involves tagging the source data to define meaning. The process typically starts with a detailed list of "points" of data that the manager has identified for recording. A point is anything we want to collect data for, and it can be physical or virtual. That could include sensors, control points, schedule status. The "points" list would typically include point names, descriptions, and units.

The list would need to be annotated to describe relationships—such as "this zone temp is fed by this AHU," and "this supply air temperature sensor is measuring supply air from this AHU." In the data modeling step, the manager is defining basic information about the units, meaning, and relationships of the points that the energy and analytics tool will analyze.

3.   **Analytic Rules/Algorithms**. With an understanding of the data available that has been identified for capture, a whiteboard session is usually done to discuss and define (in English—not programming code) the types of patterns/issues to look for, such as:
   — Economizers open when they shouldn't be;
   — AHUs, lighting and other equipment that operate outside of schedules;
   — Deviations from kW benchmarks or limits we want to track;
   — Energy performance correlated with building characteristics;
   — Short cycling;
   — Simultaneous heating and cooling;

A good pilot project typically defines 6-8 rules to start with. Start with a manageable effort to get results quickly.

To design the energy and analytics pilot project for a tool that the manager wants to evaluate, it will typically require:

Human Expertise—there are several tasks:
1.   Data: this might be the manager themselves or a CEM or project manager to lead the effort to get the above information.
2.   Systems: a systems expert to design the connectivity required to get the data. For example it will be necessary to understand how

to connect to the specific system that holds the historical data. When direct connection to a BAS is involved, this often requires some involvement from the systems integrator that implemented the system—for example a systems engineer familiar with the BAS system.

High Quality Data Access: In a case where the data are already in some type of database (i.e. SQL) then it will be necessary to have expertise/understanding of the database schema. This will require an understanding of the systems that the data come from and the ability to answer questions like:
— What do the point names mean?
— Which points are related to which equipment systems?
— What is the expected operation of the equipment systems?

Engineer/CEM knowledgeable with the analytics tool to establish the data connection (to a SQL DB for example), write the rules and determine algorithms that will be carried out.

In some cases the energy and analytics tool provider may not provide implementation services directly. This means that the manager must perform a secondary analysis of the supply channel partners, to secure the services of a company, typically a system integrator, that will provide implementations and support services for that tool.

This chapter has covered two critical topics that are very useful in selection of an energy and analytics tool: 1) best practices, and 2) the requirements for a pilot project. Once the manager has developed a set of requirements and plan, based upon this information, the next critical topic is the technology, or analytics tool itself, which will be discussed based upon the analytics architecture.

Analytics Architecture

The topic of architecture and systems has been a recurring theme throughout this book. In the evaluation of energy and analytics tools, architecture is also a critical topic. This section will cover a number of topics to provide the reader with a framework to use in developing an approach to understanding the tools themselves, and to comparing tools against one another. As part of this process the manager must also evaluate the technical requirements that may be impacted by selecting one tool over another. This content will be addressed by covering the following topics:

— Cloud and web services solutions anywhere, anytime, any device;

— BAS, middleware and device standards and solutions;

— Dashboard and API;

— Software as a service; and

— Cyber security.

CLOUD COMPUTING

Evolution of energy and analytics technology has been enabled by numerous advancements, but perhaps none more significant than cloud computing. The first article that this author wrote on the topic of analytics, then referred to as building simulation and analysis, was 30 years before the publishing of this book. At that time, the state of the art was to temporarily deploy a mini-computer in the building, outfitted with what was then an astronomical amount of data storage capability. That mini-computer was necessary to support the huge hard drive for data storage, but also to support the computing power necessary to run the algorithms. At that time the mini-computer was also necessary to physically, but temporarily, support a network containing hundreds, or even thousands, of sensors because there was no BAS standard like BACnet™. The cost of such simulation and analysis equipment and services made it inconceivable to consider deploying that kind of computing power in any building on a permanent basis.

Fast forward to today when it is possible to deploy web-based, cloud computing solutions, and interface with them at anytime from anywhere. Leveraging cloud-hosted energy and analytics solutions means that servers can be deployed online with the computing power for the analysis, and that the data storage can be scaled online and shared across numerous buildings. The internet connects those buildings to energy and analytics in the cloud, and can utilize a robust system with almost unlimited data storage capacity to scale with client needs. Cloud-based approaches can react faster to data quality or resiliency issues, and to incorporate corrective actions to compensate for missing data in real time.

SOFTWARE AS A SERVICE (SaaS) OR
DATA AS A SERVICE (DaaS)

The topic of cloud computing leads naturally to consideration of how services are priced. This book is about understanding the technology, so this topic will not be treated in any detail. It is simply important to note that, in the past, software was sold in a "shrink wrap" packaging format. The customer purchased the software, signed a license, and it belonged to them and could be used without any other costs, until an upgrade was offered at a later date. Yet products that require cloud computing, and full range of features discussed in this book, cannot be shrink wrapped, thus a new method for product offering was created call Software as a Service (SaaS). Anno Scholten, President of Connexx, has also introduced a variation on this concept in such offerings Data as a Service (DaaS), which reinforces that these approaches to technology sales are in a continual state of flux. Regarding SaaS, the intent here is not to outline the pricing models in any detail, but rather to emphasize that managers should understand how the tool is packaged and priced. This information along with an understanding of how a suite of offerings may be combined to create the best solutions for a facility's needs, are extremely help in identifying the best tool for a specific customer.

BAS, MIDDLEWARE AND HVAC-CENTRIC SOLUTIONS

Managers who are selecting tools will note that energy and analytics solutions are being offered by a host of companies. It is important for the evaluation to begin by separating the analytics tool from the rest of that company's products and services for independent analysis. Bundling is a popular approach used by companies that combine many solutions and offer them as a solution. The first thing that may become evident by conducting independent evaluations of applications, is that some companies feel compelled to have an analytics offering, and have decided to OEM (original equipment manufacturer provided) or "white label" another company's tool. This is not a bad thing, but it will help the manager decide whether the evaluation should consider a "white label tool," or eliminate that company from consideration. In the alternative, the manager may decide to consider the tool because they believe that the company's bundled offering, including the white label analytics, brings added value that makes it desirable to acquire the tool from them. The other point that may be of interest is that some HVAC manufacturers may be implementing analytics tools specific to a piece of equipment. In this case, again the manager would want to evaluate whether to implement that company's equipment-specific analytics tool, or to integrate that functionality into a more comprehensive tool. As outlined in previous chapters, highlighting BAS and middleware, the ideal energy and analytics solution will leverage standards for networking, data modeling, etc.

DASHBOARD AND API

One critical component to user friendly energy and analytics tools is "visualization." As outlined in the earlier chapter on visualization and dashboards, this technology presents an essential window into the analytics, as well as the primary interface through which to review recommendations and reports. As noted above, the dashboard can also provide the primary vehicle for prioritizing when to address analytics recommendations. Equally important to this discussion is the topic of an application programming interface (API). APIs were discussed in the chapter on middleware and are an approach to creating "glue" to enable interface between existing systems and a web services offering. It is important to understand and develop "requirements" for the analytics tool, so that the manager can determine it is necessary to enable a secure interface for enterprise applications allowing access to more of the data found in a BAS, etc. Which is a logical segue to the last topic under this heading cyber security.

Cyber Security
The 21st century marketplace utilizes the internet and web services to offer a seemingly infinite number of offers to the market. Cyber security is a topic that is inseparable from any such service. This section will not outline how a strategy might be developed for cyber security with energy and analytics tools. Rather it will make a simple point: managers should evaluate all tools in the context of existing corporate or organizational policy relating to cyber security. Such an analysis will ensure that tools meet all usual and customary customer expectations for cyber security, while providing optimum service and performance.

Chapter 17

Financing Energy Management For Buildings and Campuses

Co-Authored with Leighton Wolffe, Northbridge Energy Partners

This chapter is expanded from an article published in *Engineered Systems Magazine* in June of 2012 by Leighton Wolffe and myself. Mr. Wolffe is a thought leader in the energy technology space with three decades of experience in direct digital control, web services and demand response. He is a partner in Northbridge Energy Partners (www.northbridgeep.com). Our goal with this article was to provide insight on the many energy related services and programs to help finance capital improvement projects and infrastructure upgrades, to achieve high performance buildings. This topic is relevant to energy and analytics because the methods of delivery for these products are diverse, and coupling analytics with an energy retrofit can be very effective. It is also relevant because the outcome of energy and analytics technology will be recommendations for operational changes to the building, but inevitably these tools will drive capital programs as well. This book has not been about the sales and marketing side of energy and analytics or, in that context, a study of pricing models and market channels for the sale and service of this technology. However, this limited treatment of the financing topic is relevant as a general overview of some options, other than self-funding, that exist for building owners to deal with the overarching capital needs they will have as they pursue higher performance, energy efficient buildings.

For facility professionals every mechanism to make capital improvement projects a reality is worthy of attention. However, this has become a rather complicated formula to master, with the array of vendors, energy suppliers, service providers, demand response companies, dashboards and analytics programs, and building automation system (BAS) manufacturers all claiming to offer critical components and comprehensive service for improvements to operations and energy efficiency. While all of these offers can bring value, it is important to begin a building self-evaluation by asking questions such as:

• Which project first?

• ECMs—how to prioritize?

• How do I finance?

• What if I choose a dead-end technology?

• How does this all get integrated together?

• How do I differentiate between Vendor A and Vendor B?

• How can I avoid getting locked in to something that does not perform?

Analytics is key to answering the first two questions, and this chapter focuses primarily on the third question about financing. The other questions will be touched on briefly here; however, they should be much easier to answer after finishing this book. It is the author's hope that information provided here will make the reader better prepared than most in the industry to answer the questions above and more. These questions are just a few of the considerations important to the stakeholders responsible for finance, operations, energy procurement, labor negotiations, risk and life safety, contract management, and other departments in facilities that influence and drive the decision making process.

As every facility and energy manager knows, without an adequate operating budget, it isn't possible to maintain buildings and equipment. Hand-in-hand with the operating budget is capital, which has been harder to assemble in recent years' economic climate, but must be available to renew and upgrade infrastructure as well as invest in analytics. In this complex environment, building owners are constrained, but open to proven business models that can have positive impacts on both budgets. Using traditional channels, the justification and approval process to get funding is a time consuming and multi-hoop endeavor even in the best of times. Elevating a typical building to "high performance" is an even more complex undertaking that requires sophisticated interoperability between dissimilar equipment and systems.

As discussed in prior chapters, access to open or standard based systems in new construction, including those who incorporate BACnet™, is not always as difficult as dealing with retrofits. In either case, the first dilemma faced by owners is choosing when to upgrade a legacy BAS system, and other building technology, and move to high-performance technologies to replace equipment. Directly related to this dilemma regarding energy and analytics is the question of what data are available from the legacy system, and would more robust data be available after an upgrade? Of course these challenges go hand-in-hand with acquisition of the analytics technology itself. The economics that support this decision process are not as clear, or well defined, as the simple ROI we are all used to—efficiencies and avoided costs after project installation equals savings that pay for the project.

The concepts of 21st century energy/electricity management and access to further smart grid capabilities, introduce new issues to consider in justifying expenditures for operational and capital improvement. When renewable energy and distributed generation resources become part of the project equation, the complexities around financial modeling increase exponentially. There have been dramatic decreases in technology cost for solar photovoltaic systems in recent years, but there is also a challenge in finding vendors that can provide these diverse offerings. If one vendor cannot provide overarching service for energy efficiency, renewable energy, DG and analytics technologies, then multiple vendors must be hired. This can add to the contractual challenges of such projects, because a new general contractor (GC) or a design build integrator must step up and take full responsibility for the project, or the manager may have to deal with a fragmented project. The price and cost of aligning the vendors can quickly outweigh the benefits. In spite of these challenges there is good news.

The good news is that a growing number of companies are providing comprehensive services. These services offer end-to-end solutions now, and are expanding to include software, hardware and web services applications to provide more solutions to the customer. These solutions consider the full energy chain from supply-side strategies selling energy, to demand-side management efficiency and capital asset management. They are beginning to also offer energy and analytics as part of the bundle. With all of these options, the questions that arise are, who is the prime vendor, what technologies do we use, how does this all fit together, and how are we going to pay for it?

In terms of a business model focusing on implementation of efficiency, renewable energy resources, DG and financing vehicles for capital upgrade projects, the energy service company (ESCO) model is perhaps the best example of a comprehensive service provider. Yet ESCOs tend to stay with status-quo measures, so they may not always be the best technology providers. The ESCO financing model however has seen a great resurgence among building owners. This is particularly true for owners who have scarce capital and/or marginal credit ratings. That said, energy services is a broad topic and includes a wide range of offerings. From a financing perspective, there are also a host of alternative financing approaches that will be discussed briefly. What is particularly desirable about the model is that it entails a combination of three critical elements to provide a design/build solution. Those elements are: 1) engineering self-funding energy measures, 2) financing based upon a revenue stream (typically from savings that are calculated and, in some cases, guaranteed) and 3) implementation. The engineering and implementation/installation elements are straightforward, but highly beneficial to managers because the design is done by energy and technology experts, who tend to have much greater expertise in these areas than architects. During this time of continuing stress on capital project funding, energy services is seeing an evolution in its financing options, beyond the "plain vanilla" versions, increasingly towards what is becoming known as ESCO 2.0.

ESCO 2.0 is a variation on the proven theme that has been called performance contracting over the past three decades. Traditionally ESCOs have brought a financing partner to the table who would structure a deal that includes construction financing and long-term debt service. The construction financing is typically handled by the same financier who provides debt service. The approach is to have the customer "close" the finance agreement, and then have the financier capitalize interest over the first six months, or install duration. Payments then begin on a certain date, so the ESCO must complete the project by that time. The actual finance vehicle may vary, but one common approach is to use equipment financing in the form of a lease purchase. Many customers buy down the first cost with cash from their own budgets, or a number of other sources, which is a good segue to ESCO 2.0. The "2.0" idea comes from Web 2.0, which according to Wikipedia "is a loosely defined intersection of web application features that facilitate participatory information sharing, interoperability, user-centered design, and collaboration on the World Wide scale." With ESCO 2.0, access to the web is critical, but the "application features" in this case are designed to access new revenue streams and create larger, more exciting capital projects. So the ESCO 2.0 phenomenon seems to be upon us, and forward looking companies have embraced it by incorporating smart grid and demand response strategies to tap into positive cash flow revenue stream that is creating a 2.0 self-funding matrix. Energy service companies or "ESCOs" are those organizations that specialize in delivering this model, but of course all ESCOs are not created equal, and it is becoming much more common for other companies to offer solutions with this same model.

This chapter is intended to reacquaint the reader with the complex topic of energy services, and to cover some of the evolution that has occurred in recent years, specifically because there is such a great opportunity to use this model to acquire energy and analytics. If the reader has not kept abreast of those changes, it is time to do so, because it could make the difference between go and no-go on your next project. This chapter will revisit the history of energy services or performance contracting, address current ESCO Best Practices and describe the Next Gen ESCO 2.0 models that are a best-kept secret.

HISTORY

Energy services may be one of the most exciting concepts to hit the energy and buildings business over the last several decades. Yet this business model, and the industry that it spawned, has experienced many transitions over that time, and recent studies of performance contracting, combined with general observations of trends, indicate that many projects are doomed to languish without it. Equally important, energy services is poised for a next wave that will be characterized by broader forms of both technology applied, i.e. energy and analytics, and financing approaches used. Integral to these new elements will be traditional efficiency coupled with demand response using the OpenADR Standard to leverage more smart grid functionality, which will contribute more dollars to the financing pool. Analytics will be critical to leveraging the greatest potential value here through detailed analysis of building demand and consumption profiles. Before exploring all of these developments however, it may be helpful to revisit the origins of this model. The energy services model has been around for decades. This method of implementing energy and capital projects originated in Europe after World War II, when it was called "chauffage." Chauffage means "heat" in French, but at that time the idea was to address two major challenges: the need to rebuild and renew war-ravaged capital infrastructure, and the need to control astronomical energy costs for building owners. Chauffage was a solution that provided building owners with real value, delivered by a third party that turn keyed the engineering, facility management and financing for projects. At the same time, the model provided entrepreneurs with the opportunity to convert the risk associated with building renewal into a viable business opportunity. The term win-win could be used because building owners got problems fixed, investors made money, and the workforce got jobs.

The concept of energy services or performance contracting came to the U.S. in the late 1970s under a different name "shared savings." Shared savings is a concept that has seen some resurgence recently, in the form of power purchase agreements (PPAs) for renewable energy. Uncertainty in the energy markets, impacted by dramatic changes in oil/gas supply and energy price drops in the mid-1980s, resulted in changes to the model. As a result of unpredictable price volatility, the industry decided that it would exit the business of speculating on energy futures and focus on engineering of self-funding projects. As a result, the energy services model came into being and is sometimes referred to as performance contracting. This could be where a story reads, "And the rest is history." However, that's not the case for performance contracting because new electricity programs from rebates to demand response are positioning the industry to enter a new frontier.

A key point with performance contracting is that the ultimate technology limiters have to do with energy cost and the enabling legislation in a particular state. (Readers who want to learn more about enabling legislation in specific states may start by visiting http://www.dsireusa. org and clicking on the states of interest.) Critical aspects of the legislation, such as the term (number of years) that is enabled for such agreements and the types of energy measures that are allowed, will define the technologies that can be implemented. By the same token, the local cost of energy (particularly electricity), and the presence of utility rebates are also factors.

There are a number of other websites containing a wealth of information available for additional research on this topic. Two websites that include great data on performance contracting are for the National Association of Energy Service Companies (NASECO), (http://www. naesco.org/index.htm) and the Energy Service Coalition (ESC) (http://

www.escperform.org/). NAESCO, the major ESCO trade association, has a website offering information to better understand the process, the pitfalls and answers to many other questions. NAESCO, ESC, and the Association of Energy Engineers offer web resources and sponsor seminars throughout the year. The ESC is a national nonprofit organization composed of experts from wide-ranging organizations working, at state and local levels, to increase the number of building energy upgrades completed through performance contracting. This organization also offers sample documents like request for proposals or performance contract documents. The ESC website also has list of providers and other industry professionals. An LBNL study that also has good basic information that may be downloaded at http://eetd.lbl.gov/ea/EMS/EMS_pubs.html.

THE NEXT WAVE

The adoption of IT-related nomenclature to describe next-generation buildings represents awareness that buildings are huge consumers of both energy, particularly electricity, and information. Among many important considerations is that buildings make up as much as half of electricity consumption in the US. The Energy Information Administration (EIA) puts buildings at 17% of US energy consumption overall, but buildings alone account for 35% of electric consumption, thus the building industry is very important to electricity companies. On the flip side, EIA data also indicate that electricity represents 75% of the energy bill for commercial buildings, and presents some real impact on occupants in a number of ways. Power outages decimate productivity, and according to a 2011 report from the Galvin Electricity Initiative, electricity outages cost the U.S. economy billions of dollars per year. Power disruptions also impact the work or learning being done in buildings and detracting the facility environment, lighting, HVAC and much more.

Targeting the energy cost metric, the first ESCO wave completely focused on efficiency and third-party financing, but the next iteration is addressing new funding opportunities from the other side of the meter. This author coined the term "electricity capital" to address this new category of funding opportunities. Electricity capital has been expanding rapidly, especially in New York and California where the closing of nuclear plants is driving these programs, but around the world as well. For example, in Japan there has been a huge emphasis here, in the post-Fukushima disaster years. The availability of electricity capital has been created because electric utilities across the United States, and around the world, are creating all sorts of mechanisms to promote implementation of buildings energy projects. There are a host of drivers including renewable portfolio standards, commission mandates, and forecasts that predict electricity demand to grow as economic recovery unfolds. These programs could grow even more as a result of the Environmental Protection Agency ruling in June of 2014, requiring power plants to reduce carbon emissions by 30% by 2030.

Among the many examples of electricity capital is that many utilities, both electric and gas, offer on-bill financing for efficiency projects including BAS. More examples were covered in Chapter 7. Quite simply, the building owner may be able to buy down the equipment cost with a rebate and then finance the balance of a BAS, analytics or other efficiency measure on the utility bill. Similarly Property Assessed Clean Energy (PACE) has been reborn as a vehicle for commercial financing of efficiency and renewable energy projects. The commercial PACE implementation varies by state, but under this approach building owners can typically finance improvements equaling up to 50% of the property value for up to 20 years, and the debt is repaid through an increase to the property tax. Of particular interest to many commercial property owners is that these improvement projects often increase the property value and net operating income, plus if the owner sells the building the new buyer takes on the debt in the form of higher real estate taxes. These programs, combined with high interest in energy and sustainability, are a boon to managers with scarce capital from traditional sources. As noted above, the financing models that are applied with any energy services agreement can remove obstacles to getting projects done.

Many ESCOs are teaming with smart grid and utility rebate experts, or are developing this knowledge in-house, to provide turn-key solutions. Of course many building automation manufacturers are already ESCOs, but more contractors are also adopting this model all the time. At the heart of all these new trends are smart building technologies, energy and analytics and other cloud-based software applications to enable the building to save more and fund projects. These technologies also make it possible to visualize building conditions and metrics at all times to validate the performance.

Electricity capital also includes programs like demand response

(DR) that pay customers to respond to curtailment events through deployment of strategies in the BAS to shed load, or shut down electrical equipment. OpenADR™ is the standard developed at Lawrence Berkley Labs, which many are aware of, but exhibitors at far ranging events including AHR Expo, Niagara Summit, Realcomm/IBcon, and the World Energy Engineering Congress are touting their ability to integrate OpenADR into BAS just like BACnet™ or LON™. Some manufacturers provide pre-programmed demand response algorithms, working with customers to deploy DR creating a revenue stream to fund a BAS. One DR provider has completed projects with multi-location customers that are paying for DR enablement and a new BAS with electricity capital. Under this model the owner gets technology installed with no upfront cost and is able to finance the deployment and repay it through DR payments from the utility over time. These trends are likely to continue as coal-fired power plants are shut down.

Certainly no one disputes the ESCO 1.0 business model—efficiency investments made by building owners are "bankable" and cost effective. These investments also help utilities, but only with one of their two concerns. When considering electricity, there are two important topics; energy use and energy demand. Efficiency helps utilities with energy use, and it makes sense to optimize building energy consumption because it reduces operating cost. In addition, with the end of the recession, electric demand is again growing, as discussed under the Energy Triple Threat. At the same time, emerging electricity markets present new utility concerns, and most building owners are unaware of the financial benefits that may exist in their utility territory. Those managers with graying temples remember demand limiting, etc. from the 1980s, but that's just part of the story. It is a shock that ~25% the multi-billion dollar electric infrastructure (power plants, transmission and distribution lines, etc.) exists to keep the lights on for ~100 hours/year. That's because the monopoly electricity business model has traditionally set one price for units of power, $/kWh, no matter when it is consumed. The demand charge, $/kW, is applied to commercial bills with loads about a certain limit, but that does not begin to match wholesale electric price volatility before, during, and after periods of peak electric use. ESCO 2.0 is about tapping into fees that utilities are willing to pay the owner for developing strategies to support the utility in keeping the lights on. ESCO projects have typically generated two types of savings, "energy" and "operations and maintenance." The 2.0 model will generate a new type cash flow, which is not "savings" but "income." Demand response is an example of this income that has been widely embraced, but that is just the beginning. Utilizing the same technology that has been put in place to enable demand response, many electricity users have begun to offer capacity back to the grid at peak times... for a price. The customer is paid a price that translates to electricity income. What makes ESCO 2.0 exciting is that these income strategies combined with savings strategies can create the opportunity for larger and more exciting ESCO projects

A key point here is that the 2.0, in ESCO 2.0, is first an indicator that this is truly a next generation business model. Central to this model however, is also the deployment of next generation technologies. ESCO 2.0 will provide a mechanism to achieve smart buildings, and with the energy techno-strategies deployed by local, and cloud-based technology, such as energy and analytics. With these advanced technologies, buildings can become energy profit centers by participating in both efficiency and the electricity markets. Quite simply, ESCO 2.0 will be made up of smart buildings that use energy in clean, efficient and cost effective ways and are therefore green buildings, but more importantly they are green in the environmental sense, as well as in the economic sense. Those buildings that integrate more functionality for energy services opportunity will benefit from more robust participation. ESCO 1.0 buildings often overlooked the smart clean tech implementation, but 2.0 will start with commissioned buildings that have effectively operated BAS, electric sub-metering, dashboard technology to visualize building performance and analytics to evaluate performance over time and develop benchmarks for comparison. Buildings enabled like this can participate in demand response (DR) immediately by implementing technology to receive electronic "event notifications," via the OpenADR standard, when demand response events are called. The building then reacts to that event by modifying equipment operation to reduce an agreed upon number of kW. Programs vary in the amount of notice that customers receive, usually "day ahead," "day of" or "10-minute" notice. Programs also vary in the amount of money paid for participation but customers typically receive payments between $50 and $1,000 per kW, but it can be higher. For example, a 200 kW enrollment would net an annual payment between $10,000 and $200,000 per year. With most programs the customer gets paid whether an event is called or not, and in California the utilities will even pay to install the technology. That all sounds pretty good, but these programs are evolving and expanding. As noted above, this same smart grid/DR technology can be used to enable customers to sell back, to electric markets, electricity they agree not to use. The author has called this "day trading for energy," and it gives customers another way to leverage financial value from the electricity system. Adding this income to the arbitrage mix will create even larger projects.

At first, building owners may think this is too complicated and maybe it's not worth it. The same could have been said of many technologies that are now widely used, when they were first available. That could also be said of green building recognition systems that have become the norm. Even more compelling, customers that leverage these technologies and programs effectively, can literally spin the meter backwards, while at the same time leveraging third-party capital and making debt service with REC payments from the utility and cost reduction on energy bills while optimizing building performance and tenant comfort. The ideal scenario is when customers go farther and expand building technologies to include energy storage—thermal or battery, on-site/distributed generation, or what are now called "microgrids." The idea is to take the electric reliability challenges faced in many parts of the country, and apply entrepreneurship to turn buildings into profit centers for energy. Demand response (DR) is relatively established in many parts of the country and is paying dividends for many building owners, but the next step is to insulate the tenants from any inconvenience that might be caused by DR. This is done by leveraging automation systems to pre-cool for example, focusing strategies on shutting down nonessential equipment, and leveraging on-site generation, but numerous other options exist. Using advanced DR and OpenADR based technology, owners can also aggregate across multiple buildings and opt in or opt out based on what is going on in the building. A depiction of such a building is provided below and comes from the Electric Power Research Institutes "Green Grid" report, which may be downloaded free at: www.epri.com/abstracts/pages/productabstract.aspx?ProductID=000000000001016905. Figure 17-1 shows the myriad technologies that are being applied with buildings of all sizes.

The challenge in today's economy is finding ways to fund the technologies shown in the green grid graph, and ESCO 2.0 may well be the answer. Equally exciting is that owners can leverage the intelligence deployed in these systems to make performance repeatable, and to apply energy and analytics tools that make it possible to evaluate the project in real time, not just once a year. All of these ideas mean that ESCO 2.0

Figure 17-1

amounts to free money and no one can afford to turn that down.

The importance of the smart grid to buildings has become both real and beneficial for building managers who are getting paid to participate in demand response. Yet the smart grid, in a broader context, represents an opportunity for new building revenue streams, allowing them to become virtual power plants and energy profit centers. It is about transforming the electricity business model to unlock capital and operating cost benefits for building owners. Energy efficiency and green buildings, along with their respective benefits, have become second nature to facility professionals in the last decade, but demand response, and ultimately the smart grid, can unleash even more benefits. A great example of this fact is the launch of PEER by the United States Green Building Council, as discussed in Chapter 7. What building owners should know:

• The difference between demand response and the smart grid;

• Why it is happening;

• How buildings can benefit; and

• What it costs to play.

These questions will be answered in closing this chapter.

Figure 17-2 depicts some smart grid basics. By definition, a smart grid is an interconnected system of information and communication technologies, and electricity generation, transmission, distribution and end use technologies which will enable consumers (in this case building owners) to manage their usage and choose the most economically efficient offering, while maintaining delivery system reliability and stability enhanced by automation and environmentally optimal generation alternatives including renewable generation and energy storage. That is a bit of a mouthful, though it gets to the heart of what is underway, but why? The best way to explain this is to start with a question: What would happen if Alexander Graham Bell and Thomas Edison came back to life tomorrow and observed the industries they were instrumental in creating? If Bell were handed an iPhone™ and asked to make a call, he would not know how to do it. Edison on the other hand would be able to explain, in fairly technical detail, how every aspect of today's electric system works, even though Tesla promoted what became today's alternating current (AC)-based grid. It has not changed in ~100 years!

Bob Galvin, former chairman of Motorola and founder of the Galvin Electricity Initiative became very focused on this topic late in his

Figure 17-2

life. Mr. Galvin was instrumental in starting the cell phone industry, and he compared electricity in 2010 to telecom in the early 1980s—a monopoly business model, pent up need for innovation, and no way to unleash entrepreneurial business models. Speaking of business models, demand response (DR) and the OpenADR standard have proven to be killer aps in the buildings space. The term killer AP may be overused, but getting paid to implement a control strategy is pretty exciting. The OpenADR standard was developed at Lawrence Berkley National Laboratories, and it is in the vanguard of initial Smart Grid Standards to be mandated by the Federal Energy Regulatory Commission. More exciting, OpenADR is integral to demand response programs across the country, and as noted, utilities in states like California will even pay building owners to conduct a DR audit and then install the DR-enabling technology. In California, OpenADR is required for those projects. After technology is installed, the utility will continue to pay the customer every month to execute the strategies that are put in place... if needed. That is DR and OpenADR, but why smart grid? Because the electric industry is dangerously outdated and, equally alarming, the grid is increasingly unreliable. That is why power outages cost US businesses billions of dollars per year. August 14, 2003, was the day that brought this issue to the attention of congress and the American public. On that day the entire US eastern seaboard went dark from a massive power outage. This was not an isolated event; outages continue to occur regularly—thankfully, not on that scale— but with significant impacts. So aging infrastructure and an antiquated business model, along with escalating demand for electricity by our digital economy, all contribute to the reasons why the smart grid has been so important. If it could be said that there was anything good about the economic downturn, it was that electric providers got a reprieve from load growth, since electric use was down due to businesses closing, etc. But demand for electricity is growing again. A few years before the downturn, the Department of Energy was projecting a 40% increase in electric demand over 20 years, and that it would cost ~\$1 trillion to build new infrastructure to keep the lights on, and those investments are still needed. Utilities and state commissions will be hard pressed to justify rate increases to fund needed investments in electric infrastructure. So they will turn to energy users with new electricity programs. Demand response is one key way to hedge against the speed at which new infrastructure must be built. Regardless, the building owner is more concerned with creative ways to meet operations and capital needs, and ESCO 2.0 is a great way to support that effort.

Again the term win-win could be applied to ESCO 2.0 because it will help renew building infrastructure and enhance electricity resilience, while hedging the need to build new grid systems. ESCO 2.0 will also support transition from fossil fuels as well as cost savings from efficiency. In closing, the term "ESCO 2.0" could be replaced with "creative financing," "electricity capital," etc. The term is not important, rather the recognition that there are a host of financing alternatives that will benefit building managers.

Chapter 18

Analytics for Measurement and Verification

There are a tremendous number of applications for energy and analytics. Many such uses have been covered throughout the book, but one that is worthy of some additional discussion is measurement and verification (M&V). Given the previous chapter on ESCO 2.0 and the many other types of financing that are being used in the buildings space, M&V is critical. Of course M&V is equally as critical when building owners self-finance energy efficiency, renewable energy and other capital investments as well. The goal of this chapter is to introduce how analytics is a game changer for M&V, but equally important how the practice of M&V could morph to incorporate commissioning and become "continuous improvement for energy management." Throughout this book, there has been extensive discussion of fault detection and diagnostics (FD&D), and a host of other analytics strategies that produce cost savings, while also providing operational benefits to improve the mission of organization inside the buildings themselves. M&V represents another potential application for analytics and is a significant topic in itself. The purpose of this chapter is to explore the idea of M&V using analytics and highlight three topics:

- M&V definition and discussion of how analytics can support the effort.

- Analytics as a stimulus that could cause the science of M&V to morph with the science of commissioning, providing a science that both evaluates performance of capital investments, and optimizes the overall building and its systems performance.

- M&V/optimization in 21st century electric markets

Analytics for conventional M&V is important to managers/owners who make a capital investment and want to ensure that the products or services purchased are producing the expected results. The science of conducting analysis to evaluate such investments is called measurement and verification (M&V), and there is an international protocol on these processes. This chapter cannot cover this topic in great detail, but it can make the point that analytics is the ideal technology for conducting M&V. It is the intent here to provide some general background on M&V and provide the reader with some insight as to how energy and analytics can offer far-reaching functionality that they may not have initially realized.

MEASUREMENT AND VERIFICATION (M&V) SCIENCE

The International Performance Measurement and Verification Protocol (IPMVP) defines the science of M&V and provides an overview of best practice techniques available for verifying results of energy efficiency, water efficiency, and renewable energy projects. It may also be used by facility operators to assess and improve facility performance. The IPMVP began as an effort by the U.S. Department of Energy and Lawrence Berkley National Laboratories in 1994 to establish international consensus on methods to determine energy/water efficiency savings and thus promote third-party investment in energy efficiency projects. It was ultimately published under the name International Performance Measurement and Verification Protocol (IPMVP) in 1997, and seen several updated versions. The IPMVP organization grew and expanded its service offerings leading the board of IPMVP Inc. to change the name of the non-profit corporation to the Efficiency Valuation Organization (EVO) in 2004.

Capital investments related to energy in buildings and plants often include multiple individual projects, often called retrofits. Individual retrofit projects are often called energy conservation measures (ECMs). ECM is a term that usually describes one individual project, retrofit or activity that is completed in a building or plant, such as a lighting retrofit or replacement of an antiquated chiller with a high efficiency model. Of course the savings produced from multiple ECMs are typically cumulative, and they may include energy and operational cost reductions as well as qualitative operational factors that help improve how well the building accommodates the work being done there. In the 21st century energy marketplace that has been discussed throughout this book, the measures that are combined to form a project will likely encompass more than energy/water efficiency and renewable energy. There are a host of measures incorporated into projects today that straddle the demand and supply sides of the electricity system. Such measures include, but are not limited to, fuel saving, water efficiency, load shifting, demand response, participating in capacity markets for electricity, and energy reductions through installation or retrofit of equipment, and/or modification of operating procedures. Of course the savings typically include operational cost reductions as well as energy. Therefore EVO recommends that the design of a measurement and verification (M&V) plan must consider approaches that best align with: i) project costs and savings magnitude, ii) technology-specific requirements, and iii) risk allocation between buyer and seller, i.e., which party is responsible for installed equipment performance and which party is responsible for achieving long-term energy savings.

EVO has received extensive user feedback over the years and each updated version has sought to provide greater internal consistency, more precise definition of M&V options, and treatment of additional issues. The specific application of IPMVP is to measure and verify performance of projects improving energy or water efficiency in buildings and industrial plants. The current version of IPMVP is divided into three separate volumes: Volume I Concepts and Options for Determining Savings, Volume II Indoor Environmental Quality (IEQ) Issues, and Volume III Applications. More detail on content by volume is provide below.

- Volume I—Concepts and Options for Determining Savings
  — Defines basic M&V terminology
  — General procedures to achieve reliable and cost-effective determination of savings
  — Applicable to energy or water efficiency projects in buildings and industrial plants

- Volume II—Concepts and Practices for Improving IEQ
  — Reviews IEQ issues that can be influenced by an energy efficiency project
  — Focuses on maintaining acceptable indoor conditions under an energy efficiency project

- Volume III—Specific Applications
  — M&V of Renewable Energy Systems
  — M&V in New Construction

— Emissions Reduction from Energy Efficiency and Renewable Energy Projects

Verification of savings is then done relative to the M&V Plan for the project. The IPMVP also makes provisions for definitions to be customized for each project, with the help of other resources.

In the context of energy and analytics, what is most important to consider is the IPMVP option that is selected by the manager/owner. Table 18-1 summarizes the M&V options that may be considered.

Most energy managers believe that the utility revenue meter is the great equalizer in determining whether energy savings have been achieved. This is particularly true when law or customer circumstances require that savings are guaranteed (in energy units or dollars), and that the financial value of savings provides the necessary cash flow from savings that is necessary to meet debt payments. This balance of savings

Table 18-1. M&V Options

M&V Option	Measurement Requirements	Basis of Savings Calculations
Option A –\n\nPartially Measured\n\nRetrofit Isolation	Combination of measured & stipulated factors. Spot or short-term measurements at component or system level. Stipulated factor is supported by historical or manufacturer's data.	Engineering calculations, component or system models
Option B –\n\nRetrofit Isolation	Spot or short-term measurements at component or system level for constant loads. Based on continuous measurements taken at the component or system level for variable loads.	Engineering calculations, component or system models
Option C –\n\nWhole Facility	Based on long-term whole-building utility meter, facility level, or sub-metered data.	Regression analysis of utility billing meter data.

vs. debt service can be precarious and of course the vendors providing services cannot control utility rates. So if savings must be at or below debt service, vendors will typically base projects on 80% to 85% of calculated savings. This means that the project is designed to hedge savings and make provisions for utility rate increases, severe weather years, some variation in occupancy, etc. Bear in mind that the use of a building is in continual flux; changes in a host of operating factors, including occupancy, must be evaluated over time to determine whether they have impacted savings. This can be more complex when dealing with campus complexes, but in those cases utility consumption baselines must be developed on a building-by-building basis to form the basis for energy savings, and M&V must be conducted on each building. A final note on IPMVP and Option C is that it assumes regression analysis on bills from the utility and based upon readings from the revenue meter. The promise of energy and analytics for M&V is twofold: 1) the revenue meter data may be complemented by interval meters for demand and consumption, and 2) this analysis can be completed electronically and available on at least a monthly basis. M&V is expensive, it is highly labor intensive and generally must be done by energy engineers, so it is usually only done on an annual basis. If a project goes off the rails early in the year, and you don't find out about a problem until months later, the outcome could be catastrophic. Coupling energy and analytics with the human expertise of certified energy managers could be a significant advancement for M&V.

ENERGY AND ANALYTICS

Again there is a data quality benefit and a timing benefit offered to M&V by analytics. These benefits can be significant to energy managers in their quest to optimize performance, control cost, and find new ways to leverage greater value from that asset. Analytics is exciting because it is a technology-rich discipline which requires professionals who understand every aspect of building operations along with the complex technology deployed. As discussed, these building technologies include metering, building automation systems (BAS), dashboards, middleware, web services/energy services tools, and these are all sources of data for analytics. Of course content knowledge is critical to analytics success; this is why M&V is normally conducted by engineers. Even with more robust comparative data from direct data access to the revenue meter or sophisticated sub-metering, it takes a trained eye to pick up some anomalies. The analytics tools can be trained to identify and report on many types of anomalies, but the ultimate question remains to be answered. What caused the anomaly and how can it be corrected? Doing the research and analysis to answer these questions requires the content expert.

Energy and analytics, as a market and a technology, are in a state of rapid growth, and enhancements are occurring at a high rate of speed. One exciting thing about this technology is that it can is being enhanced on an ongoing basis. For example, if an energy meter shows a high consumption or electric demand reading for January compared to the baseline and past months, including past Januarys, that is an anomaly. Initially the analytics tool may just flag the anomaly, but enhancements would allow the system to access data on occupancy, lighting and HVAC runtime, ancillary loads such as elevators or parking lot lights and a host of other factors that could explain the anomaly. For any particular building type, the data evaluated can be tailored to the application, and then the analytics tool can be upgraded to incorporate algorithms that look for anomalies. Coppertree analytics, a leader in this market, recently reported an excellent example of such an algorithm. In a customer's facility, the tool identified a high electric meter reading and executed a series of analyses, which identified that the parking lot lights in a 200,000-sq.-ft. parking structure were on 24/7. The tool identified the problem and the cause, so that the building owner could correct it by returning the lighting to automated control.

On a broader basis, energy and analytics can be linked with continuous commissioning for HVAC and other systems for optimization, as part of the fault, diagnostics and detection application identified in Chapter 1. The intent of this strategy would be to ensure that the facility is operating as expected by the owner and tenants. Accomplishing that goal would produce a real "mission benefit." Mission benefit means that the space is providing the expected environment for the work being done by occupants, a very important thing. For example the Building Operators and Managers Association (BOMA) has conducted surveys of tenants for decades. One of the questions on the survey is, Did you move to a new space and if so, why? Usually at the top of the list or in the top 3 for tenants who move is that the building was uncomfortable. Uncomfortable buildings are usually inefficient, so using analytics drives two benefits: cost savings (energy, O&M, etc.) and mission benefits (tenant retention, etc.). The value of optimizing building operations and energy management can be huge. This is particularly true for electricity, use and cost. Electricity is the highest quality form of energy, and is essential for a 21st century quality of life, including education, business and entertainment technology. Electric energy cost also represents one of the largest controllable operation expense in commercial buildings. Combine those facts with those of a recent report from Next 10, predicting that buildings will make up 80 percent of projected growth in energy consumption between now and 2040, and it means that the time for energy and analytics is now. Regarding analytics and commissioning, the U.S. Environmental Protection Agency (EPA) EnergyStar Program published "A Retrocomissioning Guide for Building Owners" in 2007. That guide pointed out that interval data coupled with energy analytics can help to change the game for retro-commissioning. Granular consumption data can provide a detailed view into a building's energy use. Applying energy analytics to historic data can help detect opportunities related to a building's operations and systems in minutes, without ever going on-site. Many utilities are also beginning to pay rebates for this technology and service as well.

M&V IN 21ST CENTURY ELECTRIC MARKETS

The topic of M&V has broadened beyond verification of projects, in the new energy markets. First the process of establishing baselines, consumption profiles and benchmarks has taken on a new role for energy procurement including electricity and natural gas. Understanding how and when buildings consume energy is fundamental to negotiating energy purchasing contracts. Yet that is just the start in these new markets. The same tools that are used for M&V are often required for project verification with energy rebate programs. Most utilities require engineering analyses prior to approval of the rebate, but there are those that will require post-install M&V as well.

M&V techniques are also critical to demand response (DR) programs. Again it is critical with DR to understand consumption profiles, but also to track interval data on electricity demand. These data must then be analyzed together with an understanding of building operations and occupancy to determine whether to enroll in DR. The meter, as with IPMVP Option C, is the ultimate arbiter in DR programs. Utilities will pay enrolled customers at the agreed upon price, whether there is a DR event or not, but if an event is called and the customer does not respond there will be consequences. Consequences could mean a renegotiation of the contract, departure from the program or something else, but these issues are handled on a case-by-case basis. Therefore it is critical to have a robust M&V program. There are two final points on DR: 1) demand limiting and 2) fine tuning. Many energy managers believe that demand limiting is a better approach than DR. If it is possible to shed load on notice, during the highest period of consumption, shouldn't the manager do it every day? This is a philosophical question that will not be debated here, but may be worth some thought. The second point is DR fine tuning, which is the process of integrating DR with M&V of projects and other internal energy management programs. For example, if fluorescent light dimming was one of the strategies being used for DR and the facility is retrofitted to LED lighting, how does that impact DR commitments? This would be true if high efficiency chillers, BAS or other measure are installed as well. Generally speaking, it becomes harder to participate in DR as the building becomes more and more efficient.

The last topic under this heading relates to managing distributed generation (DG) and participation in electricity capacity markets. The basis for both of these activities is the same as described for DR, however there are some differences for each. With distributed generation, the first consideration is system type which could include solar photovoltaics, micro-turbines, combined heat and power (CHP), etc. and going forward the term will likely morph to encompass some form of electricity storage as well. Also of interest, recent EPA rules allow diesel-fired emergency generators to run up to 100 hours per year for DR. In any case effective management of DG requires an understanding of characteristics for the equipment types installed, plus interval data and consumption profiles to determine if the equipment is operated continuously or is started based on conditions. These are complex topics that will not be covered further here, but developing techniques using some form of M&V can be extremely valuable in planning and implementing these technologies.

It should be clear that the topics of M&V and analytics are, or should be, intertwined. These independent disciplines can inform development and enhancements for one another. The reader is encouraged to follow developments with the EVO and the IPMVP as the science of energy and analytics evolves. Knowledge in both of these domains will undoubtedly prove very useful.

Part III—Analytics Success Stories

James M. Lee, CEO Cimetrics, Inc.

Turning data into value—that has long been the promise of analytics technology. Although applying analytics to building technology is only about 15 years old, it has already reached a level of maturity where it is beginning to produce striking results. This section contains a collected cross section of examples of analytics applied to building systems. These case studies demonstrate the technology, business process and value creation that analytics applications are bringing to the field.

In the beginning, analytics applied to building systems focused primarily on energy efficiency. Over time, people realized that energy is only one of many value propositions offered by analytics, and the technology developed to include ongoing commissioning, predictive maintenance, contractual compliance (vendor management), regulatory compliance, sustainability and comfort.

As the applications for analytics expanded, it became clear that applying this technology to building systems is a classically disruptive technology, radically reshaping competition and strategy in both the construction and operation of buildings. Power is shifting from the traditional construction and operation contractors to building owners. The information allows both transparency and accountability in an industry which has traditionally been opaque. Building operators now have key performance indicators about the health of their buildings. This new technology has created a win/win situation whereby the owner/operator, automation and mechanical subcontractors and commissioning providers can all profit while improving energy efficiency, comfort and sustainable performance of the building. Owners have seen approximately a 20% energy efficiency improvement, while traditional contractors profit from making repairs and upgrades to the existing systems.

The case studies in this section demonstrate these concepts and practices, showing the potential of analytics to change the face of building construction and operation.

Chapter 19

88 Acres—
The Microsoft Energy and
Analytics Success Story

This book's author would like to thank Microsoft Corporation and Darrell Smith, Microsoft's director of facilities and energy, for allowing this document to be reprinted as a chapter here. The 88 Acres story was written by Jennifer Warnick and has been published on the internet and elsewhere, highlighting this exciting project. It has also been the topic of numerous articles, speeches and presentations demonstrating the exciting advances that the Microsoft team has made with energy, analytics and buildings. Hearty thanks are due to Jim Young and Howard Berger of Realcomm/IBcon for introducing McGowan to Darrell Smith and providing a venue to learn about the exploits achieved by the Microsoft team. As with other success stories, readers are encouraged to pursue outside research to identify recent developments.

A small, covert team of engineers at Microsoft cast aside suggestions that the company spend US$60 million to turn its 500-acre headquarters into a smart campus to achieve energy savings and other efficiency gains. Instead, applying an "Internet of Things meets Big Data" approach, the team invented a data-driven software solution that is slashing the cost of operating the campus' 125 buildings. The software, which is saving Microsoft millions of dollars, has been so successful that the company, and its partners, are now helping building managers across the world deploy the same solution. With commercial buildings consuming an estimated 40 percent of the world's total energy, the potential is huge.

THE VISIONARY

"Give me a little data and I'll tell you a little. Give me a lot of data and I'll save the world."
—*Darrell Smith, Director of Facilities and Energy, Microsoft*

"This is my office," says the sticker on Darrell Smith's laptop, and it is. With his "office" tucked under his arm, Microsoft's director of facilities and energy is constantly shuttling between meetings all over the company's 500-acre, wooded campus in Redmond, Washington.

But Smith always returns to one unique place. The Redmond Operations Center (often called "the ROC") is located in a drab, nondescript office park. Inside is something unique—a new state-of-the-art "brain" that is transforming Microsoft's 125-building, 41,664-employee headquarters into one of the smartest corporate campuses in the world.

Smith and his team have been working for more than three years to unify an incongruent network of sensors from different eras (think several decades of different sensor technology and dozens of manufacturers). The software that he and his team built strings together thousands of building sensors that track things like heaters, air conditioners, fans, and lights—harvesting billions of data points per week. That data has given the team deep insights, enabled better diagnostics, and has allowed for far more intelligent decision making. A test run of the program in 13 Microsoft buildings has provided staggering results—not only has Microsoft saved energy and millions in maintenance and utility costs, but the company now is hyper-aware of the way its buildings perform.

It's no small thing—whether a damper is stuck in Building 75 or a valve is leaky in Studio H—that engineers can now detect (and often fix with a few clicks) even the tiniest issues from their high-tech dashboard at their desks in the ROC rather than having to jump into a truck to go find and fix the problem in person.

If the facility management world were Saturday morning cartoons, Smith and his team have effectively flipped the channel from "The Flintstones" to "The Jetsons." Instead of using stone-age rocks and hammers to keep out the cold, Smith's team invented a solution that relies on data to find and fix problems instantly and remotely. "Give me a little data and I'll tell you a little," he says. "Give me a lot of data and I'll save the world."

Smith joined Microsoft in December of 2008. His previous work managing data centers for Cisco had given him big ideas about how buildings could be smarter and more efficient, but until he came to Microsoft he lacked the technical resources to bring them to life. What he found at Microsoft was support for these ideas on all sides—from his boss to a handful of savvy facilities engineers. They all knew buildings could be smarter, and together they were going to find a way to make it so.

Smith has a finger-tapping restlessness that prevents him from sitting through an entire movie. His intensity comes paired with the enthusiastic, genial demeanor of a favorite bartender or a softball buddy (and indeed, he does play first base for a company softball team, the Microsoft Misfits).

Ever punctual and an early riser, Smith lives near Microsoft headquarters and has taken to spending a few quiet hours at his desk on Sundays.

"I call it my den because I live a mile away. I come here, I make coffee, I have the building to myself," Smith says.

His family and the people who know him best understand. Smart buildings are his passion, and everything in his life has been moving toward finding ways for companies the world over to get smarter about managing their buildings (which will help them save money and reduce their energy use).

"Smart buildings will become smart cities," Smith says. "And smart cities will change everything."

88 ACRES IN A ONE-STOPLIGHT TOWN

Today Microsoft may have one of the smartest corporate campuses in the world, but in 1986, its headquarters was still a grass- and forest-covered 88-acre plot of land in Redmond, a sleepy, one-stoplight suburb of Seattle.

Back then, there wasn't even a store in town to buy underwear, and from city hall you'd have to walk to the grocery store for lunch because the nearest fast food restaurant was too far away, says Judd Black, who has worked for the Redmond planning department for 26 years.

"Redmond and Microsoft, we've grown up together, and we've learned from each other quite a bit," Black says. "We've both worked to

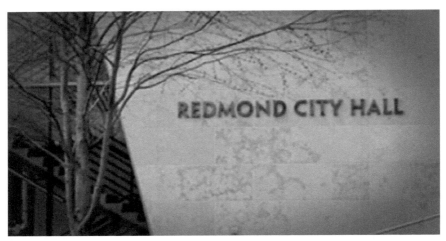

Figure 19-1

create a great place for people to work and live."

The 88 acres of land Microsoft chose for its headquarters (the code name for the project was just that: 88 Acres) was originally supposed to be a shopping center, but that plan was bagged during hard economic times. Microsoft snapped up the land and quickly constructed its first office complex—four star-shaped buildings surrounding Lake Bill (a large pond affectionately named by employees for founder and then-CEO Bill Gates).

Business was booming, and construction on campus followed—so quickly that Microsoft initially didn't have deeply defined construction standards. To meet demand, the company had to work with a variety of contractors and construction schedules, so consequently Microsoft's 125 buildings were constructed in a variety of styles and configurations. By the time Microsoft instituted comprehensive building standards in the 1990s, a large portion of the campus was already built.

Microsoft's campus would become the size of a small city—a city within a growing city. Redmond was expanding as well, and soon a quarter of its residents were Microsoft employees.

Today the campus spans 500 acres. There's a soccer field and cricket pitch, miles of wooded walking paths—and 14.9 million square feet of office space and labs that now function as one interconnected system.

It wasn't always that way.

Until recently, Microsoft was using disparate building management systems to manage 30,000 unconnected, sensor-enabled pieces of equipment. Imagine a symphony orchestra, but with every musician playing from different sheet music. Then, imagine trying to conduct that symphony—to make sure the music was on tempo, in key, and starting and stopping as it should. Microsoft's buildings were experiencing data dissonance that would make the works of Igor Stravinsky sound like a barbershop quartet.

Smith's team was on a journey to find harmony.

When Smith, Jay Pittenger (Smith's boss), and others started exploring ways to manage buildings smartly, they realized it would cost upward of $60 million to "rip and replace" enough equipment to get those 30,000 sensors to whistle the same tune.

This would not only involve costly construction and equipment replacement, but it also would mean displacing employees and losing work while teams temporarily shut down labs. Smith and team knew there had to be a less pricey, less disruptive way to achieve data harmony, but after a whole lot of looking, they couldn't find one.

So they invented one.

Smith's team enlisted the help of three vendors in the field of commercial building data systems and created a pilot program in 13 of the buildings on Microsoft's Redmond campus. The team developed an "analytical blanket" to lie on top of the diverse systems used to manage the buildings. The blanket of software finally enabled equipment and buildings to talk to each other, and to provide a wealth of data to building managers.

"It hasn't been a bowl of cherries—my hair wasn't as gray before we started," Smith says. "The challenge with building systems is that they can create a lot of chatter from multiple systems, but there's value there if you connect and capture it. It's all about the data. If you can't get data out of the buildings, you're done."

The new tool *did* get data out of the buildings—great tidal waves of data that came cascading into the ROC, telling engineers about everything from wasteful lighting schedules to hugely inefficient (but up until then, silent and undetectable) battles being waged between air conditioners and heaters to keep temperatures pleasant.

In one building garage, exhaust fans had been mistakenly left on for a year (to the tune of $66,000 of wasted energy). Within moments of coming online, the smart buildings solution sniffed out this fault and the problem was corrected.

In another building, the software informed engineers about a pressurization issue in a chilled water system. The problem took less than five minutes to fix, resulting in $12,000 of savings each year.

Those fixes were just the beginning.

Suddenly, the symphony of sensors was not only following the conductor, its musicians were all playing the same song. As buildings came online and data poured in, it created what engineers called a "target-rich environment" for problem solving. Smith and the team soon expanded the pilot to a handful of additional buildings, and by summer's end they plan to have the whole Redmond campus online.

The team now collects 500 million data transactions every 24 hours, and the smart buildings software presents engineers with prioritized lists of misbehaving equipment. Algorithms can balance out the cost of a fix in terms of money and energy being wasted with other factors such as how much impact fixing it will have on employees who work in that building. Because of that kind of analysis, a lower-cost problem in a research lab with critical operations may rank higher priority-wise than a higher-cost fix that directly affects few. Almost half of the issues the system identifies can be corrected in under a minute, Smith says.

The change has created groundbreaking opportunities for Smith and his team.

"Our conversations have changed," Smith says. "Before, the calls we got were about buildings being too hot or too cold, or about work orders. Now we're talking about data points and building faults and energy usage. We're seeing efficiencies that we never even contemplated when we started this journey."

THE LIVING, BREATHING BUILDING

Tearle Whitson and Jonathan Grove stroll across the rooftop of Microsoft's Building 88. Washington State's Cascade Mountains.

"This is one of the perks of the job," says Whitson, taking a moment to survey the scene before climbing into the whirring, dark interior of one of the roof's large, white air handlers. As nice as they can be, now rooftop field trips like this are few and far between.

Whitson and Grove have experienced a seismic shift in their workday since helping to develop Microsoft's smart buildings tool. Two years ago the two spent a lot of time climbing over rooftops, inspecting pump rooms, and peering above ceiling tiles at variable air volume (VAV) boxes.

"I used to spend 70 percent of my time gathering and compiling data and only about 30 percent of my time doing engineering," Grove says. "Our smart buildings work serves up data for me in easily consumable formats, so now I get to spend 95 percent of my time doing engineering, which is great."

Before Microsoft's buildings leapt up the IQ curve, the duo's home was on the so-called range. They'd move from building to building, camping out in each for two weeks at a time to inspect and tune it top to bottom before moving on to the next. It would take them five years to tune up all of the buildings on campus, and then they'd start the process all over again. Their tune-ups were making the buildings run more efficiently, saving the company around $250,000 annually—but the new data gold rush will help them save six times that much.

The duo now spends most of their time at the ROC, chewing on building data. Though they're no longer camping out together tuning up Microsoft's campus the old-fashioned way, the two have maintained the comfortable rapport and geeky banter they established working in the field.

Figure 19-2

Facilities engineers like Whitson and Grove think of the buildings they care for as living, breathing things. Just like the human body, buildings have a wealth of indicators that things are going well—or, in some cases, not so well. Also like the human body, small ailments can lead to much larger failures, and an ounce of prevention can lead to many pounds of cure.

And now, with the new data-driven software solution that the team built, they can do an even better job of managing the health of Microsoft's buildings—they've gone from country doctors, tapping a patient's knees with a rubber hammer, to specialists with an MRI machine who can examine every layer of the knee inside and out.

Still, Whitson says it can be a tad unnerving to take a building and its network of sensors online and watch as the software immediately discovers a host of inefficiencies.

"There is a little bit of a mindset among facilities engineers. Everybody is prideful, and they take such ownership of their buildings, that it's hard for them to find out that there was a lot that they were missing. It was a humbling lesson I had to learn early on while doing this," Whitson says. "We have to get the old-school technicians out there to understand that this is going to help them. This is not to say you've been doing it wrong—you're doing fine. But you can go farther."

Both are quick to tell you that Microsoft's smart buildings solution has revolutionized the way they and their fellow engineers work.

"We had the perfect environment and people to put all the pieces together. Our solution is a little unique to Microsoft, but very applicable industry-wide," Grove says.

ENOUGH DATA TO CHANGE THE WORLD

The ROC itself looks like an air-traffic control tower—albeit without the windows.

A bevy of large, wall-mounted displays wrap around the interior of the room, and the same monitors sit atop every desk. The smart buildings tool dashboard is splashed across many of the screens, showing off a colorful collection of maps, dials, lists, and tickers.

Engineers can get big-picture information at a glance, like how many kilowatts of energy are being consumed across Microsoft headquarters at any one moment. With a few clicks they can also zoom in on one building, one floor or office in that building, or one piece of equipment.

"Let's see how City Center building is doing today," Whitson says, and within seconds he's clicking through a wealth of information about the building—the number of employees who work there, the outside air temperature, the thermostat, what time the lights come on and go off, even a list of mechanical inefficiencies the software has detected and how much each of those faults is costing the company per year.

Once Whitson sits down in front of one of the terminals, he is suddenly connected to Microsoft's buildings. Those 500 million data transactions per day can be accessed from the dashboard at his desk rather than from crawling through pump rooms or across rooftops to get data.

Now that the smart buildings software cooks up a chuck wagon of data every day, what to do with all of that tasty information?

The software identifies issues large and small, and even puts them in prioritized order according to how much the problem is costing the company. A majority of problems they can fix right from their desks, and for the rest, the engineers issue work orders (about 32,300 per business quarter).

Apart from efficiency, the surge of data has also made for some eye-popping analytics. These are mechanical engineer Trevor Sodorff's

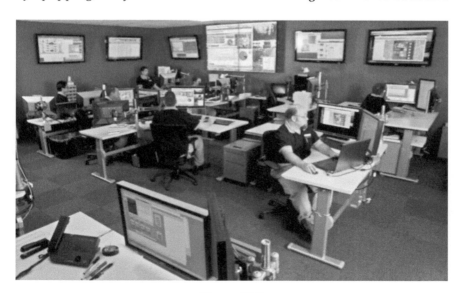

Figure 19-3

specialty. "We have good people, but without good software there are limits to what you can do," Sodorff says. "Everything lives within the context of the bigger picture."

One of Sodorff's party tricks, if you will, is whipping out algorithms to detect new mechanical faults. So during meetings that wander through stretches that don't pertain directly to him? Rather than discreetly checking his email or letting his mind wander, Sodorff writes algorithms.

At one such meeting, Sodorff announces that he's just written a new algorithm for detecting when the air in a given building is being overcooled. He projects the algorithm on a screen, and then launches into a deeply technical explanation about when a discharge air pressure set point is something-something, then the air is being overcooled by something-something for a duration of 900,000 milliseconds.

"That's 15 minutes," says Grove, his fellow engineer, translating on the fly.

Later in the meeting, Grove is talking about how the smart buildings software helps the engineers measure and validate that the energy reduction they're

Figure 19-4

Microsoft's Smart Campus

125
2,000,000

500,000,000

Protocols, Hardware, and Interfaces

Actionable Information

30,000

Graphics, Charts, and Trending Reports

48%
60 Seconds

6-10%
Per Year

32,300
Work Orders
Per Quarter

Microso

seeing is due to reduced consumption and not because it was 5 degrees cooler than yesterday. It's an important distinction for companies to make, especially when seeking a utility rebate.

"We may do an audit, and find we've done something that saves 200,000 kilowatt hours, which works out to ... uh ..." Grove says.

"Sixteen-thousand dollars," Sodorff says without missing a beat. ("I studied math for two years before I decided to be an engineer," he adds. "It's what butters my bread, if you will.")

"Never in my wildest dreams did I think I'd be presenting at the Pentagon. It was a thrill."

Darrell Smith beams at his team.

"Now you see why developing this software at this scale was a once-in-a-lifetime opportunity," Smith says. "It affords you the ability to work on some very large-scale, world-changing projects with some very smart people. It's Microsoft University."

If the smart buildings tool was developed at Microsoft University, today is graduation day. Where much of Smith's time the last few years has been spent developing the software, he now spends hours with visiting business, government and industry leaders offering enthusiastic show-and-tells. He's presented to hospitals, oil companies, automobile manufacturers, cities, and federal government agencies—even at the Pentagon and very soon, this same solution Microsoft has deployed will be available to any business.

Smith says. "It's been interesting, because I don't see myself as a salesperson. I see myself as an evangelist for the smart building industry, and what can be achieved with smarter buildings."

Office buildings, hotels, stores, schools, hospitals, malls and other such commercial buildings are responsible for up to 40 percent of the world's total energy consumption. In the U.S. alone, businesses spend about $100 billion on energy every year.

"Buildings have been built and run the same way for the last 30 to 50 years," Smith says. "This isn't a Microsoft problem, it's an industry problem."

A SMARTER FUTURE

In one memorable scene from the 1987 movie Wall Street, Michael Douglas stands on a beach, hair slick and wearing a black bathrobe, barking orders to his protégé via a brick-sized cell phone as the waves crash behind him.

It was one of the first times a mobile phone appeared in a movie, and at the time talking on the phone on the beach demonstrated the high-tech fruits of a stock broker's wealth and power. Twenty-six years later, the scene feels dated—solely for technology reasons.

That brick with an antenna that Douglas is holding? That is the current state of commercial buildings, Smith says.

"At first, all mobile phones were bricks—basically two-way radios. Now, in just a few short years, they have advanced to become a laptop in your hand," Smith says. "Buildings are still that brick phone. We want to get buildings to where phones are."

Microsoft's campus went from bricks to brains, and Smith believes all commercial buildings can follow suit.

Jessica Granderson, a commercial building and lighting research scientist at Lawrence Berkeley National Laboratory, agrees with Smith. She says smart buildings are becoming more prevalent, and the commercial real estate industry is going through a "time of rapid change and maturation."

Granderson, whose research focuses on intelligent lighting controls and building energy performance monitoring and diagnostics, says the commercial real estate industry is reaching a major tipping point as people realize the power of capturing and analyzing data from buildings.

Granderson says it's still not as easy as it should be to get data out of today's buildings.

"There are two sides to the coin really. There's data that is out there that's not put to good use, and businesses that aren't using it. The other side of the coin is that once we do become in the habit of making use of what's there, then you quickly realize the challenges of getting what you really need and want," she says.

Another challenge is having the right people in place to analyze and interpret the data and act on it.

Granderson contributed to a white paper on Microsoft's new software, "Energy-Smart Buildings: Demonstrating how information technology can cut energy use and costs of real estate portfolios." The paper investigates and evaluates Microsoft's smart building tool, which Granderson says deserves to be held up as a best practice in the industry.

"It's one of the more sophisticated implementations that I've seen," she says. "There are a lot of lessons to be learned (in what Microsoft created)."

Probably the most important take-away from Microsoft's smart buildings breakthrough is just how much money and energy businesses can save with relatively little up-front investment, says Jim Young, CEO of the commercial real estate and information technology company Realcomm.

Young has traveled all over the globe for more than a decade, visiting and studying all manner of smart buildings and smart campuses.

"Companies, even a lot of Fortune 500 companies, have these massive real estate portfolios that they're running with sledgehammers," Young says. "What Darrell and his team can do is watch their buildings at a rate no human has before. When you start connecting to the buildings, generating data, and grouping inefficiencies by cost and priority, all of a sudden you go from the sledgehammer to running buildings with laser precision."

Smith's plan to take Microsoft's smart buildings software worldwide is to adopt the role of matchmaker. His team developed the smart buildings software, with the help of vendors, exclusively with off-the-shelf Microsoft software such as Windows Azure, SQL Server and Microsoft Office.

Smith says these partners and vendors are eager to help businesses of every size, shape, and need to take their buildings from piles of bricks to data-driven brains. Some companies need only a little push—the know-how to incorporate weather data, or energy meters, or perhaps just the right connections. Others need both hands held, procedurally and technologically. Regardless, Smith and his partners can help.

"People may be bumping their heads, but they come here and get a glimpse of the potential," he says.

Young says Smith has been talking about the possibility of making buildings smarter since the two met more than a decade ago at a Realcomm conference on the collision of commercial real estate and information technology.

"He'd say, 'I'm going to figure this out.' I'd call him every few months and say, 'How are you doing, Darrell?' and he'd say, 'I'm not ready to talk to you yet.' Then, when he finally had something to show, he was like, 'Here it is,' and it blew us away," Young says.

Though Smith and his team were quiet for the years they spent developing the software, their work has already garnered serious attention in the industry.

There's now such an interest in smart buildings in general—and Microsoft's smart buildings software in particular—that Realcomm hosted a conference on smart buildings in the Seattle area in 2013. He held it there so attendees could visit Microsoft and experience one of Smith's enthusiastic show-and-tells.

"Darrell's going to be a rock star. Well, he already is in our world," Young says. "If he's not shaking the president's hand in a year then we've all done something wrong."

Unsurprisingly, Smith is more measured about his part as the leader of a team that developed a game-changing smart buildings tool. Though his team started with little more than a notion that there had to be a better way, they used Microsoft's own software, their own background and expertise, and an unyielding determination to solve an industry-wide problem. Smith played the roles of catalyst and mortar in this process, sparking the revolution but also helping to hold his small team of "ninja innovators" tightly together.

"It's not me that's great, it's our story," Smith says. "Yes I'm passionate, but you could put someone else in my place and it would still be a great story."

Figure 19-5

Chapter 20

Smart People, Smart Grid

Ron Rajecki, Contributing Editor, Contracting Business Magazine

This book's author would like to thank *Contracting Business Magazine*, and Ron Rajecki, Contributing Editor, who authored it, for allowing this article from October of 2009 to be reprinted as a chapter here. The project described here was an early implementation of technology types and approaches that have been discussed throughout this book. The reader will note how the article points out many of the challenges and obstacles that have been faced by owners of complex building systems. Equally exciting, it should be evident that the advances underway in the industry, as outlined in this book, will simplify these types of project solutions going forward with more standardized products and web services. The University of New Mexico has been an early adopter of new technology. In the interest of full disclosure, the book's author is former CEO of Energy Control, Inc., so that distinction has been made as appropriate. Further, the article appears here as written by Mr. Rajecki and published in the magazine in 2009. As a result, some of the facts, figures and government references may no longer be accurate. Particularly for future projections, the reader is encouraged to consult updated information.

An intelligent energy system at the University of New Mexico proves electric systems can be designed to be more reliable and efficient. Should there ever come a time when cities of the future are powered by "smart grids," projects such as one undertaken by Energy Control, Inc. (ECI), at the University of New Mexico (UNM), will be looked upon as one that led the way to that future. For the present time, we gladly award this project with a 2009 ContractingBusiness.com Design/Build award.

The University of New Mexico smart grid leverages smart buildings, smart meters, thermal storage, renewable energy, and distributed generation. For those not familiar with the concept of the smart grid, Jack McGowan, CEM, former CEO of ECI, is happy to provide a brief primer. After all, he was a founding member of the U.S. Department of Energy GridWise Architecture Council, and served as its chairman for two years.

"August 14, 2003, when the eastern seaboard of North America went dark, was a significant date in electric industry history that captured the attention of both the media and Capitol Hill," McGowan says. "It quickly became evident however, that the blackout was a symptom of a much larger problem, which many have begun calling the 'energy perfect storm.' This problem begins with an aging electric infrastructure that has not had major technological advancement in a nearly a half century. It is exacerbated by a U.S. Department of Energy (DOE)-projected 40% increase in electric demand over the next 20 years that will cost utilities a projected $3 trillion. That includes the impact of cap and trade, which is part of the third element of this perfect storm: climate change."

Thus was born GridWise™, an initiative created under the DOE Office of Electricity and Energy Reliability. The focus of GridWise is on stimulating the development and adoption of an intelligent energy system, or smart grid, to make the U.S. electric system more reliable and efficient.

UNM was an ideal site for a GridWise project because of ongoing technology investments the university had made. UNM had built a mechanical engineering building in the 1980s equipped with solar thermal and thermal storage, but the systems had fallen into disrepair and were not operating. In fact, Andrea Mammoli, Ph.D., professor of engineering at UNM, stepped up to lead a team of academics and facility engineers to work with ECI on the design and construction of this project. The university had also invested in a smart meter system, a district heating and cooling plant with power generation capability of eight megawatts of combined heat and power, and numerous automation and integration technology projects over several decades.

The advent of smart grid, according to McGowan, presented an opportunity for a truly cutting-edge Design/Build energy project, and the ultimate Green Building system. Using this rationale, ECI was successful in acquiring around $600,000 in pre-stimulus DOE funding, partially matched by UNM and the state of New Mexico. "This was a perfect example of the type of design/build shovel-ready projects sought under the American Reinvestment and Recovery Act," McGowan says.

Figure 20-1

This design/build energy technology project leverages existing technologies that have been implemented at UNM, with new technology and Internet-based web services. "This unique Design / Build project leveraged wide ranging relationships and skills," according to McGowan. "ECI has had a strong presence in building automation and in the smart grid market since its inception. We recognized the connection between smart buildings and smart grid, and saw how this market offered explosive opportunity for design build solutions that blend automation, system integration, mechanical/renewable energy systems, and efficiency."

AN INTUITIVE TOOL TO UNDERSTAND ENERGY USE

This Design/Build energy technology project leverages existing technologies that have been implemented at UNM, with new technology and Internet-based web services. The project touches many campus buildings with automation, metering and integration. In addition, an "energy business intelligence tool" combining energy and analytics with dashboard technology provides full information for more than 100 buildings. Energy data from the mechanical engineering building, shown here, is reported in real-time through an integration using Tridium Java Application Control Engine (JACE) and Delta Controls technology. Energy data from 84 other buildings is reported in less than 20-minute intervals and can be displayed in key performance indicators such as energy consumption or cost per square foot. The introductory graphic in this chapter was used by the DOE in a poster session to depict this project.

"This system provides an intuitive management tool for building owners to understand the impact of energy on their business and to provide for real-time management of building performance," McGowan says. "The system also integrates multiple BACnet™ and legacy automation systems to provide seamless interface to building operations. This smart campus can use this tool to manage energy use, energy cost, and its carbon footprint." ECI worked with an Analytics and Dashboard vendor and Delta controls to deploy a seamless BACnet integration between the BACnet systems in more than a dozen campus buildings and the Dashboard. A similar integration was executed between Tridium JACE and the Dashboard to access Btu energy data from systems that

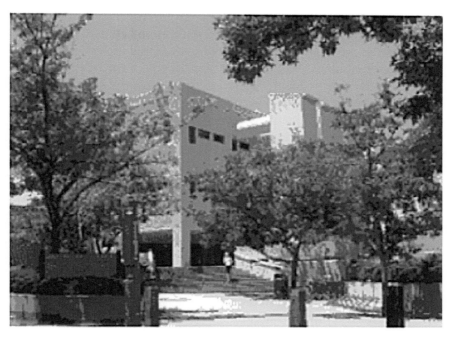

Figure 20-2

pick up this data from industrial controls on HVAC.

The project deploys automated demand response (ADR). ADR is a technology that integrates utility systems with home and building control and energy information systems. Technical development and software programming at each customer's site may include a smart thermostat or a building automation system programmed to shut down equipment and reduce electrical demand if it receives a signal to do so. A signal could also cause the start-up of an emergency generator or a CHP system to generate power on campus when the utility grid can't keep up with demand.

"The UNM project was designed to show how this level of performance data could be combined with automation and energy technology to provide a new generation of smart green building. We believe that smart buildings use energy in a clean and efficient way, to become green buildings," McGowan says. The site's "ultimate" green building is—not surprisingly—the mechanical engineering building. As part of this project, ECI's team rebuilt the solar thermal system with vacuum tube collectors and 400,000 gallons of thermal storage in the building. The project completely upgraded the system, added a 200-ton absorption chiller, and connected the building to the campus chilled water loop. As a result of the work in just this one building, the project can actually take the entire building "off the grid" for cooling, with the exception of some fan and pump loads. Centennial Engineering, the newest building on campus, was designed for optimum energy performance including a connection to the thermal storage loop from the mechanical energy building.

"The total campus project shows the next generation of smart building/smart grid strategies for energy management and load management, to support the power grid. It provides a great example of optimized Design/Build delivery," McGowan says.

INSPIRING FUTURE GENERATIONS

Mammoli says working with McGowan and the team from ECI has helped him see the real-world, practical applications of the theories that underlie the smart grid. And while no one really knows exactly what a city-wide smart grid is going to look like, or how it will ultimately function, putting one on a college campus is the right thing to do. "The campus is like a small city, so it's very exciting to look at the potential of smart grids, and to think that someday we'll say this is one of the places where it all started," Mammoli says. Mammoli is not the only one excited by the technology. "One of the things I really enjoyed about working with ECI is that doing practical things like this on buildings and energy systems really fires up students," he says.

"There are a lot of students that are really interested in this topic, and I think the interaction with ECI has been instrumental in sparking that interest. This is where the people who are going to be doing this type of work in the future are going to see it."

Chapter 21

Envision Charlotte:
Energy Big Data at Community Scale

Contributed by Tom Shircliff
Chair, Envision Charlotte and Principal, Intelligent Buildings, LLC

AUTHOR'S NOTE

An initial premise for this book has been that the technology described presents huge potential benefits for energy efficiency, but more importantly for the owners and occupants of buildings. Envision Charlotte is a great example that this is true, but more importantly that those benefits extend to the larger community that is shared by those occupants and buildings. This is one of the most exciting stories shared in this book, and I want to sincerely thank Tom Shircliff for writing such a masterful account of this city's success. Tom's work with Envision Charlotte and Intelligent Buildings, LLC, is exemplary.

INTRODUCTION

Envision Charlotte is the ultimate big data energy and analytics project that leverages millions of square feet of near real time energy usage pumped through wired and wireless networks into the cloud and back out to data bases, web sites, social media and digital signage.

However, before Envision Charlotte was associated with big data or analytics, it was considered an economic development, "smart grid" and community alignment effort. In this case the community was up-town Charlotte, NC, which is a well defined urban business district comprised of 65 office buildings totaling 25 million square feet, dense residential towers, retail and other use-types with a weekday population of approximately 75,000.

329

The big idea was simple: connect and measure energy as a community with a single number and work together leveraging behavioral science to drive down usage. This concept of connect, measure and move the needle was so understandable and powerful it was accepted as a Clinton Global Initiative that subsequently exceeded it's three-year goals for energy reduction according to the North Carolina utilities commission[1].

The effort was borne from a long-term economic development planning process that sought a way to use energy and sustainability to drive economic activity as well as attract and keep talent. It would demonstrate a progressive, cooperative and innovative spirit in the city that is creating excitement and a new dimension to branding.

This revolutionary approach is changing the way we look at urban business districts and adds great context to how big data and analytics can facilitate and measure energy, sustainability, community engagement and economic development.

This has become the elusive definition of a "smart city," which is a focused, measured effort that has a combination of stakeholder alignment, technology and a unifying purpose.

A COMMUNITY MODEL

Along with unprecedented sustainability, economic and quality-of-life improvements Envision Charlotte is creating the model for how community stakeholders can work together including government, business, real estate owners, utilities and academia as well as solution partners. While Charlotte has a history of cooperation to achieve big things, this offered a programmatic and repeatable model based on the unifying theme of energy and sustainability being leveraged for economic development.

Envision Charlotte solution partners have made substantial investments totaling over $5MM—for good business reasons—and their results and reactions speak for themselves.

Cisco CEO John Chambers says "With Envision Charlotte we can completely transform a city... suddenly we see a model for the rest of the nation and the rest of the world"

This community model is built to be manageable, measurable and replicable by approaching cites and regions one sub-market at a time for fast implementation and clearly measurable results. The first sub-market was the downtown urban core, which is a place that is described as "small enough to manage but big enough to matter." That means there is a nimble structure for fast-decision making, innovation and actual implementation—but with 75,000 people, 25 million square feet, multiple corporate headquarters, city and county government, professional sports venues, a transportation hub for buses and light rail, world class hotels and fine restaurants there are all the elements of any world-class, urban community.

The concept of connect, measure and move the needle was so simple and powerful there was a movement to expand beyond energy to include air, water and waste. Thus a non-profit was formed that has developed a similar water program and likewise waste and air quality programs are being formed.

The approach is very business-like requiring all efforts to "plug in" and measure whatever it is that is being measured not only in energy but in the other three pillars of air, water and waste. You can't manage what you can't measure and if you are serious about sustainability, business and economic development you have to measure like that by capturing and analyzing the data.

Envision Charlotte also engaged or communicated with leading experts from MIT, Wake Forest, University of Pennsylvania, UNC-Charlotte and sustainability, behavior and economic experts from around the country to hone the approach and results.

A BUSINESS MODEL

The base business model was an innovative approach to the existing utility incentive program. Unlike many other Smart community initiatives that implore or require private building owners to invest capital infrastructure in their buildings as part of a coordinated effort, Envision Charlotte took a different approach. Since the goal was 100% participation of the building owner community there would be no capital investment requirement from them. The only request was that they allow the Energy data from their buildings into the program and that they allow some equipment be installed in their building and the lobby. Additionally, there would be some coordination required other facility management staff. The Capital investments required for this program would come from the electric utility Duke Energy. Duke energy would get cost recovery and a return based on the avoided cost of energy generation equal to the energy that the program saved. Awareness and behavior programs have been tried all over the country with varying results and very few successes at a scale like this. The challenge has been getting accurate measurement and verification results usually because of a very wide geography or and inability to get actual data. The foundational attributes of this approach that enabled accurate measurement are limited geography, limited use type and hard, real-time data acquisition from the buildings with a combination of technologies.

Technology and Program

Big data is a general term that can imply many different technology components based on the application. In this case there was a powerful combination of the cloud wide-area networking, local area network wired, and wireless Smart grid technologies and analytics. Duke energy leveraged key partners including Cisco Systems Verizon wireless and intelligent buildings LLC (contributing author). Duke energy implemented various smart grid technologies including smart electrical meters for near real-time Energy Data, as well as their secure and private customer information software systems. Verizon wireless offered flexible fast wireless connectivity required to connect dozens of buildings in a dense permanent environment. Cisco Systems provided the networking gear as well as Digital media infrastructure and equipment such as large interactive touch screens and related equipment. Intelligent buildings focused on the overall architecture, program approach and real estate owner perspective.

Differentiation

Envision Charlotte studied and met with many of the highest quality and best-known efforts such as Austin's Pecan Street Project, The Portland Sustainability Institute, Greenworks Philadelphia, Denver Living City Block and others where a great deal was learned from their successes and challenges. Envision Charlotte gained clarity on several key differentiators in its approach including:

1.   Data: Connecting and measuring with the detail, scale and data points

2.   Focus: Laser focus of geography and use-type

3.   Business: Depth of involvement with the business community and economic development purpose

Results

The results from Envision Charlotte have exceeded expectations both objectively and subjectively. These are just some of the documented numbers in this growing effort:

- 98% building owner participation

- 6.2% net savings from awareness and behavior

- 8.4% net savings from awareness/behavior and ECMs[1] (two years remaining)

- Over 1,000 "energy champions" trained

- $10MM in energy operating expense savings

From the beginning it was clear that Envision Charlotte was meant to be a true community program, which required 100% or at least very high participation from building owners. Some other so-called smart community programs asked a limited number of building owners to make capital improvements and highlighted them as examples. However, this does not have broad enough impact or representation to be called "community."

Therefore, a deep understanding of the real estate culture and decision-making process is necessary joined with a program that would gain acceptance from all points of view. The formal participation rate of 98% is perhaps one of the most significant accomplishments and a beacon for other similar community efforts.

The hard numbers for both overall and awareness and behavior energy savings have been marked as a milestone for the awareness and behavior industry. There have been many types of attempts across the country and the world but few that have assembled the components to connect and create hard measure for such a large number of people and square footage.

At the heart of the community are the tens of thousands of building occupants who impact energy and also take the training and experience of Envision Charlotte with them wherever they go. The over 1,000 energy champions, many more that connect through social media, the facility mangers participating in training and town hall meetings and the various other interactions all redound to a convening power and connectivity that will have lasting affects.

Underneath all of the aforementioned numbers, perhaps the most sustaining figure is the more than $10 million dollars in real estate operating expenses that have been saved through this program. This creates financial incentive, economic attractiveness and reinvestment opportunities that will attract and keep business and talent in Charlotte.

Reference
1.   NC Utilities Commission filing 5/13/2014 Document number F-E-20140513-016

Chapter 22

Medical Center Energy and Analytics Case Study

Jim Lee, President/CEO, Cimetrics Inc.
David Landman, Chief Energy Engineer, Cimetrics Inc.

Cimetrics, Inc. is an industry leader in energy and analytics. This case study in a medical center is an excellent example of how the technology that has been discussed throughout this book can be applied to critical care environments.

INTRODUCTION

In the past 15 years since Cimetrics introduced automated monitoring based commissioning and automatic fault detection and diagnostics to the buildings industry, there have been many innovations and new entrants into the market. Through the fog of marketing rhetoric, it has become difficult for building owners to understand what analytics are and their importance to building commissioning. This case study will introduce analytics and fault detection as applied to building operations and demonstrate how the technology and applications deliver value.

Analytika is the process of extracting value-adding insights from data. Insights can come from understanding what has happened in the past and from predicting what is likely to happen in the future.

Historically, manual analysis has been performed; temperatures and pressures have been monitored and occasionally, trend analysis has been applied to building automation data. What is new is the ability to gather and process much more physical data than in the past. By using modern big data approaches, which apply algorithms to system models, the effectiveness of monitoring based commissioning is greatly increased.

Cimetrics Inc. through its analytika brand provides ongoing commissioning software and services to owners and occupants of commercial, institutional and industrial buildings. Analytika collects real-time data from a client's BASs and sub-meters, integrates information from multiple facilities, and applies over 1,000 proprietary algorithms to the data. Analytika identifies opportunities to reduce energy, environmental, maintenance, operations and regulatory costs; uncovers potential equipment problems; points to profitable retrofit projects; improves occupant comfort; and enhances facility operations and uptime. By correlating control system data with data from networked switchgear and meters, analytika also enables demand response programs, studying mechanical, electrical and control systems' behavior to select and optimize the sheddable load in buildings without compromising mission-critical activities. The analysis of actual building performance during demand response events over time can improve the buildings' response to such events.

After connecting to a building automation system, data relevant to the analysis are transmitted over a secure internet connection to the analytika data center. Cimetrics' energy, electrical and mechanical engineers use proprietary algorithms and software to analyze building efficiency. Analytika algorithms apply static data (equipment specs, system topography) and weather information to the operational data collected on each piece of HVAC equipment as well as the entire building's mechanical system. The algorithms have been designed based on standard energy engineering techniques (such as bin analysis) and academic research which provide an independent measurement of building system efficiencies. The purpose of the analysis is to identify, quantify and prioritize viable energy and operational cost savings opportunities for all aspects of a facility: control systems, HVAC systems, lighting, electrical distribution, metering, operational and other equipment, and scheduling procedures. Figure 22-2 shows a screen shot from the tool with one example of such energy savings calculations.

An analysis of the facility is made including investigation of electrical power usage of motors, air delivery from fans, combustion efficiency of boilers, lighting intensity, etc. The analysis also includes interviewing appropriate administrative and maintenance personnel regarding equipment usage and operating schedules. These data are used to model the facility for analysis. Definitions of building shape, size, construction, occupancy, lighting, temperatures, schedules, controls, weather locale and other details are used to create a computer model to optimize cost saving opportunities for the facility. Figure 22-3 shows an overall summary of analysis conducted and opportunities identified from the analytika dashboard.

Figure 22-1

Analytika Pro

Energy savings and impact analysis

Energy savings calculations and assumptions:

Potential energy savings calculations from installing a VFD, not using the bypass valve, and reducing DP and the associated assumptions are shown below.

Methodology and assumptions:

- TMY2 hours for BOS > 28 F = 7,906
- Pump = 23 BHP (from mechanical plans)
- 0.746 kW/hp
- Controls info indicates sized for 20 psi DP, not 40 psi
- Savings based on using VFD instead of DP valve and reducing the hot water loop differential pressure setpoint from 40 psi to 25 psi. Resetting the hot water loop setpoint results in lowering the pump motor speed. Pump head = 150 ft. - from mechanical plans
- Use the Pump law relationship between Power and Pressure

$$\frac{PWR\_ELEC}{PWR\_ELEC_{Full}} = (\frac{HEAD}{HEAD_{Full}})^2$$

- 1 HP = 0.746 kW
- Assume 90% pump motor efficiency
- Blended electric rate of $0.115/kWh

Annual Cost Savings: $18,359

Annual kWh savings: 159,641

Annual CO_2 Savings: 83.25 Metric-Tons

ANALYTIKA Confidential

Figure 22-2

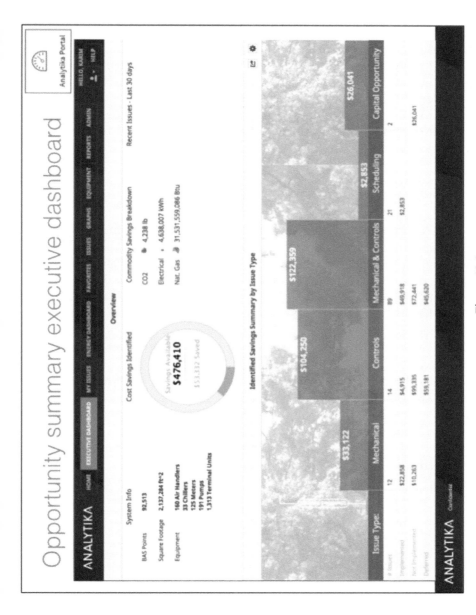

Figure 22-3

To illustrate these concepts in a real world example, consider the case study information provided below.

Medical Center Saves $1.3 Million in
Annual Energy Costs While Improving Patient Comfort

This medical center (MC)* is a 500-bed academic medical center providing pediatrics, primary and advanced medical care. MC is a large provider of trauma care and is affiliated with a prestigious university. The medical center has almost 1 million outpatient visits per year and the medical center campus includes over 2.5 million square feet located in the northeastern United States.

THE CHALLENGE

According to the EPA: "Health care organizations spend over $6.5 billion on energy each year to meet patient needs. Every dollar that a nonprofit health care organization saves on energy is equivalent to generating new revenues of $20 for hospitals or $10 for medical offices."

MC's guiding principles include efficiency and sustainability through a goal to reduce CO_2 emissions by 20% by 2020. To this end, MC was interested in implementing targeted energy conservation measures and technologies, which help achieve the sustainability goals while taking into account MC's specific needs.

MC also committed to the Healthier Hospitals Leaner Energy Challenge. The Healthier Hospitals Initiative (HHI) is "a national campaign to implement a completely new approach to improving environmental health and sustainability in the health care sector."

As a result of these goals and efforts, here is a summary of MC's achievements:

- Financial summary
  — Total energy savings: $1.3 million (annual)
  — Simple payback: 0.3 years
  — Net present value: $1,221,237

- Operational benefits
  — Sustainability and environmental stewardship: Achieved

---

*Due to confidentiality agreements, we are not able to provide the client name. We will refer to the organization as MC throughout this case study.

3,400+ metric tons in annual CO_2 emissions reduction, which is the equivalent of taking 715 cars off the road.

— Utility metering: Provided campus wide metering data by building and submeters which assisted fault detection and internal billing.

— Reporting: Assisted in joint commission reporting by providing analysis of specific zone conditions, including airflows, relative humidity levels, and temperatures for the operating rooms.

Cimetrics was selected to provide its Analytika Pro solution for 5 buildings comprising over 800,000 square feet including inpatient and outpatient care, medical offices, and the central plant. Cimetrics collaborated with MC, JCI and Siemens, their building automation system providers, to connect to and collect sensor and actuator data from over 9,400 physical points. Data were collected every 15 minutes, 24 hours a day, 365 days a year, totaling more than 900,000 data samples per day. The following systems were monitored: 41 air handling units, 19 hot water pumps, 11 chillers, 35 chilled water/condenser water pumps, 10 heat exchangers, 125 exhaust fans, 1,000 terminal units, 116 fume hoods, and other miscellaneous equipment. In addition, 2 chilled water meters, 1 condensate return meter, 52 electric meters, 17 steam meters, and 24 water meters were monitored.

Over 1,000 analytika software algorithms then analyzed the data to identify opportunities to reduce energy consumption, improve environmental conditions and reduce operations and maintenance costs. Analytika also uncovered potential equipment problems, quantified improved patient comfort, improved operating room zone conditions, and provided opportunities for profitable retrofit projects.

Experienced Cimetrics engineers leveraged analytika software to identify opportunities, determine root cause, and calculate annual savings impact. Actionable recommendations were documented and provided to the client both through online and offline channels. Cimetrics' role didn't end with providing recommendations; Cimetrics engineers engaged with the client team on a regular basis to help answer questions, coordinate implementation, and provide regular feedback on progress

Here is an example of an individual analytika issue—excess hours of operation for air handling units:

Four large air handling units (AHUs) serve an outpatient building. All were operating 24/7. However, there was no patient care at night and minimal building usage on weekends. The AHUs were left on 24/7 to serve magnetic resonance imaging (MRI) equipment and other high heat gain loads in the building. This issue was not detected because there were no temperature complaints; however, it was identified with analytika.

MRI machines and other hospital equipment can create substantial, unwarranted energy consumption if HVAC equipment is not specifically designed to exclusively serve that equipment.

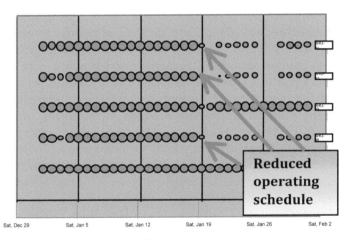

Figure 22-4

SOLUTION

Cimetrics worked with MC staff and the controls vendor to change the AHU sequence of operation to limit the equipment run times to only occupied hours and allow for override of the AHUs to maintain zones within the required temperature and relative humidity range.

Annual energy savings achieved: **$261,278**
Annual carbon emissions reduction: **605 metric tons**

Index